The Ultimate

DIABETIC

COOKBOOK

FOR BEGINNERS

800 Foolproof, Delicious recipes for the Newly Diagnosed Diabetic With a 28-day Meal Plan

Kathleen S. Lamberth

Table of Content

Chapter 5: Meatless Mains and Seafood 51

Chapter 8: Pork, Beef, and Lamb 105

Chapter 9: Soups and Stews 120

Chapter 10: Poultry 129

Chapter 11: Dinner Recipes: Salads 145

Chapter 12: Snacks and Appetizers 154

Chapter 13: Desserts 162

Chapter 14: Sauces, Dips, and Dressing 174

Introduction

A diabetes diagnosis can undoubtedly be scary, especially when you are first diagnosed. Over the years, much of the fear comes from the unknown and from stories of complications that can be caused by long periods of time with uncontrolled blood sugar. It is true that people living with uncontrolled diabetes have a higher risk of complications such as heart disease, stroke, vision loss, depression, kidney failure, and other problems. But this doesn't have to be your story. It's vital to understand that it is absolutely possible for you to control your blood sugar levels and never be a part of any of the scary statistics you may have heard. And it's likely a lot easier than you may think. Well-controlled blood sugar is the goal, as this will prevent any further diabetes-related health problems. In fact, as you begin to follow the nutrition and lifestyle habits you'll learn in this book, it's very likely you will find yourself feeling better than you have in years, and with normal, healthy blood sugar levels. While some people may need medications, the good news is that many people can manage their diabetes with lifestyle changes alone. That includes losing weight if you are overweight, exercising regularly, and eating a healthy diet.

The Healthy Diet recipe in this book is simple and keeps in mind the availability and state of preparedness of a beginner. Every recipe carefully submits the nutrient chart that will help the reader to understand the nutrient intake and understand their food better. Careful consideration is also given to the language of the book, by making it a healthy abode and not a medical prescription booklet. The recipes in the book are easy to make and not repetitive. Most of the recipes are designed to ensure that the person does not get bored with being monotonous.   The book is committed to working to enhance the lives of people affected with diabetes and are looking to manage their diet plan. Whether it is about managing your diabetes, of someone in your family, the book can be of great help for someone beginning to fight diabetes and also anyone looking for a refreshing change to their lifestyle and diet. Every recipe in the book is guaranteed to offer healthy living and extra attention and diligence to overcome diabetes. Sticking with the right lifestyle, medical support, and healthy food habits and lead to controlling diabetes. The book brings interesting recipes as a method to inspire you to control the disease while also enjoys the pleasure of cooking fresh. The recipes are easy to contain and be ferried away. The recipes in the book use ingredients that are easy to find from your closest grocery store and are prepared without consuming a lot of time or special types of equipment. Happy Cooking..!

Chapter 1: Understanding Diabetics

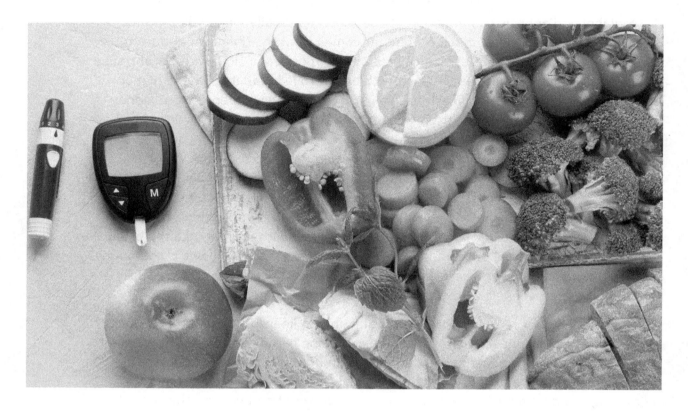

What is Diabetics?

Primarily diabetes is of three kinds, however, the majority of diabetes patients are the cases are type 2 and are preventable with careful deliberation between medication and food habit.

Diabetes mellitus (DM), Diabetes is a disease that is a result of high blood glucose in the human body. In a diabetic patient, the insulin that helps transform glucose in our body to be used for energy, at times does not produce enough insulin. This, therefore, prevents the glucose to reach our cells resulting in diabetes. Though diabetes is not curable, if the disease left untreated, diabetes can cause various bodily complications in the patients. Diabetic ketoacidosis, hyperosmolar hyperglycemic state are some of the acute complications produced by diabetes. Symptoms of diabetes include frequent urination, increased thirst, and increased hunger rate, extreme weakness or fatigue, unusual irritability, nausea, vomiting and abdominal pain, Unpleasant breath. Diabetes can also lead to a few serious long-term complications in patients. These include cardiovascular disease, chronic kidney disease, heart stroke, foot ulcers, damaged nerves, and weakening of eyesight.

Types of diabetes

Primarily diabetes is of three kinds, however, the majority of diabetes patients are the cases are type 2 and are preventable with careful deliberation between medication and food habit.

The three most common kinds of diabetes are, Type 1 diabetes (pancreas's failure to produce enough insulin), Type 2 diabetes (cells failing to respond to insulin diligently), and Gestational diabetes (pregnant women diabetes history developing high blood sugar levels).

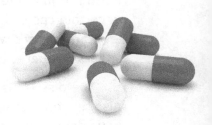

What is Type 1 Diabetes?

The most feared of them all, Type 1 diabetes is also called as the 'juvenile diabetes' as it tends to develop in both children and adults. In Type 1 diabetes, the body of the patient stops producing insulin, an essential substance required to break sugar in the body. This results in the weakening of the patients' immune system. The disease attacks the beta cells in the pancreas, responsible for making insulin. Once the body stops producing insulin, the patient with Type 1 diabetes is bound to take insulin every day to sustain life. The loss of beta cells is caused by the autoimmune response; the cause of this response is still unknown. Some theories, however, suggest that Type 1 diabetes may be influenced by genetic factors. A family member with a similar condition may be a carrier of the risk.

Since there is no way to cure the disease, the patient suffering from Type 1 diabetes has to be administered with insulin shots via injection just under the skin or through an insulin pump. The patient has to be on a strict diet throughout and exercise regime throughout life.

What is Type 2 Diabetes?

This is the most common type of diabetes type found today. Type 2 diabetes is very prevalent among the young and adults of today. One of the main reasons behind this is the nature of lifestyle and lack of physical exercise. The disease occurs due to obesity and lack of exercise. People with the genetic history of the diseases are at times also vulnerable to attracting Type 2 diabetes. What used to be usually found in people over 35 years old in age, Type 2 diabetes is today radically found in the youngsters as well. At least 90 percent of diabetic patients are found to be carrying traits od Type 2 diabetes.

This is a non-insulin type of disease, which means that, although the patient has a condition of high blood sugar but is not required taking insulin shots regularly. The body of the patients with Type 2 diabetes produces insulin but is not enough to break glucose. The prevention of Type 2 diabetes depends on checking one's weight, regular physical exercise, and following a healthy diet and lifestyle. This should be enough to regulate the smooth flow of blood sugar levels. In case, the patient still cannot control the level, medication is usually prescribed by the doctor. The symptoms of type 2 diabetes include are not very noticeable as those for type 1 diabetes. However, should always be careful not to put extra weight or give up on physical exercise.

What is Gestational diabetes?

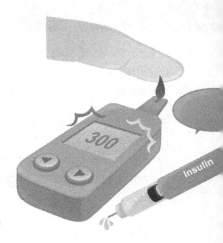

This type of diabetes is found to develop in women, mostly during or just after pregnancy. In Gestational Diabetes, the women in certain cases during pregnancy develop diabetes high blood sugar levels. Pregnant women without any prior history of high blood sugars/ diabetes are also found to develop Gestational diabetes.

The disease is also seen to have vanished after the child is born. Also, in some cases, after the child is born the women are seen to have developed the signs and symptoms of Type 2 diabetes. Women who develop Gestational diabetes during their pregnancy period are believed to have a higher probability of developing Type 2 diabetes in the later stages of life. Hard to identify the symptoms of Gestational diabetes and increase the possibility of pre-eclampsia, depression, cesarean section delivery.

It is advised to properly treat the pregnant mother during the pregnancy period. Mothers who have a history of any illness or are negligent, have a tendency to develop risk to the delivery of the normal child. In certain cases, the child born may be prone to low blood sugar after birth, and jaundice. The children born also have a greater risk of developing type 2 diabetes in the later stages of their lives.

The patient suffering from Gestational diabetes should observe a healthy lifestyle and food habits.

Prevention and Control of Diabetes

One of the foremost ways to prevent or control diabetes is by bringing changes to your lifestyle and food habits. Once an ailment, usually found in people over 35-year old, diabetes is creeping into our lives and affecting the health of young and teens of today. Obesity and lack of physical exercise are the prime reasons to attract diabetes.

- **Patients with Type 1 diabetes-** need to rely on insulin shots, either injected or through a pump to maintain the insulin level in their body. Besides this, a high maintained diet, usually prescribed by the doctor should be strictly followed to counter the damage done by Type 1 diabetes.

- **Heart strokes-**diabetes also attacks the heart by damaging the blood vessels that could lead to various heart-related diseases and cause stroke. The patient should maintain a permissible blood sugar level at all times and quit smoking.

- **Hypoglycemia-**is a condition of low blood glucose levels. Diabetic patients suffering from low blood glucose levels should consult a doctor for medicine and follow a strict diet plan.

- **Other pertinent diseases-** that might affect a diabetic patient are chronic kidney disease, heart stroke, foot ulcers, damaged nerves, and weakening of eyesight.

Preventing diabetes requires lifestyle management, the best remedy to a diabetes patient.

Diabetes Prevention: 5 Tips for Taking Control

When it comes to type 2 diabetes — the most common type of diabetes — prevention is very important. It's especially important to make diabetes prevention a priority if you're at increased risk of diabetes, such as if you're overweight or you have a family history of the disease or you have been diagnosed with prediabetes (also known as impaired fasting glucose).Diabetes prevention is as basic as eating more healthfully, becoming more physically active and losing a few extra pounds. It's never too late to start. Making a few simple changes in your lifestyle now may help you avoid the serious health complications of diabetes in the future, such as nerve, kidney and heart damage. Consider these diabetes prevention tips from the American Diabetes Association.

1. Get more physical activity: There are many benefits to regular physical activity. Exercise can help you:

- **Lose weight**
- **Lower your blood sugar**
- **Boost your sensitivity to insulin — which helps keep your blood sugar within a normal range**

Research shows that aerobic exercise and resistance training can help control diabetes. The greatest benefit comes from a fitness program that includes both.

2. Get plenty of fiber: Fiber may help you:

- **Reduce your risk of diabetes by improving your blood sugar control**
- **Lower your risk of heart disease**
- **Promote weight loss by helping you feel full**

Foods high in fiber include fruits, vegetables, beans, whole grains and nuts.

3. Go for whole grains: It's not clear why, but whole grains may reduce your risk of diabetes and help maintain blood sugar levels. Try to make at least half your grains whole grains. Many foods made from whole grains come ready to eat, including various breads, pasta products and cereals. Look for the word "whole" on the package and among the first few items in the ingredient list.

4. Lose extra weight: If you're overweight, diabetes prevention may hinge on weight loss. Every pound you lose can improve your health, and you may be surprised by how much. Participants in one large study who lost a modest amount of weight — around 7 percent of initial body weight — and exercised regularly reduced the risk of developing diabetes by almost 60 percent.

5. Skip fad diets and just make healthier choices: Low-carb diets, the glycemic index diet or other fad diets may help you lose weight at first. But their effectiveness at preventing diabetes and their long-term effects aren't known. And by excluding or strictly limiting a particular food group, you may be giving up essential nutrients and often craving such foods. Instead, make variety and portion control part of your healthy-eating plan.

Understanding Nutrients in Diet

Think of your body like a car: You want to fill it up with quality fuel to make sure it runs optimally. If you have type 2 diabetes, feeding your body with healthy nutrients will help control blood sugar, aid with weight management, decrease your risk of complications, and promote overall health. Carbohydrates, proteins, and fats are the three macronutrients your body needs. Carbohydrates have the most significant impact on blood sugar levels. Fats and protein have little or no effect on blood sugar. So here is a crash course in nutrition.

• Protein

Protein is used for building and repairing tissues, as well as making enzymes, hormones, and other body chemicals. It can also help make you feel more full and satisfied at meals. Research has shown that the body uses protein best when you space your intake throughout the day, rather than eating a large amount just once a day. Protein comes from animal products, including meat, poultry, eggs, dairy, fish, seafood, and protein powder. Vegan sources of protein include soy products (such as tofu, tempeh, and edamame), seitan, legumes (beans, nuts, peas, and lentils), and seeds— and again, some protein powders.

• Carbohydrates

Carbohydrates are your body's main source of energy Carbohydrates are the sugars, starches and fiber found in fruits, grains, vegetables and milk products. Though often maligned in trendy diets, carbohydrates — one of the basic food groups — is important to a healthy diet.

While all carbs break down into glucose, the best carbs for your health are the ones you'll eat in their closest-to-nature state as possible: vegetables, fruit, pulses, legumes, unsweetened dairy products, and 100% whole grains, like brown rice, quinoa, wheat, and oats

• Fats

Fats are important for maintaining cell membranes and facilitating vitamin absorption, as well as other functions. Eating fat at meals can also help promote feelings of fullness. There are four major kinds of fat: monounsaturated, polyunsaturated, saturated, and trans fats. Generally speaking, you should choose the unsaturated types, limit saturated fats, and avoid Tran's fats.

Unsaturated fats, which are found in the Mediterranean diet, may actually reduce the risk of cardiovascular disease and improve glucose metabolism. A diet high in saturated fat is linked to elevated LDL (bad) cholesterol levels. There is some conflicting research on whether or not saturated fat increases the risk of heart disease. At this time, though, most experts still recommend that saturated fat intake be limited.

• Fiber

Fiber is the indigestible part of plants. It's found in vegetables, fruit, whole grains, legumes, and nuts. Despite the fact that most of it doesn't get digested, fiber does a lot of good things in the body. It contributes to digestive health and helps keep you feeling full longer. The soluble fiber (it absorbs water to form a gel) found in foods such as beans, lentils, and nonstarchy vegetables helps lower cholesterol and regulate blood sugar.

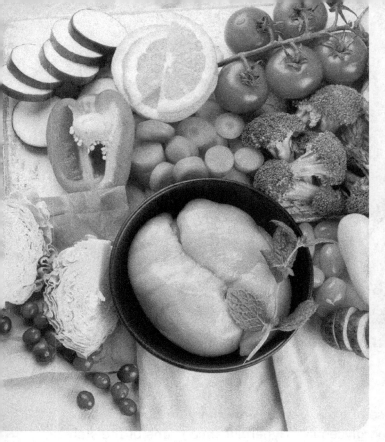

Healthy Diet for Diabetic

People with diabetes often think they need to become strictly focused on avoiding sugar or carbohydrates, and neglect to consider the nutritional quality of their diet. While it's true that carbohydrates have the greatest impact on blood sugar, it is the diet as a whole that contributes to health, weight management, and blood sugar control. Strictly limiting carbohydrates found in fruit and whole grains while eating a diet high in saturated fat and sodium will not promote optimal health.

Focusing on healthy foods, portion control of carbohydrates, and losing weight if you are overweight are the three most important things you can do to manage type 2 diabetes from a nutritional standpoint. And do not feel that you have to get to an unrealistically low weight—even losing 5 to 7 percent of your body weight can help lower blood sugar and reduce the need for diabetic medications. While the exact recommended servings will vary from person to person, here are some guidelines for a healthy diet:

- Eat a variety of fruits and vegetables.

- Include whole grains

- Aim for two or three servings of fish a week.

- Include heart-healthy fats such as olive oil, canola oil, nuts and nut butters, seeds, and avocado

- Consume fewer than 2,300 milligrams of sodium per day.

- Limit your intake of added sugars, which are found in sweetened beverages and many processed foods

• Sodium

Sodium is a mineral that helps maintain your electrolyte balance, as well as performing other functions in the body. However, excessive amounts may increase the risk for developing serious medical conditions such as high blood pressure, heart disease, and stroke. Since cardiovascular disease is the number one cause of illness and death in people with diabetes, it is especially important to limit your sodium intake. The majority of people's sodium intake comes from processed foods and restaurant meals—not the salt shaker.

People with diabetes should limit their sodium consumption to 2,300 milligrams (mg) a day. Lowering your sodium intake even more, to 1,500 mg a day, may benefit blood pressure in certain circumstances. The American Heart Association recommends 1,500 mg a day for African Americans; people diagnosed with hypertension, diabetes, or chronic kidney disease; and people over 51 years of age.

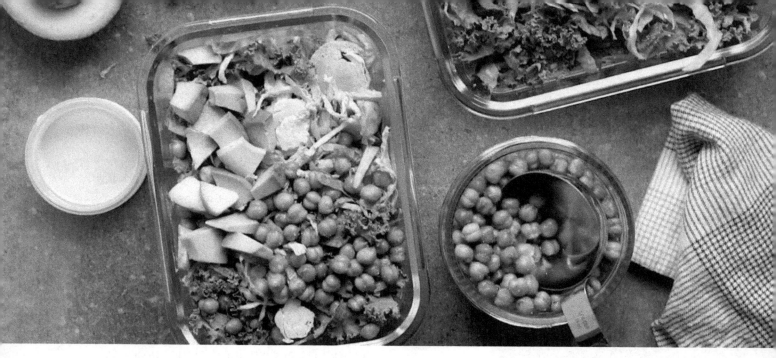

10 Tips for Healthy Diet with Diabetes

Sugar is not always sweet. Consider a case of excess sugar entering your bloodstream, also known as 'high blood sugar level' or "hyperglycemia". Hyperglycemia is one of the state's leading to Diabetes. Diabetes mellitus is a chronic disorder caused by hereditary or non-standard eating habits and a sedentary lifestyle leading to volatility in blood sugar levels. There are different types of diabetes; no two people with diabetes have similar complications. Hence, a 'one-size-fits-all' diabetes diet is unthinkable for people suffering from diabetes. Further, this type of diet helps manage blood glucose (sugar), control blood pressure, and regulate cholesterol levels. Further, a self-disciplined diet regime as prescribed by a doctor/nutritionist lowers body weight and reduces the risk of diabetes complications i.e. heart problems and strokes, organ degenerative health conditions including certain types of cancers.

Here are 10 tips to revolutionize the lifestyle of a diabetic patient.

Tip #1: Three meals and three snacks per day: Your everyday food consumption should be distributed across 3 major meals (i.e. breakfast, lunch, and dinner) and 3 healthy snacks in-between meals to resist hunger pangs. The quantity of snacks should not be equal to any of the 3 meals rather it should be fewer portions. A healthy bedtime snack helps a diabetic patient to overcome mid-night or early morning hypoglycemia (low blood sugar level).

Tip #2: Consume more of complex carbohydrates: Complex CHO (carbohydrates) is significantly better than simple CHO. As simple CHO (i.e. sugar, honey, jaggery, sweets, chocolates, muffins, fruit juice, carbonated beverages, plain rice, maida, sabudana or tapioca, etc.) does not contain any fiber so the absorption is fast leading to a spike in blood sugar level. Foods like wheat, fruits with skin and pulp, rice with vegetables, salads, any kind of vegetables, wheat bread, wheat noodles, wheat pasta, etc. are complex carbs that are rich in fiber content (i.e. thereby digestion and absorption period are longer than usual.

Tip #3: Reduce added sugar: We love sugar in our foods and it's difficult to resist or cut down sugar/sugar variants at the beginning. Therefore, practical substitutes of sugar are a good starting point. For example low-sugar or '0' sugar labeled drinks, zero-calorie energy drink, coconut water, plain milk, buttermilk, different types of flavored tea, and coffee without refined/natural sugar added and cut fruits with skin are healthy substitutes for sugar.

Moreover, consumption of low or zero-calorie sweeteners (i.e. artificial sweeteners) moderates our blood glucose levels and body weight. Most of the sweeteners available in the stores may harm more than do good to our body. Comparatively, stevia leaves as a sweetener are safer to switch to. In the case of diabetes treatment, there are few conditions of 'hypoglycemia' (hypo) where sugary drinks can be used in moderation for treatment. For this special case, it is important not to cut down sugar intake as part of your diabetes management. However, if there is prolonged hypoglycemia (i.e. low blood sugar level), consult with your doctor and diabetes management team on the diet plan.

Tip #4: Eat good quality and quantity of protein: Indian diet lacks in both quality and quantity of protein. It is advised to have a sizable portion of 1st class of protein such as lean meat, eggs, egg, chicken, fish, etc. in your diet if you are non-vegetarian. However, a vegetarian plate must have protein from plant and dairy sources such as broccoli, home-made paneer, low-fat cheese, different pulses and legumes, soybeans, mushrooms, tofu, etc.

Tip #5: Healthier fat eases your blood flow: Fat generates energy in our bodies. Vitamins and minerals are absorbed in our body with the help of fat molecules to provide us with energy and immunity strength. Are you aware that there are different types of fats that positively or negatively impact our health? Daily cooking oil (e.g. rice bran oil, sunflower oil, sesame oil, canola oil, soya oil, corn oil, olive oil), unsalted nuts, seeds, avocados, oily fish are sources of healthy fats providing for good cholesterol in our body. In contrast, saturated fats increase the amount of bad cholesterol in the blood, thereby causing heart ailments and arterial blockage. Found primarily in animal products and processed foods like red and processed meat, ghee, butter, 'vanaspati', mayonnaise, biscuits, cakes, pies, and pastries. A life-long fit-tip would be cut down on using oils in general for cooking, instead, try to grill steam or baked foods.

Tip #6: Fulfill your daily dairy consumption: Dairy products such as curd, cheese, milk, buttermilk, or home-made paneer are enough to meet the daily dietary calcium intake for your body. When it comes to a diabetic patient, his or her average daily dairy product consumption should be ~500 ml.

Tip #7: Fiber creates magic with your blood sugar: Fiber has a key role in diabetic diet management to suppress blood sugar levels. When it comes to a diabetic person, his or her average daily dietary fiber requirement is ~25-35 gm from normal consumed food (excluding any supplements). The best sources of dietary fiber are raw and cooked vegetables, whole fruits with pulp and whole grains, and legumes. Thus, vegetable or lightly cooked leafy vegetables across 3 major meals with whole fruits for snacks can provide an adequate amount of fiber in your diet.

Tip #8: Light and tasty snacks are a smart choice: We all love tasty snacks. But, one should always select snacks that not only tasty but also healthy at the same time. For example, low-fat yogurts, unsalted nuts (almonds and walnuts), flax/pumpkin seeds, fruits and vegetables, sprouts salads, makhana (lotus seeds) instead of fried crisps, potato or banana chips, biscuits, and chocolates. Portion size is sacrosanct and needs our self-control. Therefore, the snacks portion should be little as compared to your basic meals.

Tip #9: Consume alcohol responsibly: Alcohol has a high calorific value, so drinking in moderation is recommended to lose bodyweight. Hence, restrict your alcohol consumption to a maximum of 1 ounce per week. Guard your urge to binge drinking, and practice surviving for several days a week without consuming alcohol. If you are administered with insulin dose and or periodic diabetes medications, avoid alcohol on an empty stomach as it may lead to a serious condition of hypoglycemia. Instead, you may consume alcohol (always in moderation) either during dinner or after dinner.

Tip #10: The body is water, so keep yourself hydrated: Generally, water is never considered as a nutrient in our diet. Did you know that up to 60% of the human adult body is water? Our body uses water to nourish all its cells, organs, and tissues. Water is depleted from our body through various actions including involuntary functions like breathing, sweating, and digestion. Drinking water can be practiced throughout the daylight hours, however, water should be consumed before major meals. Additionally, there should be a time interval after a meal to recommence drinking water. Hence, it is pertinent to re-hydrate ourselves by drinking enough water, non-sugar fluids, and eating foods that contain natural water or freshly squeezed juices along with pulp (instead of packaged or processed juices) as it helps lower our body temperature and systematically maintains other body functions.

Best and Worst Foods for Diabete

Nothing is completely off-limits. Even items that you might think as the worst could be occasional treats in tiny amounts. But they won't help you nutrition-wise, and it's easiest to manage your diabetes if you mainly stick to the "best" options.

The prime objective of any food plan for a diabetic patient is to control the blood sugar levels of the person. Here's a list of foods that the patient should opt for and avoid during their course to control diabetes are:

Starches	
Best Choices	**Worst Choices**
• Whole grains, such as brown rice, oatmeal, quinoa, millet, or amaranth	• Processed grains, such as white rice or white flour
• Baked sweet potato	• Cereals with little whole grains and lots of sugar
• Items made with whole grains and no (or very little) added sugar	• White bread
	• French fries
	• Fried white-flour tortillas

Vegetables

Best Choices	Worst Choices
• Fresh veggies, eaten raw or lightly steamed, roasted, or grilled	• Canned vegetables with lots of added sodium
• Plain frozen vegetables, lightly steamed	• Veggies cooked with lots of added butter, cheese, or sauce
• Greens such as kale, spinach, and arugula	• Pickles, if you need to limit sodium. Otherwise, pickles are OK.
• Low sodium or unsalted canned vegetables	• Sauerkraut, for the same reason as pickles.
• dark greens, red or orange (think of carrots or red peppers),	
• whites (onions) and even purple (eggplants)	

Fruits

Best Choices	Worst Choices
• Fresh fruit	• Canned fruit with heavy sugar syrup
• Plain frozen fruit or fruit canned without added sugar	• Chewy fruit rolls
• Sugar-free or low-sugar jam or preserves	• Regular jam, jelly, and preserves
• No-sugar-added applesauce	• Sweetened applesauce
	• Fruit punch, fruit drinks, fruit juice drinks

Protein

Best Choices	Worst Choices
• Plant-based proteins such as beans, nuts, seeds, or tofu	• Fried meats
• Fish and seafood	• Higher-fat cuts of meat, such as ribs
• Chicken and other poultry (Choose the breast meat if possible.)	• Pork bacon
• Eggs and low-fat dairy	• Regular cheeses
	• Poultry with skin
	• Deep-fried fish
	• Deep-fried tofu
	• Beans prepared with lard

Dairy

Best Choices	Worst Choices
• 1% or skim milk	• Whole milk
• Low-fat yogurt	• Regular yogurt
• Low-fat cottage cheese	• Regular cottage cheese
• Low-fat or nonfat sour cream	• Regular sour cream
	• Regular ice cream
	• Regular half-and-half

Fats, Oils, and Sweets

Best Choices	Worst Choices
• Natural sources of vegetable fats, such as nuts, seeds, or avocados	• Anything with trans-fat in it. It's bad for your heart. Check the ingredient list for anything that's "partially hydrogenated," even if the label says it has 0 grams of trans fat.
• Foods that give you omega-3 fatty acids, such as salmon, tuna, or mackerel	
• Plant-based oils, such as canola, grape seed, or olive oils	• Big portions of saturated fats, which mainly come from animal products but also are in coconut oil and palm oil. Ask your doctor what your limit should be, especially if you have heart disease as well as diabetes.

Drinks

Best Choices	Worst Choices
• When you down a favourite drink, you may get more calories, sugar, salt, or fat than you bargained for. Read the labels so you know what's in a serving.	• Regular sodas
	• Regular beer, fruity mixed drinks, dessert wines
• Unflavoured water or flavoured sparkling water	• Sweetened tea
• Unsweetened tea with or without a slice of lemon	• Coffee with sugar and cream
	• Flavoured coffees and chocolate drinks
• Light beer, small amounts of wine, or non-fruity mixed drinks	• Energy drinks
• Coffee, black or with added low-fat milk and sugar substitute	

Chapter 2: Diabetic Diet Action Plan

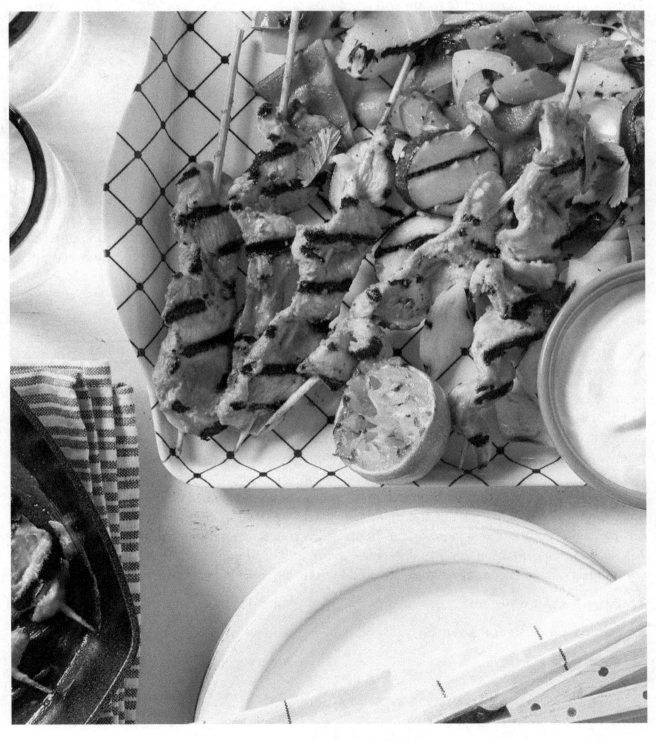

Pantry Stock for the 28-Day Meal Plan

Keeping your pantry supplied with these diabetes-friendly foods can make mealtimes easier while helping to keep your blood sugars in a healthy range. These convenient ingredients follow the principles of a diabetes-friendly diet, so what you'll see are heart-healthy fats (like olive oil), high-fiber whole grains and legumes, lean protein, low-salt seasonings, healthy fruit-based sweet treats and plenty of shelf-stable fruits and veggies. This list will take the guesswork out of what to buy and with the simple recipe ideas to go with each item, it'll be easy to know what to make, too.

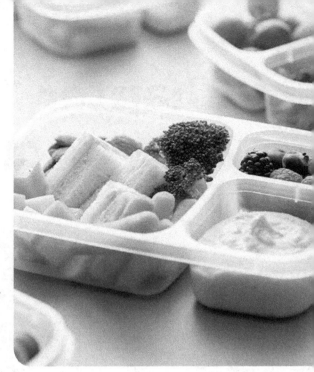

No-Salt Seasonings: No-salt seasonings and many store-bought spices blends are great for enhancing the flavor of a dish, without the need for too much salt. Spice mixes are convenient ingredients to have on hand as they can quickly and easily turn a bland recipe into something super flavorful with just a few shakes. You can still use salt when you cook but by adding it yourself, you have better control over how much you use. Few basic spice blends to keep handy

- **Italian seasoning**
- **Curry powder**
- **Taco or fajita seasoning**
- **Lemon pepper**

Vinegars & Heart-Healthy Oils: Some examples of heart-healthy oils include olive oil, sesame oil and canola oil. Made from plants, these oils are low in (or free of) , which tends to harm our heart when eaten too often. Different oils impart different flavors and also have different uses in cooking. Olive oil is great in and medium-heat cooking, where canola oil is often used for higher-heat applications, like frying. (You can read more about what oils to use when .) Infused olive oils are also a nice option—try lemon-infused olive oil (citron oil) drizzled over fish, chicken, vegetables or salad greens for a burst of flavour without adding salt.Vinegar is the other part of the equation—it can be used in combination with one of these oils to create yummy dressings, or can be mixed with water and herbs to make quick-pickles. Just like the oils, each oil imparts different flavors and are used in different ways. Here are some basic oils and vinegar to keep stocked in your kitchen:

- **Extra-virgin olive oil**
- **Canola oil or grape seed oil**
- **Sesame oil**
- **Balsamic vinegar**
- **Red-wine vinegar**
- **Rice vinegar**

Nuts & Seeds: and Seeds are great sources of heart-healthy fats and they also deliver a small dose of fiber and protein. Nuts and seeds make for a great snack or salad topper and when turned into a nut butter, it can top toast, add flavor in an (and help keep it from falling apart) and make your morning smoothie extra creamy. The combination of healthy fats, plus a little fiber and protein, will help keep you feeling fuller for longer and will help prevent your blood sugars from going too high, too quickly. Go for the unsalted versions to cut back on added sodium. Here are a few versatile staples to keep in your kitchen:

- Almonds
- Walnuts
- Cashews
- Chia seeds
- Sesame seeds
- Pepitas (pumpkin seeds)

No-salt-added canned beans: such as white, black, kidney, and chickpeas—are full of fiber, protein, vitamins and minerals. Canned beans are very versatile, which means you won't get bored of using the same beans over and over again. Drain and rinse the beans to get rid of the excess liquid before adding to salads, blending into a dip or mixing into soups. Or go with an even easier option and pick up a few cans of low-sodium for a ready-to-eat meal. Stir in vegetables and lean meats with your canned soup for a semi-homemade meal that delivers extra nutrients and satisfying protein. Here are some beans and soups to keep in your kitchen:

- Black beans
- White beans (or cannellini beans)
- Chickpeas
- Kidney beans
- Pinto beans
- Minestrone soup
- Tuscan-style white bean soup
- Bean and barley soup

Canned Tuna, Salmon & Chicken: Canned , salmon and chicken are great protein add-ons for soups, salads, casseroles and sandwiches—no cooking needed! Keeping a few cans of each of these healthy proteins on hand means you can make a delicious and nutritious meal in minutes.

- Skinless, boneless canned salmon
- Canned chicken, packed in water
- Canned albacore tuna, packed in water

Whole Grains: Whole grains, like whole-wheat bread and pasta, brown rice, quinoa and oatmeal are key components of a healthy diet for diabetes. Whereas refined grains (like white pasta and bread) are processed in a way that removes most of the fiber, whole grains deliver a hefty dose of fiber, which has so many amazing health benefits and in particular plays a important role in blood-sugar management. Fiber slows down digestion which in turn slows down how quickly the glucose from the carbs enters your blood stream. So, by going with whole grains, your blood sugar is less likely spike too high, too quickly. Here are some healthy whole grains to keep on hand:

- Old-fashioned oats
- Whole-wheat bread
- Whole-wheat pastas
- Brown rice
- Quinoa
- Whole-wheat couscous

28-Day Meal Plan

Day	Breakfast	Lunch	Dinner	Snack/ Dessert	Motivational Quotes
1	Classic Morning Berry Smoothie	Easy Cheesy Pan Cake with Bean Mixture	Rise and Shine Veggie Salad	Low Carb Butter Milk Cauliflower Cake	Life changes very quickly, in a very positive way, if you let it.
2	Cinnamon Walnut Breakfast Bowl	Green Lentils Salad Bowl with Pine Nuts	Homemade Red & Green Cabbage Slaw	Buttery Mashed Cauliflower Puree	Food can be both enjoyable and nourishing.
3	Breakfast Pita Bacon with Pepper	Brown Rice Bowl with Egg and Avocado	Best Ever Green Salad with Honeyed Black Berry	Southern Vanilla Banana Pudding Casserole	I am a better person when I have less on my plate
4	Wheat Apple Bake	Chicken Broth Wild Rice Perfect Bowl	Delicious Scallions and Three Bean Salad	Delicious Vanilla Carrot Banana Muffins	If I don't eat junk, I don't gain weight.
5	Low Carb Oatmeal Milk Bowl	Low Fat Pepper Pilaf with basil	Honeyed Rainbow Fruit Baby Spinach Salad	Delicious Vanilla Carrot Banana Muffins	Keep an open mind and a closed refrigerator.
6	Spiced Spinach Omelet	Spicy Veggie Black Bean Bowl with yogurt	Crunchy Kale and Chickpea Salad Recipe	Easy Step by Step Potato and Salmon Fish	Start where you are. Use what you have. Do what you can.
7	Zucchini Egg Bake	Wheat Couscous with Scallions & Pecans	Lettuce Walnut Salad with Honey	Buttery Almond Biscuits	The hard days are what make you stronger.
8	5 Ingredient Cheese Pancakes with fruits	Veggie Quinoa Zucchini Bowl	High Protein Kidney Bean Cucumber Salad	Baked Cinnamon Banana Bread	My body is less judgmental of my diet than my mind is.
9	Vanilla flavoured Oat Flat cake	Low Sodium Chicken Coconut Quinoa	Nutty Fruity Spinach Chicken Salad	Appetizing Buttery Tomato Waffles	Let food be thy medicine and medicine be thy food.

10	Healthy Whole Wheat Pumpkin Waffles	Veggie Pasta with Pesto & Parmesan	Kale, Cantaloupe, and Chicken Salad	Buffalo Chicken Celery Rolls	New meal; fresh start.
11	Mom's Special Milk Berry Crêpes	Spicy Peppery Wax Beans Bowl	Best Ever Honey Cobb Salad	No Bake Chocolate Peanut Butter Balls	You didn't gain all your weight in one day; you won't lose it in one day. Be patient with yourself.
12	Oyster Mushroom Omelette	Navy Bean Tomato Bowl with Feta cheese	Traditional Spinach Sofrito Steak Salad	Oven baked Stevia Almonds	Ability is what you're capable of doing. Motivation determines what you do. Attitude determines how well you do it.
13	Special Greek Yogurt Nut Bowl	Baked Navy Bean Oregano Mix	Strawberry Farro Salad with Almonds	Easy Cinnamon Roasted Pumpkin Seeds	I always believed if you take care of your body it will take care of you.
14	Cheesy Vanilla Crêpe Cakes	Lemony Black-Eyed Peas Dish	Broccoli Barley Salad with Balsamic Vinaigrette	Instant Bacon Shrimps Lettuce Wraps	Looking after my health today gives me a better hope for tomorrow.
15	Spinach Tortillas with Scallions and Avocado	Tomato Green chillies Soup with Lime Yogurt	Autumn Pear Walnut Salad	Cheddar Cheese Baked Broccoli	You may be disappointed if you fail, but you are doomed if you don't try.
16	Maple flavoured Chicken Mushroom Omelette	Perfect Corn Salad with Paprika Dressing	Citrusy Seafood Fruit Salad	Ginger Sesame Grilled Tofu with Marinade	Fitness is like marriage; you can't cheat on it and expect it to work.
17	Low Carb Spinach Egg Sandwiches	Veggie Salsa Fritters	Fresh and Easy Fettuccini Noodles Salad	Crispy Garlic Kale Chips	Exercise should be regarded as a tribute to the heart.
18	Shrimp Scallion Breakfast Bowl	Low Sodium Veggie Greens with Black Beans	Best Ever Scallion Slaw	Classic Peppery Eggs	If it doesn't challenge you, it doesn't change you.
19	One Pan Zucchini Banana Bake	Classy Chicken Black Bean Soup	Asparagus Egg Salad with Vinaigrette	Cinnamon Apple Wheat Pitas	It's going to be a journey. It's not a sprint to get in shape.

20	Breakfast Ground Corn Fruit Bowl	Spicy Brown Rice with Red Pepper & Paprika	Italian Tomato Mozzarella Salad	Nutty Butter Cake	Just believe in yourself. Even if you don't, pretend that you do and, at some point, you will.
21	Bacons with Eggs and Cheese	Chicken Rice with Almond Cranberry Salad	Crunchy Dates with Maple Shallot Vinaigrette	Coconut Almond Margarine Cookies	Nobody is perfect, so get over the fear of being or doing everything perfectly. Besides, perfect is boring.
22	Asparagus Onion Quiche Bowl	Spicy Cheesy Zucchini Macaroni Pie	Baked Chicken Avocado Salad	3 Ingredient Low Carb Almond Cookies	The secret of change is to focus all of your energy not on fighting the old, but on building the new.
23	Cinnamon Farro Bowl with Berries	Chickpea Wraps for Quesadillas	Raw Veggie Salad	Sticky and Crispy Soy Chicken Wings	You get what you focus on, so focus on what you want.
24	Almond Cranberry Morning Bowl	Eggs and Snap Peas Fried Rice	Feel Cool Watermelon Mint Salad	Vanilla flavoured Banana-Walnut Cookies	Yes, I can.
25	Chilled Three Berry Smoothie	Baked Margarine Cheesy Fish	Holiday Special Pomegranate Almonds Salad	Bacon Cucumber Lettuce Salad	Don't stop until you're proud.
26	Mashed Avocado Bread with Crumbled Bacon	The Best Ever Veggie Fajitas	Blue Cheese Mixed Green Salad	Pepper Cauliflower with Hot Sauce	A little progress each day adds up to big results.
27	Cinnamon Cereal with Dried Cherries	Weeknight Chickpea Spaghetti Bolognese	Berry Pumpkin Seed Salad Bowl	Quick and Easy Butter Pecan Bowl	It has to be hard so you'll never ever forget
28	Vanilla flavoured Yogurt Smoothie	Fat free Sofrito Dumplings	Simple Pickled Onion Salad	Tahini Cauliflower Bowl with Favourite Veggies	The groundwork of all happiness is health

Chapter 3: Breakfast

Classic Morning Berry Smoothie

Prep time: 5 minutes | Cook time: 0 minutes | Serves 2

½ cup mixed berries (blueberries, strawberries, blackberries)
1 tablespoon ground flaxseed
2 tablespoons unsweetened coconut flakes
½ cup unsweetened plain coconut milk
½ cup leafy greens (kale, spinach)
¼ cup unsweetened vanilla nonfat yogurt
½ cup ice

1. In a blender jar, combine the berries, flaxseed, coconut flakes, coconut milk, greens, yogurt, and ice.
2. Process until smooth. Serve.

Per serving
Calories: 182 | fat: 14.9g | protein: 5.9g | carbs: 8.1g | fiber: 4.1g | sugar: 2.9g | sodium: 25mg

Low Carb Turkey Thyme Patties

Prep time: 10 minutes | Cook time: 10 minutes | Serves 8 (1 patty each)

1 pound (454 g) lean ground turkey
½ teaspoon dried thyme
½ teaspoon dried sage
½ teaspoon salt
½ teaspoon freshly ground black pepper
¼ teaspoon ground fennel seeds
1 teaspoon extra-virgin olive oil

1. Mix the ground turkey, thyme, sage, salt, pepper, and fennel in a large bowl, and stir until well combined.
2. Form the turkey mixture into 8 equal-sized patties with your hands.
3. In a skillet, heat the olive oil over medium-high heat. Cook the patties for 3 to 4 minutes per side until cooked through.
4. Transfer the patties to a plate and serve hot.

Per Serving
Calories: 91 | fat: 4.8g | protein: 11.2g | carbs: 0.1g | fiber: 0.1g | sugar: 0g | sodium: 155mg

Veggie Cheesy Tomato Toast

Prep time: 5 minutes | Cook time: 0 minute | Serves 2

½ cup cottage cheese
½ avocado, mashed
1 teaspoon Dijon mustard
Dash hot sauce
(optional)
2 slices whole-grain bread, toasted
2 slices tomato

1. In a small bowl, mix together the cottage cheese, avocado, mustard, and hot sauce, if using, until well mixed.
2. Spread the mixture on the toast.
3. Top each piece of toast with a tomato slice.

Per Serving
Calories: 179 | fat: 8g | protein: 11g | carb: 17g | fiber: 4g | sugar: 9.54g | sodium: 327mg

Whole-Wheat Bread with Peppery Egg

Prep time: 5 minutes | Cook time: 5 minutes | Serves 2

2 tablespoons butter
2 slices whole-wheat bread
2 large eggs
Sea salt to taste
Freshly ground black pepper

1. In a medium nonstick skillet over medium heat, heat the butter until it bubbles.
2. As the butter heats, cut a 3-inch hole in the middle of each piece of bread. Discard the centers.
3. Place the bread pieces in the butter in the pan. Carefully crack an egg into the hole of each piece of bread.
4. Cook until the bread crisps and the egg whites set, about 3 minutes.
5. Flip and cook just until the yolk is almost set, 1 to 2 minutes more.
6. Season to taste with the salt and pepper.

Per Serving
Calories: 241 | fat: 17g | protein: 10g | carbs: 12g | fiber: 2g | sugar: 0.21g | sodium: 307mg

Homemade Yogurt Cashew Bowl

Prep time: 5 minutes | Cook time: 0 minutes | Serves 1

¾ cup Low-fat Greek yogurt
¼ cup mixed berries (blueberries, strawberries, blackberries)
2 tablespoons cashew,

walnut, or almond pieces
1 tablespoon ground flaxseed
2 fresh mint leaves, shredded

1. Pour the yogurt into a tall parfait glass and scatter the top with the berries, cashew pieces, and flaxseed.
2. Sprinkle the mint leaves on top for garnish and serve chilled.

Per Serving
Calories: 238 | fat: 11.2g | protein: 20.9g | carbs: 15.8g | fiber: 4.1g | sugar: 8.9g | sodium: 63mg

Oatmeal Porridge Bowl with Peanut Butter

Prep time: 5 minutes | Cook time: 5 minutes | Serves 2

1½ cups unsweetened vanilla almond milk
¾ cup rolled oats
1 tablespoon chia seeds
2 tablespoons natural

peanut butter
¼ cup fresh berries, divided (optional)
2 tablespoons walnut pieces, divided (optional)

1. Add the almond milk, oats, and chia seeds to a small saucepan and bring to a boil.
2. Cover and continue cooking, stirring often, or until the oats have absorbed the milk.
3. Add the peanut butter and keep stirring until the oats are thick and creamy.
4. Divide the oatmeal into two serving bowls. Serve topped with the berries and walnut pieces, if desired.

Per Serving
Calories: 260 | fat: 13.9g | protein: 10.1g | carbs: 26.9g | fiber: 7.1g | sugar: 1.0g | sodium: 130mg

Moms' Special Nutty Fruity Oats Bowl

Prep time: 5 minutes | Cook time: 0 minute | Serves 1

⅓ Cup unsweetened almond milk
⅓ Cup rolled oats (use gluten-free if necessary)
¼ apple, cored and

finely chopped
2 tablespoons chopped walnuts
½ teaspoon cinnamon
Pinch sea salt to taste

1. In a single-serving container or Mason jar, combine all of the ingredients and mix well.
2. Cover and refrigerate overnight.

Per Serving
Calories: 242 | fat: 12g | protein: 6g | carb: 30g | fiber: 6g |sugar: 12.31 g | sodium: 97mg

Cheese Muffin Topped with Fried Egg

Prep time: 5 minutes | Cook time: 0 minute | Serves 2

1 whole-grain English muffin, split and toasted
2 teaspoons Dijon mustard
2 slices tomato

4 thin slices deli ham
½ cup shredded Cheddar cheese
2 large eggs, fried (optional)

1. Preheat the oven broiler on high.
2. Spreads each toasted English muffin half with 1 teaspoon of mustard, and place them on a rimmed baking sheet, cut-side up.
3. Top each with a tomato slice and 2 slices of ham. Sprinkle each with half of the cheese.
4. Broil in the preheated oven until the cheese melts, 2 to 3 minutes.
5. Serve immediately, topped with a fried egg, if desired.

Per Serving
Calories: 234 | fat: 13g | protein: 16g | carb: 16g | fiber: 3g |sugar: 1.78 g | sodium: 97mg

Milky Steel-Cut Oatmeal in Vanilla Flavor

Prep time: 5 minutes | Cook time: 40 minutes | Serves 4

4 cups water
Pinch sea salt to taste
1 cup steel-cut oats

¾ cup skim milk
2 teaspoons pure vanilla extract

1. In a large pot over high heat, bring the water and salt to a boil.
2. Reduce the heat to low and stir in the oats.
3. Cook the oats for about 30 minutes to soften, stirring occasionally.
4. Stir in the milk and vanilla and cook until your desired consistency is reached, about 10 more minutes.
5. Remove the cereal from the heat. Serve topped with sunflower seeds, chopped peaches, fresh berries, sliced almonds, or flaxseeds.

Per Serving
Calories: 186 | fat: 0g | protein: 9g | carbs: 30g | fiber: 5g | sugar: 2g| sodium: 36mg

Instant Buckwheat Porridge with Nuts

Prep time: 5 minutes | Cook time: 35 minutes | Serves 4

2 cups raw buckwheat groats
3 cups water

Pinch sea salt
1 cup unsweetened almond milk

1. Put the buckwheat groats, water, and salt in a medium saucepan over medium-high heat.
2. Bring the mixture to a boil, and then reduce the heat to low.
3. Cook until most of the water is absorbed, about 20 minutes. Stir in the milk and cook until very soft, about 15 minutes.
4. Serve the porridge with your favourite toppings such as chopped nuts, sliced banana, or fresh berries.

Per Serving
Calories: 122 | fat: 1g | protein: 6g | carbs: 22g | fiber: 3g | sugar: 4g| sodium: 48mg

Stomach Friendly Ginger Carrot Smoothie

Prep time: 10 minutes | Cook time: 0 minutes | Serves 2

2 carrots, peeled and grated
1 ripe pear, unpeeled, cored and chopped
2 teaspoons grated fresh ginger
Juice and zest of 1

lime
1 cup water
½ teaspoon ground cinnamon
¼ teaspoon ground nutmeg

1. Put the carrots, pear, ginger, lime juice, lime zest, water, cinnamon, and nutmeg in a blender and blend until smooth.
2. Pour into two glasses and serve.

Per Serving
Calories: 74 | fat: 0g | protein: 1g | carbs: 19g | fiber: 4g | sugar: 11g| sodium: 43mg

Bell pepper Egg Tortillas

Prep time: 10 minutes | Cook time: 15 minutes | Serves 4

8 ounces bulk pork breakfast sausage
½ onion, chopped
1 green bell pepper, seeded and chopped
8 large eggs, beaten

4 (6-inch) low-carb tortillas
1 cup shredded pepper Jack cheese
½ cup prepared salsa (optional, for serving)

1. In a large non-stick skillet on medium-high heat, cook the sausage, crumbling it with a spoon, until browned, about 5 minutes.
2. Add the onion and bell pepper. Cook, stirring, until the veggies are soft, about 3 minutes.
3. Add the eggs and cook, stirring, until eggs are set, about 3 minutes more.
4. Spoon the egg mixture onto the 4 tortillas. Top each with the cheese and fold into a burrito shape.
5. Serve.

Per Serving
Calories: 486 | fat: 36g | protein: 32g | carbs: 13g | fiber: 8g | sugar: g| sodium: 810mg

Gluten Free Pumpkin Smoothie Bowl

Prep time: 5 minutes | Cook time: 0 minute | Serves 2

1 cup Low-fat Greek yogurt
½ cup canned pumpkin purée (not pumpkin pie mix)
1 teaspoon pumpkin pie spice

2 (1-gram) packets stevia
½ teaspoon vanilla extract
Pinch sea salt
½ cup chopped walnuts

1. In a bowl, whisk together the yogurt, pumpkin purée, pumpkin pie spice, stevia, vanilla, and salt (or blend in a blender).
2. Spoon into two bowls. Serve topped with the chopped walnuts.

Per Serving
Calories: 292 | fat: 23g | protein: 9g | carb: 15g | fiber: 4g |sugar: 12.86g | sodium: 85mg

Breakfast Pork Sausage Cheesy Wrap

Prep time: 10 minutes | Cook time: 15 minutes | Serves 4

8 ounces (227 g) bulk pork breakfast sausage
½ onion, chopped
1 green bell pepper, seeded and chopped
8 large eggs, beaten
4 (6-inch) low-carb

tortillas
1 cup shredded pepper Jack cheese
½ cup sour cream (optional, for serving)
½ cup prepared salsa (optional, for serving)

1. In a large nonstick skillet on medium-high heat, cook the sausage, crumbling it with a spoon, until browned, about 5 minutes.
2. Add the onion and bell pepper. Cook, stirring, until the veggies are soft, about 3 minutes. Add the eggs and cook, stirring, until eggs are set, about 3 minutes more.
3. Spoon the egg mixture onto the 4 tortillas. Top each with the cheese and fold into a burrito shape.
4. Serve with sour cream and salsa, if desired.

Per Serving
Calories: 487 | fat: 36.1g | protein: 31.8g | carbs: 13.1g | fiber: 7.9g | sugar: 5.1g | sodium: 811mg

Special Greek Yogurt Nut Bowl

Prep time: 5 minutes | Cook time: 0 minutes | Serves 2

1½ cups plain low-fat Greek yogurt
2 kiwis, peeled and sliced
2 tablespoons shredded unsweetened coconut flakes

2 tablespoons halved walnuts
1 tablespoon chia seeds
2 teaspoons honey, divided (optional)

1. Divide the yogurt between two small bowls.
2. Top each serving of yogurt with half of the kiwi slices, coconut flakes, walnuts, chia seeds, and honey (if using).

Per Serving
Calories: 261 | fat: 9.1g | protein: 21.1g | carbs: 23.1g | fiber: 6.1g | sugar: 14.1g | sodium: 84mg

Easy Creamy Coconut Kiwi Dessert

Prep time: 5 minutes | Cook time: 0 minutes | Serves 2

7 ounces (198 g) light coconut milk
¼ cup chia seeds
3 to 4 drops liquid stevia

1 clementine
1 kiwi
Shredded coconut (unsweetened)

1. Start by taking a mixing bowl and adding in the light coconut milk. Add in the liquid stevia to sweeten the milk. Mix well.
2. Add the chia seeds to the milk and whisk until well-combined. Set aside.
3. Peel the clementine and carefully remove the skin from the wedges. Set aside.
4. Also, peel the kiwi and dice it into small pieces.
5. Take a glass jar and assemble the pudding. For this, place the fruits at the bottom of the jar; then add a dollop of chia pudding. Now spread the fruits and then add another layer of chia pudding.
6. Finish by garnishing with the remaining fruits and shredded coconut.

Per Serving
Calories: 486 | fat: 40.5g | protein: 8.5g | carbs: 30.8g | fiber: 15.6g | sugar: 11.6g | sodium: 24mg

Cinnamon Walnut Breakfast Bowl

Prep time: 10 minutes | Cook time: 30 minutes | Serves 16

4 cups rolled oats
1 cup walnut pieces
½ cup pepitas
¼ teaspoon salt
1 teaspoon ground cinnamon
1 teaspoon ground ginger

½ cup coconut oil, melted
½ cup unsweetened applesauce
1 teaspoon vanilla extract
½ cup dried cherries

1. Preheat the oven to 350ºF (180ºC). Line a baking sheet with parchment paper.
2. In a large bowl, toss the oats, walnuts, pepitas, salt, cinnamon, and ginger.
3. In a large measuring cup, combine the coconut oil, applesauce, and vanilla. Pour over the dry mixture and mix well.
4. Transfer the mixture to the prepared baking sheet. Cook for 30 minutes, stirring about halfway through. Remove from the oven and let the granola sit undisturbed until completely cool. Break the granola into pieces, and stir in the dried cherries.
5. Transfer to an airtight container, and store at room temperature for up to 2 weeks.

Per Serving
Calories: 225 | fat: 14.9g | protein: 4.9g | carbs: 20.1g | fiber: 3.1g | sugar: 4.9g | sodium: 31mg

Zucchini Egg Bake

Prep time: 20 minutes | Cook time: 50 minutes | Serves 4

2 teaspoons extra-virgin olive oil
½ sweet onion, finely chopped
2 teaspoons minced garlic
½ small eggplant, peeled and diced
1 green zucchini, diced
1 yellow zucchini, diced
1 red bell pepper, seeded and diced

3 tomatoes, seeded and chopped
1 tablespoon chopped fresh oregano
1 tablespoon chopped fresh basil
Pinch red pepper flakes
Sea salt and freshly ground black pepper, to taste
4 large eggs

1. Preheat the oven to 350ºF (180ºC).
2. Place a large ovenproof skillet over medium heat and add the olive oil.
3. Sauté the onion and garlic until softened and translucent, about 3 minutes. Stir in the eggplant and sauté for about 10 minutes, stirring occasionally. Stir in the zucchini and pepper and sauté for 5 minutes.
4. Reduce the heat to low and cover. Cook until the vegetables are soft, about 15 minutes.
5. Stir in the tomatoes, oregano, basil, and red pepper flakes, and cook 10 minutes more. Season the ratatouille with salt and pepper.
6. Use a spoon to create four wells in the mixture. Crack an egg into each well.
7. Place the skillet in the oven and bake until the eggs are firm, about 5 minutes.
8. Remove from the oven. Serve the eggs with a generous scoop of vegetables.

Per Serving
Calories: 148 | fat: 7.9g | protein: 9.1g | carbs: 13.1g | fiber: 4.1g | sugar: 7.1g | sodium: 99mg

Yogurt Bowl with Macadamia Nuts

Prep time: 10 minutes | Cook time: 5 minute | Serves 2

1 cup fresh pineapple chunks
1 cup Low-fat Greek yogurt
¼ cups canned coconut milk

¼ cup flaxseed
2 tablespoons unsweetened toasted coconut flakes
2 tablespoons chopped macadamia nuts

1. Preheat the oven broiler on high.
2. Spread the pineapple chunks in a single layer on a rimmed baking sheet.
3. Broil until the pineapple begins to brown, 4 to 5 minutes.
4. In a small bowl, whisk together the yogurt, coconut milk, and flaxseed. Spoon the mixture into two bowls. Top with the pineapple chunks.
5. Serve with the coconut flakes and chopped macadamia nuts sprinkled over the top.

Per Serving
Calories: 402 | fat: 31g | protein: 10g | carbs: 26g | fiber: 9g | sugar: 69.6g | sodium: 71mg

My Favorite Butter Pancakes

Prep time: 10 minutes | Cook time: 10 minutes | Serves 2

1 cup almond flour
½ teaspoon baking soda
Pinch sea salt
2 large eggs
¼ cup sparkling water
(plain, unsweetened)
2 tablespoons canola oil, plus more for cooking
4 tablespoons peanut butter

1. Heat a nonstick griddle over medium-high heat.
2. In a small bowl, whisk together the almond flour, baking soda, and salt.
3. In a glass measuring cup, whisk together the eggs, water, and oil.
4. Pour the liquid ingredients into the dry ingredients, and mix gently until just combined.
5. Brush a small amount of canola oil onto the griddle.
6. Using all of the batter, spoon four pancakes onto the griddle.
7. Cook until set on one side, about 3 minutes. Flip with a spatula and continue cooking on the other side.
8. Before serving, spread each pancake with 1 tablespoon of the peanut butter.

Per Serving
Calories: 454 | fat: 41g | protein: 17g | carbs: 8g | fiber: 3g | sugar: 12.53g | sodium: 408mg

Healthy Whole Wheat Pumpkin Waffles

Prep time: 10 minutes | Cook time: 20 minutes | Serves 6

2¼ cups whole-wheat pastry flour
2 tablespoons granulated sweetener
1 tablespoon baking powder
1 teaspoon ground cinnamon
1 teaspoon ground
nutmeg
4 eggs
1¼ cups pure pumpkin purée
1 apple, peeled, cored, and finely chopped
Melted coconut oil, for cooking

1. In a large bowl, stir together the flour, sweetener, baking powder, cinnamon, and nutmeg.
2. In a small bowl, whisk together the eggs and pumpkin.
3. Add the wet ingredients to the dry and whisk until smooth.
4. Stir the apple into the batter.
5. Cook the waffles according to the waffle maker manufacturer's directions, brushing your waffle iron with melted coconut oil, until all the batter is gone.
6. Serve immediately.

Per Serving
Calories: 232 | fat: 4.1g | protein: 10.9g | carbs: 40.1g | fiber: 7.1g | sugar: 5.1g | sodium: 52mg

Breakfast Pita Bacon with Pepper

Prep time: 5 minutes | Cook time: 15 minutes | Serves 2

1 (6-inch) whole-grain pita bread
3 teaspoons extra-virgin olive oil, divided
2 eggs
2 Canadian bacon slices
Juice of ½ lemons
1 cup micro greens
2 tablespoons crumbled goat cheese
Freshly ground black pepper, to taste

1. Heat a large skillet over medium heat. Cut the pita bread in half and brush each side of both halves with ¼ teaspoon of olive oil (using a total of 1 teaspoon oil). Cook for 2 to 3 minutes on each side, and then remove from the skillet.
2. In the same skillet, heat 1 teaspoon of oil over medium heat. Crack the eggs into the skillet and cook until the eggs are set, 2 to 3 minutes. Remove from the skillet.
3. In the same skillet, cook the Canadian bacon for 3 to 5 minutes, flipping once.
4. In a large bowl, whisk together the remaining 1 teaspoon of oil and the lemon juice. Add the micro greens and toss to combine.
5. Top each pita half with half of the micro greens, 1 piece of bacon, 1 egg, and 1 tablespoon of goat cheese. Season with pepper and serve.

Per Sserving
Calories: 251 | fat: 13.9g | protein: 13.1g | carbs: 20.1g | fiber: 3.1g | sugar: 0.9g | sodium: 400mg

Spiced Spinach Omelet

Prep time: 10 minutes | Cook time: 15 minutes | Serves 4

2 tablespoons extra-virgin olive oil
½ sweet onion, chopped
1 red bell pepper, seeded and chopped
½ teaspoon minced garlic
¼ teaspoon sea salt
½ teaspoons freshly

ground black pepper
8 egg whites
2 cups shredded spinach
½ cup crumbled low-sodium feta cheese
1 teaspoon chopped fresh parsley, for garnish

1. Preheat the oven to 375ºF (190ºC).
2. Place a heavy ovenproof skillet over medium-high heat and add the olive oil.
3. Sauté the onion, bell pepper, and garlic until softened, about 5 minutes. Season with salt and pepper.
4. Whisk together the egg whites in a medium bowl, then pour them into the skillet and lightly shake the pan to disburse.
5. Cook the vegetables and eggs for 3 minutes, without stirring.
6. Scatter the spinach over the eggs and sprinkle the feta cheese evenly over the spinach.
7. Put the skillet in the oven and bake, uncovered, until cooked through and firm, about 10 minutes.
8. Loosen the edges of the frittata with a rubber spatula, then invert it onto a plate.
9. Garnish with the chopped parsley and serve.

Per Serving
Calories: 146 | fat: 10.1g | protein: 10.1g | carbs: 3.9g | fiber: 1.0g | sugar: 2.9g | sodium: 292mg

Cheesy Vanilla Crêpe Cakes

Prep time: 5 minutes | Cook time: 20 minutes | Serves 4

Avocado oil cooking spray
4 ounces (113 g) reduced-fat plain cream cheese, softened

2 medium bananas
4 large eggs
½ teaspoon vanilla extract
⅛ teaspoon salt

1. Heat a large skillet over low heat. Coat the cooking surface with cooking spray, and allow the pan to heat for another 2 to 3 minutes.
2. Meanwhile, in a medium bowl, mash the cream cheese and bananas together with a fork until combined. The bananas can be a little chunky.
3. Add the eggs, vanilla, and salt, and mix well.
4. For each cake, drop 2 tablespoons of the batter onto the warmed skillet and use the bottom of a large spoon or ladle to spread it thin. Let it cook for 7 to 9 minutes.
5. Flip the cake over and cook briefly, about 1 minute.

Per Serving
Calories: 176 | fat: 9.1g | protein: 9.1g | carbs: 15.1g | fiber: 2.1g | sugar: 8.1g | sodium: 214mg

5 Ingredient Cheese Pancakes with Fruits

Prep time: 10 minutes | Cook time: 20 minutes | Serves 4

2 cups low-fat cottage cheese
4 egg whites
2 eggs

1 tablespoon pure vanilla extract
1½ cups almond flour
Nonstick cooking spray

1. Place the cottage cheese, egg whites, eggs, and vanilla in a blender and pulse to combine.
2. Add the almond flour to the blender and blend until smooth.
3. Place a large nonstick skillet over medium heat and lightly coat it with cooking spray.
4. Spoon ¼ cup of batter per pancake, 4 at a time, into the skillet. Cook the pancakes until the bottoms are firm and golden, about 4 minutes.
5. Flip the pancakes over and cook the other side until they are cooked through, about 3 minutes.
6. Remove the pancakes to a plate and repeat with the remaining batter.
7. Serve with fresh fruit.

Per Serving
Calories: 345 | fat: 22.1g | protein: 29.1g | carbs: 11.1g | fiber: 4.1g | sugar: 5.1g | sodium: 560mg

Vanilla flavoured Oat Flat cake

Prep time: 5 minutes | Cook time: 20 minutes | Serves 4

1 cup 2 percent Low-fat Greek yogurt	granulated sweetener
3 eggs	1 teaspoon baking powder
1½ teaspoons pure vanilla extract	1 teaspoon ground cinnamon
1 cup rolled oats	Pinch ground cloves
1 tablespoon	Nonstick cooking spray

1. Place the yogurt, eggs, and vanilla in a blender and pulse to combine.
2. Add the oats, sweetener, baking powder, cinnamon, and cloves to the blender and blend until the batter is smooth.
3. Place a large nonstick skillet over medium heat and lightly coat it with cooking spray.
4. Spoon ¼ cup of batter per pancake, 4 at a time, into the skillet. Cook the pancakes until the bottoms are firm and golden, about 4 minutes.
5. Flip the pancakes over and cook the other side until they are cooked through, about 3 minutes.
6. Remove the pancakes to a plate and repeat with the remaining batter.
7. Serve with fresh fruit.

Per Serving
Calories: 244 | fat: 8.1g | protein: 13.1g | carbs: 28.1g | fiber: 4.0g | sugar: 3.0g | sodium: 82mg

Vanilla flavoured Berry Muffins

Prep time: 10 minutes | Cook time: 25 minutes | Serves 18 muffins

2 cups whole-wheat pastry flour	Pinch sea salt
1 cup almond flour	2 eggs
½ cup granulated sweetener	1 cup skim milk, at room temperature
1 tablespoon baking powder	¾ cup 2 percent Low-fat Greek yogurt
2 teaspoons freshly grated lemon zest	½ cups melted coconut oil
¾ teaspoon baking soda	1 tablespoon freshly squeezed lemon juice
¾ teaspoon ground nutmeg	1 teaspoon pure vanilla extract
	1 cup fresh blueberries

1. Preheat the oven to 350ºF (180ºC).
2. Line 18 muffin cups with paper liners and set the tray aside.
3. In a large bowl, stir together the flour, almond flour, sweetener, baking powder, lemon zest, baking soda, nutmeg, and salt.
4. In a small bowl, whisk together the eggs, milk, yogurt, coconut oil, lemon juice, and vanilla.
5. Add the wet ingredients to the dry ingredients and stir until just combined.
6. Fold in the blueberries without crushing them.
7. Spoon the batter evenly into the muffin cups. Bake the muffins until a toothpick inserted in the middle comes out clean, about 25 minutes.
8. Cool the muffins completely and serve.
9. Store leftover muffins in a sealed container in the refrigerator for up to 3 days or in the freezer for up to 1 month.

Per Serving
Calories: 166 | fat: 9.1g | protein: 3.9g | carbs: 18.1g | fiber: 2.1g | sugar: 6.9g | sodium: 75mg

Chilled Three Berry Smoothie

Prep time: 10 minutes | Cook time: 0 minutes | Serves 2

½ cup mixed berries (blueberries, strawberries, blackberries)	½ cup unsweetened plain coconut milk
½ cup leafy greens (kale, spinach)	2 tablespoons unsweetened coconut flakes
¼ cup unsweetened vanilla nonfat yogurt	1 tablespoon ground flaxseed
	½ cup ice

1. Process the mixed berries, leafy greens, yogurt, coconut milk, coconut flakes, flaxseed, and ice in a blender until all ingredients are combined into a smooth mixture. Pour the mixture into two smoothie glasses.
2. Serve chilled or at room temperature.

Per Serving
Calories: 183 | fat: 15.3g | protein: 6.2g | carbs: 8.2g | fiber: 4.1g | sugar: 3.2g | sodium: 26mg

Low Carb Oatmeal Milk Bowl

Prep time: 10 minutes | Cook time: 35 minutes | Serves 6

2 cups rolled oats
¼ cup shredded unsweetened coconut
1 teaspoon baking powder
½ teaspoon ground cinnamon
¼ teaspoon sea salt
2 cups skim milk
¼ cup melted coconut oil, plus extra for greasing the baking

dish
1 egg
1 teaspoon pure vanilla extract
2 cups fresh blueberries
⅛ cup chopped pecans, for garnish
1 teaspoon chopped fresh mint leaves, for garnish

1. Preheat the oven to 350ºF (180ºC).
2. Lightly oil a baking dish and set it aside.
3. In a medium bowl, stir together the oats, coconut, baking powder, cinnamon, and salt.
4. In a small bowl, whisk together the milk, oil, egg, and vanilla until well blended.
5. Layer half the dry ingredients in the baking dish, top with half the berries, then spoon the remaining half of the dry ingredients and the rest of the berries on top.
6. Pour the wet ingredients evenly into the baking dish. Tap it lightly on the counter to disperse the wet ingredients throughout.
7. Bake the casserole, uncovered, until the oats are tender, about 35 minutes.
8. Serve immediately, topped with the pecans and mint.

Per serving
Calories: 296 | fat: 17.1g | protein: 10.2g | carbs: 26.9g | fiber: 4.1g | sugar: 10.9g | sodium: 154mg

Breakfast Ground Corn Fruit Bowl

Prep time: 5 minutes | Cook time: 35 minutes | Serves 8

1 cup teff
1 cup stone-ground corn grits
1 cup quinoa
¼ teaspoon whole cloves
1 tablespoon sunflower

seed oil
5 cups water
2 cups roughly chopped fresh fruit
2 cups unsalted crushed nuts

1. In an electric pressure cooker, combine the teff, grits, quinoa, and cloves.

2. Add the oil and water, mixing together with a fork.
3. Close and lock the lid, and set the pressure valve to sealing.
4. Select the Porridge setting, and cook for 20 minutes.
5. Once cooking is complete, allow the pressure to release naturally. Carefully remove the lid.
6. Serve each portion with ¼ cup fresh fruit and ¼ cup nuts of your choice.

Per Serving
Calories: 418 | fat: 19.1g | protein: 13.2g | carbs: 49.1g | fiber: 9.1g | sugar: 5.1g | sodium: 6mg

Maple flavoured Chicken Mushroom Omelet

Prep time: 10 minutes | Cook time: 15 minutes | Serves 4

Avocado oil cooking spray
1 cup roughly chopped Portobello mushrooms
1 medium green bell pepper, diced
1 medium red bell pepper, diced

8 large eggs
¾ cup half-and-half
¼ cup unsweetened almond milk
6 links maple-flavored chicken or turkey breakfast sausage, cut into ¼-inch pieces

1. Preheat the oven to 375ºF (190ºC).
2. Heat a large, oven-safe skillet over medium-low heat. When hot, coat the cooking surface with cooking spray.
3. Heat the mushrooms, green bell pepper, and red bell pepper in the skillet. Cook for 5 minutes.
4. Meanwhile, in a medium bowl, whisk the eggs, half-and-half, and almond milk.
5. Add the sausage to the skillet and cook for 2 minutes.
6. Pour the egg mixture into the skillet, then transfer the skillet from the stove to the oven, and bake for 15 minutes, or until the middle is firm and spongy.

Per Serving
Calories: 281 | fat: 17.1g | protein: 20.9g | carbs: 10.1g | fiber: 2.1g | sugar: 7.1g | sodium: 445mg

Low Carb Spinach Egg Sandwiches

Prep time: 10 minutes | Cook time: 0 minutes | Serves 4

8 large hardboiled eggs
3 tablespoons plain low-fat Greek yogurt
1 tablespoon mustard
½ teaspoons freshly ground black pepper
1 teaspoon chopped fresh chives
4 slices 100% whole-wheat bread
2 cups fresh spinach, loosely packed

1. Peel the eggs and cut them in half.
2. In a large bowl, mash the eggs with a fork, leaving chunks.
3. Add the yogurt, mustard, pepper, and chives, and mix.
4. For each portion, layer 1 slice of bread with one-quarter of the egg salad and spinach.

Per Serving
Calories: 278 | fat: 12.1g | protein: 20.1g | carbs: 23.1g | fiber: 2.9g | sugar: 3.1g | sodium: 365mg

Mom's Special Milk Berry Crêpes

Prep time: 20 minutes | Cook time: 20 minutes | Serves 5

1½ cups skim milk
3 eggs
1 teaspoon extra-virgin olive oil, plus more for the skillet
1 cup buckwheat flour
½ cup whole-wheat
flour
½ cup 2 percent Low-fat Greek yogurt
1 cup sliced strawberries
1 cup blueberries

1. In a large bowl, whisk together the milk, eggs, and 1 teaspoon of oil until well combined.
2. Into a medium bowl, sift together the buckwheat and whole-wheat flours. Add the dry ingredients to the wet ingredients and whisk until well combined and very smooth.
3. Allow the batter to rest for at least 2 hours before cooking.
4. Place a large skillet or crêpe pan over medium-high heat and lightly coat the bottom with oil.
5. Pour about ¼ cup of batter into the skillet. Swirl the pan until the batter completely coats the bottom.
6. Cook the crêpe for about 1 minute, and then flip it over. Cook the other side of the crêpe for another minute, until lightly browned. Transfer the cooked crêpe to a plate and cover with a clean dish towel to keep warm.
7. Repeat until the batter is used up; you should have about 10 crêpes.
8. Spoon 1 tablespoon of yogurt onto each crêpe and place two crêpes on each plate. Top with berries and serve.

Per Serving (2 Crêpes)
Calories: 330 | fat: 6.9g | protein: 15.9g | carbs: 54.1g | fiber: 7.9g | sugar: 11.1g | sodium: 100mg

Oyster Mushroom Omelet

Prep time: 10 minutes | Cook time: 15 minutes | Serves 4

8 large eggs
½ cup skim milk
¼ teaspoon ground nutmeg
Sea salt and freshly ground black pepper, to taste
2 teaspoons extra-
virgin olive oil
2 cups sliced oyster mushrooms
½ red onion, chopped
1 teaspoon minced garlic
½ cup goat cheese, crumbled

1. Preheat the broiler.
2. In a medium bowl, whisk together the eggs, milk, and nutmeg until well combined. Season the egg mixture lightly with salt and pepper and set it aside.
3. Place an ovenproof skillet over medium heat and add the oil, coating the bottom completely by tilting the pan.
4. Sauté the mushrooms, onion, and garlic until translucent, about 7 minutes.
5. Pour the egg mixture into the skillet and cook until the bottom of the frittata is set, lifting the edges of the cooked egg to allow the uncooked egg to seep under.
6. Place the skillet under the broiler until the top is set, about 1 minute.
7. Sprinkle the goat cheese on the frittata and broil until the cheese is melted, about 1 minute more.
8. Remove from the oven. Cut into 4 wedges to serve.

Per Serving
Calories: 227 | fat: 15.1g | protein: 17.1g | carbs: 5.1g | fiber: 0.9g | sugar: 4.1g | sodium: 224mg

Shrimp Scallion Breakfast Bowl

Prep time: 15 minutes | Cook time: 20 minutes | Serves 6 to 8

1½ cups fat-free milk
1½ cups water
2 bay leaves
1 cup stone-ground corn grits
¼ cup seafood broth
2 garlic cloves, minced
2 scallions, white and green parts, thinly

sliced
1 pound (454 g) medium shrimp, shelled and deveined
½ teaspoon dried dill
½ teaspoon smoked paprika
¼ teaspoon celery seeds

1. In a medium stockpot, combine the milk, water, and bay leaves and bring to a boil over high heat.
2. Gradually add the grits, stirring continuously.
3. Reduce the heat to low, cover, and cook for 5 to 7 minutes, stirring often, or until the grits are soft and tender. Remove from the heat and discard the bay leaves.
4. In a small cast iron skillet, bring the broth to a simmer over medium heat.
5. Add the garlic and scallions, and sauté for 3 to 5 minutes, or until softened.
6. Add the shrimp, dill, paprika, and celery seeds and cook for about 7 minutes, or until the shrimp is light pink but not overcooked.
7. Plate each dish with ¼ cup of grits, topped with shrimp.

Per Serving
Calories: 198 | fat: 1.0g | protein: 20.1g | carbs: 24.9g | fiber: 1.0g | sugar: 3.1g | sodium: 204mg

Breakfast Cheesy Eggs with Broccoli Stalk Slaw

Prep time: 10 minutes | Cook time: 35 minutes | Serves 12 to 15

Nonstick cooking spray
6 medium brown eggs
8 medium egg whites
1 green bell pepper, chopped
½ small yellow onion, chopped
1 zucchini, finely

grated, with water pressed out
1 cup shredded reduced-fat Cheddar cheese
1 teaspoon paprika
½ teaspoon garlic powder

1. Preheat the oven to 350ºF (180ºC). Spray a large cast iron skillet with cooking spray.
2. In a medium bowl, whisk the eggs and egg whites together.
3. Add the bell pepper, onion, zucchini, cheese, paprika, and garlic powder, mix well, and pour into the prepared skillet.
4. Transfer the skillet to the oven, and bake for 35 minutes. Remove from the oven, and let rest for 5 minutes before serving with Broccoli Stalk Slaw.

Per Serving
Calories: 79 | fat: 4.1g | protein: 8.1g | carbs: 2.1g | fiber: 1.1g | sugar: 1.2g | sodium: 133mg

One Pan Zucchini Banana Bake

Prep time: 15 minutes | Cook time: 45 minutes | Serves 24

1½ cups gluten-free all-purpose flour
1 cup almond meal
½ cup chickpea flour
1 teaspoon salt
1 teaspoon baking powder
1 teaspoon baking soda
½ teaspoon ground nutmeg
½ teaspoon ground

cinnamon
3 medium brown eggs
¼ cup sunflower seed oil
2 ripe bananas, mashed
2 zucchini, grated, with water squeezed out
2 teaspoons almond extract

1. Preheat the oven to 350ºF (180ºC). Line a baking pan with parchment paper.
2. In a large bowl, use a fork or whisk to combine the gluten-free flour, almond meal, chickpea flour, salt, baking powder, baking soda, nutmeg, and cinnamon.
3. In a separate large bowl, beat the eggs, oil, bananas, zucchini, and almond extract together well.
4. Fold the dry ingredients into the wet ingredients, stir until well combined, and pour into the prepared pan.
5. Transfer the pan to the oven, and bake for 40 to 45 minutes, or until a butter knife inserted into the center comes out clean. Remove from the oven, and let the bread rest for 15 minutes before serving.

Per Serving
Calories: 204 | fat: 11.1g | protein: 6.1g | carbs: 21.1g | fiber: 4.1g | sugar: 4.1g | sodium: 324mg

Healthy Sweet Waffles with Greens & Onion

Prep time: 15 minutes | Cook time: 40 minutes | Serves 8

2 cups low-fat buttermilk
½ cup crushed tomato
1 medium egg
2 medium egg whites
1 cup gluten-free all-purpose flour
½ cup almond flour
½ cup coconut flour
2 teaspoons baking powder
½ teaspoon baking soda
½ teaspoon dried chives
Nonstick cooking spray

1. Heat a waffle iron.
2. In a medium bowl, whisk the buttermilk, tomato, egg, and egg whites together.
3. In another bowl, whisk the all-purpose flour, almond flour, coconut flour, baking powder, baking soda, and chives together.
4. Add the wet ingredients to the dry ingredients.
5. Lightly spray the waffle iron with cooking spray.
6. Gently pour ¼- to ½-cup portions of batter into the waffle iron. Cook time for waffles will vary depending on the kind of waffle iron you use, but it is usually 5 minutes per waffle. (Note: Once the waffle iron is hot, the cooking process is a bit faster.) Repeat until no batter remains.
7. Enjoy the waffles warm with Dandelion Greens with Sweet Onion.

Per Serving
Calories: 144 | fat: 4.1g | protein: 7.1g | carbs: 21.2g | fiber: 5.1g | sugar: 2.9g | sodium: 171mg

Mom's Special Chicken Turkey Mixed Sausage

Prep time: 15 minutes | Cook time: 15 minutes | Serves 10

½ red bell pepper, minced
½ orange bell pepper, minced
½ jalapeño pepper, minced
1 cup roughly chopped tomatoes
1 garlic clove, minced
1 pound (454 g)
ground chicken
1 pound (454 g) ground turkey
¼ teaspoon smoked paprika
¼ teaspoon ground cumin
1 tablespoon Worcestershire sauce

1. Preheat the oven to 350ºF (180ºC).
2. In a large bowl, combine the red bell pepper, orange bell pepper, jalapeño pepper, tomatoes, garlic, chicken, turkey, paprika, cumin, and Worcestershire sauce. Gently fold together until well mixed.
3. With clean hands, take about ⅓-cup portions, and shape into balls about the size of a golf ball.
4. Gently press the balls into flat disks, and place on a rimmed baking sheet in a single layer at least 1 inch apart. Repeat with the remaining meat. You should have 10 patties.
5. Transfer the baking sheet to the oven and cook for 5 to 7 minutes.
6. Flip the patties and cook for 5 to 7 minutes, or until the juices run clear.
7. Serve with Not-So-Traditional Gravy and Veggie Hash.

Per Serving
Calories: 125 | fat: 5.1g | protein: 19.1g | carbs: 2.1g | fiber: 0g | sugar: 1.1g | sodium: 70mg

Mashed Avocado Bread with Crumbled Bacon

Prep time: 10 minutes | Cook time: 5 minutes | Serves 2

2 slices whole-wheat bread, thinly sliced
½ avocado
2 tablespoons goat cheese, crumbled
Salt, to taste
2 slices of crumbled bacon, for topping (optional)

1. Toast the bread slices in a toaster for 2 to 3 minutes on each side until golden brown.
2. Using a large spoon, scoop the avocado flesh out of the skin and transfer to a medium bowl. Mash the flesh with a potato masher or the back of a fork until it has a spreadable consistency.
3. Spoon the mashed avocado onto the bread slices and evenly spread it all over.
4. Scatter with crumbled goat cheese and lightly season with salt.
5. Serve topped with crumbled bacon, if desired.

Per Serving
Calories: 140 | fat: 6.2g | protein: 5.2g | carbs: 18.2g | fiber: 5.1g | sugar: 0g | sodium: 197mg

Tender Zucchini with Okra

Prep time: 15 minutes | Cook time: 30 minutes | Serves 6 t0 8

2 tablespoons extra-virgin olive oil
2 garlic cloves, minced
1 small yellow onion, finely chopped
4 russet potatoes cut into 1-inch cubes
2 tablespoons Creole sseasoning

¼ cup low-sodium broth
1 zucchini, roughly chopped
1 green bell pepper, roughly chopped
2 cups okra, cut into 1-inch rounds

1. Heat the olive oil in a skillet over medium-low heat.
2. Toss in the garlic and onion and sauté for 4 minutes, or until the onion is translucent.
3. Add the potatoes, Creole sseasoning, and broth and stir well.
4. Cover, and cook for about 15 minutes, or until the potatoes are pierced easily with the tip of a sharp knife.
5. Add the zucchini, bell pepper, and okra into the skillet. Mix well, and cook uncovered for 7 to 10 minutes, stirring frequently, or until the zucchini is fork-tender.
6. Remove from the heat and serve on plates.

Per Serving
Calories: 168 | fat: 2.3g | protein: 6.7g | carbs: 30g | fiber: 5.5g | sugar: 3.7g | sodium: 286mg

Hot and Creamy Milk Corn Grits

Prep time: 5 minutes | Cook time: 7 minutes | Serves 4

1 cup fat-free milk
2 cups water

1 cup stone-ground corn grits

1. Pour the milk and water into a saucepan over medium heat, and then bring to a simmer until warmed through.
2. Add the corn grits and stir well. Reduce the heat to low and cook covered for 5 to 7 minutes, whisking continuously, or until the grits become tender.
3. Remove from the heat and serve warm.

Per Serving
Calories: 168 | fat: 1.1g | protein: 6.2g | carbs: 33.8g | fiber: 1.1g | sugar: 2.8g | sodium: 33mg

Vanilla flavoured Yogurt Smoothie

Prep time: 5 minutes | Cook time: 0 minutes | Serves 4

2 cups frozen berries of choice
1 cup plain low-fat Greek yogurt

1 cup unsweetened vanilla almond milk
½ cup natural almond butter

1. In a blender, add the berries, almond milk, yogurt, and almond butter. Process until fully mixed and creamy. Pour into four smoothie glasses.
2. Serve chilled or at room temperature.

Per Serving
Calories: 279 | fat: 18.2g | protein: 13.4g | carbs: 19.1g | fiber: 6.1g | sugar: 11.1g | sodium: 138mg

Almond Milk Egg Muffins

Prep time: 10 minutes | Cook time: 20 to 25 minutes | Serves 8 (1 egg bite each)

6 eggs, beaten
¼ cup unsweetened plain almond milk
¼ cup crumbled goat cheese
½ cup sliced brown mushrooms
1 cup chopped spinach

¼ cup sliced sun-dried tomatoes
1 red bell pepper, diced
Salt and freshly ground black pepper, to taste
Nonstick cooking spray

Special Equipment :
An 8-cup muffin tin

1. Preheat the oven to 350ºF (180ºC). Grease an 8-cup muffin tin with nonstick cooking spray.
2. Make the egg bites: Mix together the beaten eggs, almond milk, cheese, mushroom, spinach, tomatoes, bell pepper, salt, and pepper in a large bowl, and whisk to combine.
3. Spoon the mixture into the prepared muffin cups, filling each about three-quarters full.
4. Bake in the preheated oven for 20 to 25 minutes, or until the top is golden brown and a fork comes out clean.
5. Let the egg bites sit for 5 minutes until slightly cooled. Remove from the muffin tin and serve warm.

Per Serving
Calories: 68 | fat: 4.1g | protein: 6.2g | carbs: 2.9g | fiber: 1.1g | sugar: 2.0g | sodium: 126mg

Cut Oats Bowl with Peaches & Mango Chunks

Prep time: 5 minutes | Cook time: 20 minutes | Serves 4

1 cup steel cut oats
1 cup unsweetened almond milk
2 cups coconut water or water
¾ cup frozen chopped peaches
¾ cup frozen mango chunks
1 (2-inch) vanilla bean, scraped (seeds and pod)
Ground cinnamon
¼ cup chopped unsalted macadamia nuts

1. In the electric pressure cooker, combine the oats, almond milk, coconut water, peaches, mango chunks, and vanilla bean seeds and pod. Stir well.
2. Close and lock the lid of the pressure cooker. Set the valve to sealing.
3. Cook on high pressure for 5 minutes.
4. When the cooking is complete, allow the pressure to release naturally for 10 minutes, then quick release any remaining pressure. Hit Cancel.
5. Once the pin drops, unlock and remove the lid.
6. Discard the vanilla bean pod and stir well.
7. Spoon the oats into 4 bowls. Top each serving with a sprinkle of cinnamon and 1 tablespoon of the macadamia nuts.

Per Serving
Calories: 126 | fat: 7.1g | protein: 1.9g | carbs: 14.2g | fiber: 2.9g | sugar: 8.1g | sodium: 166mg

Cinnamon Cereal with Dried Cherries

Prep time: 10 minutes | Cook time: 30 minutes | Serves 16

4 cups rolled oats
½ cup pepitas
1 cup walnut pieces
1 teaspoon ground ginger
1 teaspoon ground cinnamon
¼ teaspoon salt
½ cup melted coconut oil
½ cup unsweetened applesauce
1 teaspoon vanilla extract
½ cup dried cherries

1. Preheat the oven to 350ºF (180ºC) and line a baking sheet with parchment paper. Set aside.
2. Mix together the oats, pepitas, walnut pieces, ginger, cinnamon, and salt in a large bowl. Gently toss to combine well.
3. In a separate bowl, whisk together the melted coconut oil, applesauce, and vanilla extract until completely mixed. Pour into the bowl of dry mixture and stir until the oats are coated in the oil mixture.
4. Spread out the mixture on the prepared baking sheet. Bake in the preheated oven for 30 minutes, stirring once halfway through, or until the oats are toasted.
5. Remove the granola from the oven to a wire rack. Allow to sit undisturbed until completely cooled.
6. When cooled, break the granola into small pieces. Stir in the dried cherries, and serve.

Per Serving
Calories: 194 | fat: 13.5g | protein: 6g | carbs: 12.2g | fiber: 4.5g | sugar: 1.8g | sodium: 39mg

Almond Cranberry Morning Bowl

Prep time: 10 minutes | Cook time: 15 minutes | Serves 5

¾ cup stone-ground grits or polenta (not instant)
½ cup unsweetened dried cranberries
Pinch kosher salt
1 tablespoon half-and-half
¼ cup sliced almonds, toasted

1. In the electric pressure cooker, stir together the grits, cranberries, salt, and 3 cups of water.
2. Close and lock the lid. Set the valve to sealing.
3. Cook on high pressure for 10 minutes.
4. When the cooking is complete, hit Cancel and quick release the pressure.
5. Once the pin drops, unlock and remove the lid.
6. Stir until the mixture is creamy, adding more half-and-half if necessary.
7. Spoon into serving bowls and sprinkle with almonds.

Per Serving
Calories: 219 | fat: 10.2g | protein: 4.9g | carbs: 32.1g | fiber: 4.1g | sugar: 6.9g | sodium: 30mg

Almond Walnut Berry Bowl

Prep time: 5 minutes | Cook time: 40 minutes | Serves 7

½ cup steel cut oats
½ cup short-grain brown rice
½ cup millet
½ cup barley
⅓ cup wild rice
¼ cup corn grits or polenta (not instant)
3 tablespoons ground flaxseed
½ teaspoon salt
Ground cinnamon (optional)
Unsweetened almond milk (optional)
Berries (optional)
Sliced almonds or chopped walnuts (optional)

1. In the electric pressure cooker, combine the oats, brown rice, millet, barley, wild rice, grits, flaxseed, salt, and 8 cups of water.
2. Close and lock the lid of the pressure cooker. Set the valve to sealing.
3. Cook on high pressure for 20 minutes.
4. When the cooking is complete, hit Cancel and allow the pressure to release naturally for 15 minutes, then quick release any remaining pressure.
5. Once the pin drops, unlock and remove the lid. Stir.
6. Serve with any combination of cinnamon, almond milk, berries, and nuts (if using).

Per Serving
Calories: 265 | fat: 3.1g | protein: 7.9g | carbs: 50.9g | fiber: 7.1g | sugar: 0.5g | sodium: 141mg

Cinnamon Farro Bowl with Berries

Prep time: 8 minutes | Cook time: 15 minutes | Serves 6

1 cup farro, rinsed and drained
1 cup unsweetened almond milk
¼ teaspoon kosher salt
½ teaspoon pure vanilla extract
1 teaspoon ground cinnamon
1 tablespoon pure maple syrup
1½ cups fresh blueberries, raspberries, or strawberries (or a combination)
6 tablespoons chopped walnuts

1. In the electric pressure cooker, combine the faro, almond milk, 1 cup of water, salt, vanilla, cinnamon, and maple syrup.

2. Close and lock the lid. Set the valve to sealing.
3. Cook on high pressure for 10 minutes.
4. When the cooking is complete, allow the pressure to release naturally for 10 minutes, then quick release any remaining pressure. Hit Cancel.
5. Once the pin drops, unlock and remove the lid.
6. Stir the farro. Spoon into bowls and top each serving with ¼ cup of berries and 1 tablespoon of walnuts.

Per Serving
Calories: 190 | fat: 4.9g | protein: 5.1g | carbs: 31.9g | fiber: 2.9g | sugar: 6.0g | sodium: 112mg

Vanilla Cheese Pancakes with Sugar-free Jam

Prep time: 5 minutes | Cook time: 10 minutes | Serves 2

½ cup low-fat cottage cheese
¼ cup oats
⅓ cup egg whites (about 2 egg whites)
1 tablespoon stevia
1 teaspoon vanilla extract
Olive oil cooking spray
Berries or sugar-free jam, for topping (optional)

1. Add the cottage cheese, oats, egg whites, stevia and vanilla extract to a food processor. Pulse into a smooth and thick batter.
2. Coat a large skillet with cooking spray and place it over medium heat.
3. Slowly pour half of the batter into the pan, tilting the pan to spread it evenly. Cook for about 2 to 3 minutes until the pancake turns golden brown around the edges.
4. Gently flip the pancake with a spatula and cook for 1 to 2 minutes more.
5. Transfer the pancake to a plate and repeat with the remaining batter.
6. Top with the berries or sugar-free jam and serve, if desired.

Per Serving
Calories: 188 | fat: 1.6g | protein: 24.6g | carbs: 18.9g | fiber: 1.9g | sugar: 2g | sodium: 258mg

Healthy Morning Oats Banana Pancakes

Prep time: 10 minutes | Cook time: 15 minutes | Serves 6

1 cup quick cooking oats
1½ teaspoons baking powder
2 eggs
⅓ cup mashed banana (about ½ medium bananas)
⅓ cup skim milk
½ teaspoon vanilla extract
2 tablespoons chopped pecans
1 tablespoon canola oil

1. Pulse the oats in a food processor until they are ground into a powder-like consistency.
2. Transfer the ground oats to a small bowl, along with the baking powder. Mix well.
3. Whisk together the eggs, mashed banana; skim milk, and vanilla in another bowl.
4. Pour into the bowl of dry ingredients, and stir with a spatula just until well incorporated. Add the chopped pecans and mix well.
5. In a large nonstick skillet, heat the canola oil over medium heat.
6. Spoon ¼ cup of batter for each pancake onto the hot skillet, swirling the pan so the batter covers the bottom evenly.
7. Cook for 1 to 2 minutes until bubbles form on top of the pancake. Flip the pancake and cook for an additional 1 to 2 minutes, or until the pancake is browned and cooked through. Repeat with the remaining batter.
8. Remove from the heat and serve on a plate.

Per Serving (1 Pancake)
Calories: 131 | fat: 6.9g | protein: 5.2g | carbs: 13.1g | fiber: 2.0g | sugar: 2.9g | sodium: 120mg

Yogurt Berry Smoothie Bowl

Prep time: 5 minutes | Cook time: 0 minute | Serves 2

½ cup frozen blackberries
1 cup Low-fat Greek yogurt
1 cup baby spinach
½ cup unsweetened
almond milk
½ teaspoon peeled and grated fresh ginger
¼ cup chopped pecans

1. In a blender or food processor, combine the blackberries, yogurt, spinach, almond milk, and ginger. Blend until smooth.
2. Spoon the mixture into two bowls.
3. Top each bowl with 2 tablespoons of chopped pecans and serve.

Per Serving
Calories: 202 | fat: 15g | protein: 7g | carbs: 15g | fiber: 4g | sugar: 31.1g | sodium: 566mg

Honey Almond Muffins

Prep time: 15 minutes | Cook time: 15 minutes | Serves 8

Dry Ingredients:
2½ cups finely ground almond flour
½ teaspoon baking powder
½ teaspoon ground
cardamom
¾ teaspoon ground cinnamon
¼ teaspoon salt

Wet Ingredients:
2 large eggs
4 tablespoons avocado or coconut oil
1 tablespoon raw honey
¼ teaspoon vanilla extract
Grated zest and juice of 1 medium orange

Special Equipment:
An 8-cup muffin tin

1. Preheat the oven to 375ºF (190ºC) and line an 8-cup muffin tin with paper liners.
2. Stir together the almond flour, baking powder, cardamom, cinnamon, and salt in a large bowl. Set aside.
3. Whisk together the eggs, oil, honey, vanilla, zest and juice in a medium bowl. Pour the mixture into the bowl of dry ingredients and stir with a spatula just until incorporated.
4. Pour the batter into the prepared muffin cups, filling each about three-quarters full.
5. Bake in the preheated oven for 15 minutes, or until the tops are golden and a toothpick inserted in the center comes out clean.
6. Let the muffins cool for 10 minutes before serving.

Per Serving
Calories: 287 | fat: 23.5g | protein: 7.9g | carbs: 15.8g | fiber: 3.8g | sugar: 9.8g | sodium: 96mg

Fried Eggs and Garlicky Brussels Sprouts

Prep time: 10 minutes | Cook time: 15 minutes | Serves 4

3 teaspoons extra-virgin olive oil, divided
1 pound (454 g) Brussels sprouts, sliced
2 garlic cloves, thinly sliced
¼ teaspoon salt
Juice of 1 lemon
4 eggs

1. Heat 1½ teaspoons of olive oil in a large skillet over medium heat.
2. Add the Brussels sprouts and sauté for 6 to 8 minutes until crispy and tender, stirring frequently.
3. Stir in the garlic and cook for about 1 minute until fragrant. Sprinkle with the salt and lemon juice.
4. Remove from the skillet to a plate and set aside.
5. Heat the remaining oil in the skillet over medium-high heat. Crack the eggs one at a time into the skillet and fry for about 3 minutes. Flip the eggs and continue cooking, or until the egg whites are set and the yolks are cooked to your liking.
6. Serve the fried eggs over the crispy Brussels sprouts.

Per Serving
Calories: 157 | fat: 8.9g | protein: 10.1g | carbs: 11.8g | fiber: 4.1g | sugar: 4.0g | sodium: 233mg

Sugarless Almond Milk Pancakes

Prep time: 5 minutes | Cook time: 15 minutes | Serves 4

½ cup coconut flour
1 teaspoon baking powder
½ teaspoon ground cinnamon
⅛ Teaspoon salt
8 large eggs
⅓ cup unsweetened almond milk
2 tablespoons avocado or coconut oil
1 teaspoon vanilla extract

1. Stir together the flour, baking powder, cinnamon, and salt in a large bowl. Set aside.
2. Beat the eggs with the almond milk, oil, and vanilla in a medium bowl until fully mixed.

3. Heat a large nonstick skillet over medium-low heat.
4. Make the pancakes: Pour ⅓ cup of batter into the hot skillet, tilting the pan to spread it evenly.
5. Cook for 3 to 4 minutes until bubbles form on the surface.
6. Flip the pancake with a spatula and cook for about 3 minutes, or until the pancake is browned around the edges and cooked through.
7. Repeat with the remaining batter.
8. Serve the pancakes on a plate while warm.

Per Serving
Calories: 269 | fat: 17.8g | protein: 13.9g | carbs: 10.1g | fiber: 5.1g | sugar: 1.9g | sodium: 324mg

Spinach Goat Cheese Bake

Prep time: 10 minutes | Cook time: 35 minutes | Serves 8

1 (10-ounce / 284-g) package frozen spinach, thawed and drained
1 (14-ounce / 397-g) can artichoke hearts, drained
¼ cup finely chopped red bell pepper
8 eggs, lightly beaten
¼ cup unsweetened plain almond milk
2 garlic cloves, minced
½ teaspoon salt
½ teaspoons freshly ground black pepper
½ cup crumbled goat cheese
Nonstick cooking spray

1. Preheat the oven to 375ºF (190ºC). Spray a baking dish with nonstick cooking spray and set aside.
2. Mix the spinach, artichoke hearts, bell peppers, beaten eggs, almond milk, garlic, salt, and pepper in a large bowl, and stir to incorporate.
3. Pour the mixture into the greased baking dish and scatter the goat cheese on top.
4. Bake in the preheated oven for 35 minutes, or until the top is lightly golden around the edges and eggs are set.
5. Remove from the oven and serve warm.

Per Serving
Calories: 105 | fat: 4.8g | protein: 8.9g | carbs: 6.1g | fiber: 1.7g | sugar: 1.0g | sodium: 486mg

Pepper Jack Cheesed Egg Scramble

Prep time: 5 minutes | Cook time: 10 minutes | Serves 2

2 tablespoons extra-virgin olive oil
½ red onion, finely chopped
1 green bell pepper, seeded and finely chopped
8 large egg whites (or

4 whole large eggs), beaten
½ teaspoon sea salt
2 ounces grated pepper Jack cheese
Salsa (optional, for serving)

1. In a medium nonstick skillet over medium-high heat, heat the olive oil until it shimmers.
2. Add the onion and bell pepper and cook, stirring occasionally, until the vegetables begin to brown, about 5 minutes.
3. Meanwhile, in a small bowl, whisk together the egg whites and salt.
4. Add the egg whites to the pan and cook, stirring, until the whites set, about 3 minutes. Add the cheese. Cook, stirring, 1 minute more.
5. Serve topped with salsa, if desired.

Per Serving
Calories: 314 | fat: 23g | protein: 22g | carbs: 6g | fiber: 1g | sugar: 4.46g | sodium: 977mg

Spiced Mushroom Tofu

Prep time: 5 minutes | Cook time: 10 minutes | Serves 2

2 tablespoons extra-virgin olive oil
½ red onion, finely chopped
8 ounces mushrooms, sliced
1 cup chopped kale
8 ounces tofu, cut into

pieces
2 garlic cloves, minced
Pinch red pepper flakes
½ teaspoon sea salt
⅛ teaspoon freshly ground black pepper

1. In a medium nonstick skillet over medium-high heat, heat the olive oil until it shimmers.
2. Add the onion, mushrooms, and kale. Cook, stirring occasionally, until the vegetables begin to brown, about 5 minutes.
3. Add the tofu. Cook, stirring, until the tofu starts to brown, 3 to 4 minutes more.

4. Add the garlic, red pepper flakes, salt, and pepper. Cook, stirring constantly, for 30 seconds more.

Per Serving
Calories: 234 | fat: 16g | protein: 13g | carbs: 12g | fiber: 6.9g | sugar: 13g | sodium: 673mg

Berried Buckwheat Crêpes with Yogurt

Prep time: 20 minutes | Cook time: 20 minutes | Serves 5

1½ cups skim milk
3 eggs
1 teaspoon extra-virgin olive oil, plus more for the skillet
1 cup buckwheat flour
½ cup whole-wheat

flour
½ cup 2 per cent Low-fat Greek yogurt
1 cup sliced strawberries
1 cup blueberries

1. In a large bowl, whisk together the milk, eggs, and 1 teaspoon of oil until well combined.
2. Into a medium bowl, sift together the buckwheat and whole-wheat flours. Add the dry ingredients to the wet ingredients and whisk until well combined and very smooth.
3. Allow the batter to rest for at least 2 hours before cooking.
4. Place a large skillet or crêpe pan over medium-high heat and lightly coat the bottom with oil.
5. Pour about ¼ cup of batter into the skillet. Swirl the pan until the batter completely coats the bottom.
6. Cook the crêpe for about 1 minute, and then flip it over. Cook the other side of the crêpe for another minute, until lightly browned. Transfer the cooked crêpe to a plate and cover with a clean dish towel to keep warm.
7. Repeat until the batter is used up; you should have about 10 crêpes.
8. Spoon 1 tablespoon of yogurt onto each crêpe and place two crêpes on each plate. Top with berries and serve.

Per Serving
Calories: 329 | fat: 7g | protein: 16g | carbs: 54g | fiber: 8g | sugar: 11g| sodium: 102mg

Mushroom Onion Omelet

Prep time: 5 minutes | Cook time: 10 minutes | Serves 4

2 tablespoons extra-virgin olive oil
½ onion, finely chopped
1 cup broccoli florets
1 cup sliced shiitake mushrooms
1 garlic clove, minced
8 large eggs, beaten
½ teaspoon sea salt
½ cup grated Parmesan cheese

1. Preheat the oven broiler on high. In a medium ovenproof skillet over medium-high heat, heat the olive oil until it shimmers.
2. Add the onion, broccoli, and mushrooms, and cook, stirring occasionally, until the vegetables start to brown, about 5 minutes.
3. Add the garlic and cook, stirring constantly, for 30 seconds. Arrange the vegetables in an even layer on the bottom of the pan.
4. While the vegetables cook, in a small bowl, whisk together the eggs and salt. Carefully pour the eggs over the vegetables.
5. Cook without stirring, allowing the eggs to set around the vegetables. As the eggs begin to set around the edges, use a spatula to pull the edges away from the sides of the pan.
6. Tilt the pan and allow the uncooked eggs to run into the spaces. Cook 1 to 2 minutes more, until it sets around the edges. The eggs will still be runny on top.
7. Sprinkle with the Parmesan and place the pan in the broiler. Broil until brown and puffy, about 3 minutes.
8. Cut into wedges to serve.

Per Serving
Calories: 280 | fat: 21g | protein: 19g | carbs: 7g | fiber: 2g | sugar: g| sodium: 654mg

Bacon Hot Sauce Cheesy Muffins

Prep time: 5 minutes | Cook time: 20 minutes | Serves 6

Cooking spray (for greasing)
6 large slices Canadian bacon
12 large eggs, beaten
1 teaspoon Dijon mustard
½ teaspoon sea salt
Dash hot sauce
1 cup shredded Swiss cheese

1. Preheat the oven to 350°F (176.67°C). Spray 6 non-stick muffin cups with cooking spray.
2. Line each cup with 1 slice of Canadian bacon.
3. In a bowl, whisk together the eggs, mustard, salt, and hot sauce. Fold in the cheese. Spoon the mixture into the muffin cups.
4. Bake until the eggs set, about 20 minutes.

Per Serving
Calories: 259 | fat: 17g | protein: 6g | carbs: 3g | fiber: 0g | sugar: g| sodium: 781mg

Morning Special Baked Eggs with Vegetables

Prep time: 20 minutes | Cook time: 50 minutes | Serves 4

2 teaspoons extra-virgin olive oil
½ sweet onion, finely chopped
2 teaspoons minced garlic
½ small eggplant, peeled and diced
1 green zucchini, diced
1 yellow zucchini, diced
1 red bell pepper, seeded and diced
3 tomatoes, seeded and chopped
1 tablespoon chopped fresh oregano
1 tablespoon chopped fresh basil
Pinch red pepper flakes
Sea salt to taste
Freshly ground black pepper
4 large eggs

1. Preheat the oven to 350°F (176.6°C).
2. Place a large ovenproof skillet over medium heat and add the olive oil.
3. Sauté the onion and garlic until softened and translucent, about 3 minutes. Stir in the eggplant and sauté for about 10 minutes, stirring occasionally. Stir in the zucchini and pepper and sauté for 5 minutes.
4. Reduce the heat to low and cover. Cook until the vegetables are soft, about 15 minutes.
5. Stir in the tomatoes, oregano, basil, and red pepper flakes, and cook 10 minutes more. Season the ratatouille with salt and pepper.
6. Use a spoon to create four wells in the mixture. Crack an egg into each well.
7. Place the skillet in the oven and bake until the eggs are firm, about 5 minutes.
8. Remove from the oven. Serve the eggs with a generous scoop of vegetables.

Per Serving
Calories: 147 | fat: 8g | protein: 9g | carbs: 13g | fiber: 4g | sugar: 7g| sodium: 98mg

Bacons with Eggs and Cheese

Prep time: 12 minutes | Cook time: 20 minutes | Serves 4

Nonstick cooking spray
1 slice whole grain bread, toasted
½ cup shredded smoked Gouda cheese
3 slices Canadian bacon, chopped
6 large eggs
¼ cup half-and-half
¼ teaspoon kosher salt
¼ teaspoons freshly ground black pepper
¼ teaspoon dry mustard

1. Spray a cake pan with cooking spray, or if the pan is nonstick, skip this step. If you don't have a 6-inch cake pan, any bowl or pan that fits inside your pressure cooker should work.
2. Crumble the toast into the bottom of the pan. Sprinkle with the cheese and Canadian bacon.
3. In a medium bowl, whisk together the eggs, half-and-half, salt, pepper, and dry mustard.
4. Pour the egg mixture into the pan. Loosely cover the pan with aluminum foil.
5. Pour 1½ cups water into the electric pressure cooker and insert a wire rack or trivet. Place the covered pan on top of the rack.
6. Close and lock the lid of the pressure cooker. Set the valve to sealing.
7. Cook on high pressure for 20 minutes.
8. When the cooking is complete, hit Cancel and quick release the pressure.
9. Once the pin drops, unlock and remove the lid.
10. Carefully transfer the pan from the pressure cooker to a cooling rack and let it sit for 5 minutes.
11. Cut into 4 wedges and serve.

Per Serving
Calories: 248 | fat: 15.1g | protein: 20.1g | carbs: 7.9g | fiber: 1.2g | sugar: 1.1g | sodium: 718mg

Asparagus Onion Quiche Bowl

Prep time: 15 minutes | Cook time: 15 minutes | Serves 2

Nonstick cooking spray
4 asparagus spears cut into ½-inch pieces
2 tablespoons finely chopped onion
3 ounces (85 g) smoked salmon
(skinless and boneless), chopped
3 large eggs
2 tablespoons 2% milk
¼ teaspoon dried dill
Pinch ground white pepper

1. Pour 1½ cups of water into the electric pressure cooker and insert a wire rack or trivet.
2. Lightly spray the bottom and sides of the ramekins with nonstick cooking spray. Divide the asparagus, onion, and salmon between the ramekins.
3. In a measuring cup with a spout, whisk together the eggs, milk, dill, and white pepper. Pour half of the egg mixture into each ramekin. Loosely cover the ramekins with aluminum foil.
4. Carefully place the ramekins inside the pot on the rack.
5. Close and lock the lid of the pressure cooker. Set the valve to sealing.
6. Cook on high pressure for 15 minutes.
7. When the cooking is complete, hit Cancel and quick release the pressure.
8. Once the pin drops, unlock and remove the lid.
9. Carefully remove the ramekins from the pot. Cool, covered, for 5 minutes.
10. Run a small silicone spatula or a knife around the edge of each ramekin. Invert each quiche onto a small plate and serve.

Per Serving
Calories: 182 | fat: 9.1g | protein: 20.1g | carbs: 2.9g | fiber: 1.0g | sugar: 1.1g | sodium: 645mg

Chapter 4: Lunch Recipes: Grains, Beans, and Legumes

Chicken Cabbage Salad

Prep time: 10 minutes | Cook time: 0 minutes | Serves 1

1 cup shredded cooked rotisserie chicken meat
1 cups shredded cabbage or coleslaw mix
1 Asian pear, cored, peeled, and julienned

2 scallions, white and green parts, sliced on the bias (cut diagonally into thin slices)
¼ cup Asian Vinaigrette

1. In a large bowl, combine the chicken, cabbage, pear, and scallions.
2. Toss with the vinaigrette just before serving.

Per Serving
Calories: 297 | fat: 20g | protein: 16g | carbs: 16g | fiber: 5g | sugar: 15.7g | sodium: 392mg

Low Sodium Veggie Greens with Black Beans

Prep time: 10 minutes | Cook time: 15 minutes | Serves 4

1 tablespoon olive oil
½ Vidalia onion, thinly sliced
1 bunch dandelion greens cut into ribbons
1 bunch beet greens, cut into ribbons
½ cup low-sodium

vegetable broth
1 (15-ounce / 425-g) can no-salt-added black beans
Salt and freshly ground black pepper, to taste

1. Heat the olive oil in a nonstick skillet over low heat until shimmering.
2. Add the onion and sauté for 3 minutes or until translucent.
3. Add the dandelion and beet greens, and broth to the skillet. Cover and cook for 8 minutes or until wilted.
4. Add the black beans and cook for 4 minutes or until soft. Sprinkle with salt and pepper. Stir to mix well.
5. Serve immediately.

Per Serving
Calories: 161 | fat: 4.0g | protein: 9.0g | carbs: 26.0g | fiber: 10.0g |sugar:1.0g| sodium: 224mg

Green Lentils Salad Bowl with Pine Nuts

Prep time: 15 minutes | Cook time: 0 minutes | Serves 4

3 tablespoons extra-virgin olive oil
2 tablespoons balsamic vinegar
2 teaspoons chopped fresh basil
1 teaspoon minced garlic
Sea salt and freshly ground black pepper, to taste
2 (15-ounce / 425-

g) cans sodium-free green lentils, rinsed and drained
½ English cucumber, diced
2 tomatoes, diced
½ cup halved Kalamata olives
¼ cup chopped fresh chives
2 tablespoons pine nuts

1. Whisk together the olive oil, vinegar, basil, and garlic in a medium bowl. Season with salt and pepper.
2. Stir in the lentils, cucumber, tomatoes, olives, and chives.
3. Top with the pine nuts, and serve.

Per Serving
Calories: 400 | fat: 15.1g | protein: 19.8g | carbs: 48.8g | fiber: 18.8g | sugar: 7.1g | sodium: 439mg

Apple and Almond butter spread Pita

Prep time: 10 minutes | Cook time: 0 minutes | Serves 2

½ apple, cored and chopped
¼ cup almond butter

½ teaspoon cinnamon
1 whole-wheat pita, halved

1. In a medium bowl, stir together the apple, almond butter, and cinnamon.
2. Spread with a spoon into the pita pocket halves.

Per Serving
Calories: 313 | fat: 20g | protein: 8g | carbs: 31g | fiber: 7g | sugar: g | sodium: 174mg

Pepperoni Cheesed Pita

Prep time: 10 minutes | Cook time: 0 minutes | Serves 2

½ cup tomato sauce
½ teaspoon oregano
½ teaspoon garlic powder
½ cup chopped black olives
2 canned artichoke hearts, drained and

chopped
2 ounces pepperoni, chopped
½ cup shredded mozzarella cheese
1 whole-wheat pita, halved

1. In a medium bowl, stir together the tomato sauce, oregano, and garlic powder.
2. Add the olives, artichoke hearts, pepperoni, and cheese. Stir to mix.
3. Spoon the mixture into the pita halves.

Per Serving
Calories: 376 | fat: 23g | protein: 17g | carbs: 27g | fiber: 6g | sugar: 17.8g | sodium: 107mg

Hot Wilted Greens with Pistachios & Thyme

Prep time: 10 minutes | Cook time: 15 minutes | Serves 6

1 teaspoon extra-virgin olive oil
½ sweet onion, finely chopped
1 teaspoon minced garlic
2 cups cooked barley
2 cups chopped kale

2 cups cooked butternut squash, cut into ½-inch cubes
2 tablespoons chopped pistachios
1 tablespoon chopped fresh thyme
Sea salt, to taste

1. Place a large skillet over medium heat and add the oil.
2. Sauté the onion and garlic until softened and translucent, about 3 minutes.
3. Add the barley and kale, and stir until the grains are heated through and the greens are wilted, about 7 minutes.
4. Stir in the squash, pistachios, and thyme.
5. Cook until the dish is hot, about 4 minutes, and season with salt.

Per Serving
Calories: 160 | fat: 1.9g | protein: 5.1g | carbs: 32.1g | fiber: 7.0g | sugar: 2.0g | sodium: 63mg

Chestnut Lettuce Wraps

Prep time: 10 minutes | Cook time: 0 minutes | Serves 2

1 tablespoon freshly squeezed lemon juice
1 teaspoon curry powder
1 teaspoon reduced-sodium soy sauce
½ teaspoon sriracha (or to taste)

½ cup canned water chestnuts, drained and chopped
2 (2.6-ounce/73.7 g) package tuna packed in water, drained
2 large butter lettuce leaves

1. In a medium bowl, whisk together lemon juice; curry powder, soy sauce, and sriracha.
2. Add the water chestnuts and tuna. Stir to combine.
3. Serve wrapped in the lettuce leaves.

Per Serving
Calories: 271 | fat: 14g | protein: 19g | carbs: 18g | fiber: 3g | sugar: 8.1g | sodium: 627mg

Perfect Corn Salad with Paprika Dressing

Prep time: 10 minutes | Cook time: 0 minutes | Serves 6

Salad:
1 ear fresh corn, kernels removed
1 cup cooked lima beans
1 cup cooked black-eyed peas
Dressing:
3 tablespoons apple cider vinegar
1 teaspoon paprika

1 red bell pepper, chopped
2 celery stalks, chopped
½ red onion, chopped

2 tablespoons extra-virgin olive oil

1. Combine the corn, beans, peas, bell pepper, celery, and onion in a large bowl. Stir to mix well.
2. Combine the vinegar, paprika, and olive oil in a small bowl. Stir to combine well.
3. Pour the dressing into the salad and toss to mix well. Let sit for 20 minutes to infuse before serving.

Per Serving
Calories: 170 | fat: 5.0g | protein: 10.0g | carbs: 29.0g | fiber: 10.0g | sugar: 4.0g | sodium: 20mg

Spicy Peppery Wax Beans Bowl

Prep time: 5 minutes | Cook time: 15 minutes | Serves 4

2 pounds (907 g) wax beans
2 tablespoons extra-virgin olive oil

Sea salt and freshly ground black pepper, to taste
Juice of ½ lemons

1. Preheat the oven to 400ºF (205ºC).
2. Line a baking sheet with aluminum foil.
3. In a large bowl, toss the beans and olive oil. Season lightly with salt and pepper.
4. Transfer the beans to the baking sheet and spread them out.
5. Roast the beans until caramelized and tender, about 10 to 12 minutes.
6. Transfer the beans to a serving platter and sprinkle with the lemon juice.

Per Serving

Calories: 99 | fat: 7.1g | protein: 2.1g | carbs: 8.1g | fiber: 4.2g | sugar: 3.9g | sodium: 814mg

Vegetable Broth Kidney Beans Veggie Bowl

Prep time: 10 minutes | Cook time: 8 to 12 minutes | Serves 8

2 tablespoons olive oil
1 medium yellow onion, chopped
1 cup crushed tomatoes
2 garlic cloves, minced
2 cups low-sodium canned red kidney

beans, rinsed
1 cup roughly chopped green beans
¼ cup low-sodium vegetable broth
1 teaspoon smoked paprika
Salt, to taste

1. Heat the olive oil in a nonstick skillet over medium heat until shimmering.
2. Add the onion, tomatoes, and garlic. Sauté for 3 to 5 minutes or until fragrant and the onion is translucent.
3. Add the kidney beans, green beans, and broth to the skillet. Sprinkle with paprika and salt, then sauté to combine well.
4. Cover the skillet and cook for 5 to 7 minutes or until the vegetables are tender. Serve immediately.

Per Serving

Calories: 187 | fat: 1.0g | protein: 13.0g | carbs: 34.0g | fiber: 10.0g | sugar: 4.0g | sodium: 102mg

Chicken Broth Wild Rice Perfect Bowl

Prep time: 15 minutes | Cook time: 45 minutes | Serves 4

1 tablespoon extra-virgin olive oil
½ sweet onion, chopped
2½ cups sodium-free chicken broth
1 cup wild rice, rinsed

and drained
Pinch sea salt
½ cup toasted pumpkin seeds
½ cup blueberries
1 teaspoon chopped fresh basil

1. Place a medium saucepan over medium-high heat and add the oil.
2. Sauté the onion until softened and translucent, about 3 minutes.
3. Stir in the broth and bring to a boil.
4. Stir in the rice and salt and reduce the heat to low. Cover and simmer until the rice is tender, about 40 minutes.
5. Drain off any excess broth, if necessary. Stir in the pumpkin seeds, blueberries, and basil.
6. Serve warm.

Per Serving

Calories: 259 | fat: 9.1g | protein: 10.8g | carbs: 37.1g | fiber: 3.9g | sugar: 4.1g | sodium: 543mg

Lettuce Tomato Salad

Prep time: 15 minutes | Cook time: 0 minutes | Serves 4

4 cups chopped iceberg lettuce
1 cucumber, chopped
10 cherry tomatoes, halved
1 cup crumbled feta cheese

1 cup pitted black olives
½ red onion, thinly sliced
½ cup Greek Vinaigrette

1. In a large bowl, combine the lettuce, cucumber, tomatoes, feta, olives, and onion. Toss to combine.
2. Toss with the dressing just before serving.

Per Serving

Calories: 337 | fat: 29g | protein: 8g | carbs: 13g | fiber: 3g | sugar: 14.5g | sodium: 904mg

Low Sodium Chicken Coconut Quinoa

Prep time: 15 minutes | Cook time: 25 minutes | Serves 4

2 teaspoons extra-virgin olive oil
1 sweet onion, chopped
1 tablespoon grated fresh ginger
2 teaspoons minced garlic

1 cup low-sodium chicken broth
¼ cup coconut milk
1 cup quinoa, well rinsed and drained
Sea salt, to taste
¼ cup shredded, unsweetened coconut

1. Place a large saucepan over medium-high heat and add the oil.
2. Sauté the onion, ginger, and garlic until softened, about 3 minutes.
3. Add the chicken broth, coconut milk, and quinoa.
4. Bring the mixture to a boil, and then reduce the heat to low and cover. Simmer the quinoa, stirring occasionally, until the quinoa is tender and most of the liquid has been absorbed, about 20 minutes.
5. Season the quinoa with salt, and serve topped with the coconut.

Per Serving
Calories: 355 | fat: 21.1g | protein: 9.1g | carbs: 35.1g | fiber: 6.1g | sugar: 4.0g | sodium: 33mg

Eggs and Snap Peas Fried Rice

Prep time: 5 minutes | Cook time: 15 minutes | Serves 8

2 cups sugar snap peas
2 egg whites
1 egg
1 cup instant brown

rice, cooked according to directions
2 tablespoons lite soy sauce

1. Add the peas to the cooked rice and mix to combine.
2. In a small skillet, scramble the egg and egg whites.
3. Add the rice and peas to the skillet and stir in soy sauce.
4. Cook, stirring frequently, about 2 to 3 minutes, or until heated through. Serve.

Per Serving
Calories: 108 | fat: 1.0g | protein: 4.1g | carbs: 20.1g | fiber: 1.0g | sugar: 1.0g | sodium: 151mg

Kale & Carrot Veggie Soup

Prep time: 10 minutes | Cook time: 15 minutes | Serves 2

2 tablespoons extra-virgin olive oil
1 onion, finely chopped
1 carrot, chopped
1 cup chopped kale (stems removed)
3 garlic cloves, minced
1 cup canned lentils, drained and rinsed

1 cups unsalted vegetable broth
2 teaspoons dried rosemary (or 1 tablespoon chopped fresh rosemary)
½ teaspoon sea salt
¼ teaspoons freshly ground black pepper

1. In a large pot over medium-high heat, heat the olive oil until it shimmers.
2. Add the onion and carrot and cook, stirring, until the vegetables begin to soften, about 3 minutes.
3. Add the kale and cook for 3 minutes more. Add the garlic and cook, stirring constantly, for 30 seconds.
4. Stir in the lentils, vegetable broth, rosemary, salt, and pepper. Bring to a simmer. Simmer, stirring occasionally, for 5 minutes more.

Per Serving
Calories: 160 | fat: 7g | protein: 6g | carbs: 19g | fiber: 6g | sugar: 15g | sodium: 187mg

Egg Pea Mix wrapped in Kale Leaves

Prep time: 10 minutes | Cook time: 0 minutes | Serves 2

1 teaspoon Dijon mustard
1 tablespoon chopped fresh dill
½ teaspoon sea salt
¼ teaspoon paprika
4 hard-boiled large

eggs, chopped
1 cup shelled fresh peas
2 tablespoons finely chopped red onion
2 large kale leaves

1. In a medium bowl, whisk together mustard, dill, salt, and paprika.
2. Stir in the eggs, peas, and onion.
3. Serve wrapped in kale leaves.

Per Serving
Calories: 295 | fat: 18g | protein: 17g | carbs: 18g | fiber: 4g | sugar: 3.7g | sodium: 620mg

Navy Bean Tomato Bowl with Feta cheese

Prep time: 20 minutes | Cook time: 0 minutes | Serves 4

2½ cups cooked navy beans
1 tomato, diced
½ red bell pepper, seeded and chopped
¼ jalapeño pepper, chopped
1 scallion, white and green parts, chopped

1 teaspoon minced garlic
1 teaspoon ground cumin
½ teaspoon ground coriander
½ cup low-sodium feta cheese

1. Put the beans, tomato, bell pepper, jalapeño, scallion, garlic, cumin, and coriander in a medium bowl and stir until well mixed.
2. Top with the feta cheese and serve.

Per Serving
Calories: 225 | fat: 4.1g | protein: 14.1g | carbs: 34.1g | fiber: 13.1g | sugar: 3.9g | sodium: 165mg

Spicy Veggie Black Bean Bowl with yogurt

Prep time: 15 minutes | Cook time: 15 minutes | Serves 6

1 tablespoon extra-virgin olive oil
½ onion, chopped
½ red bell pepper, seeded and chopped
½ green bell pepper, seeded and chopped
2 small zucchini, chopped
3 garlic cloves, minced
1 (15-ounce / 425-g) can low-sodium black beans, drained and rinsed
1 (10-ounce / 283-g) can low-sodium

enchilada sauce
1 teaspoon ground cumin
¼ teaspoon salt
¼ teaspoons freshly ground black pepper
½ cup shredded Cheddar cheese, divided
2 (6-inch) corn tortillas cut into strips
Chopped fresh cilantro, for garnish
Plain yogurt, for serving

1. Heat the broiler to high.
2. In a large oven-safe skillet, heat the oil over medium-high heat.
3. Add the onion, red bell pepper, green bell pepper, zucchini, and garlic to the skillet, and cook for 3 to 5 minutes until the onion softens.
4. Add the black beans, enchilada sauce, cumin, salt, pepper, ¼ cup of cheese, and tortilla strips, and mix together. Top with the remaining ¼ cup of cheese.
5. Put the skillet under the broiler and broil for 5 to 8 minutes until the cheese is melted and bubbly. Garnish with cilantro and serve with yogurt on the side.

Per Serving
Calories: 172 | fat: 7.1g | protein: 8.1g | carbs: 20.9g | fiber: 6.9g | sugar: 3.0g | sodium: 566mg

Low Fat Pepper Pilaf with Basil

Prep time: 10 minutes | Cook time: 30 minutes | Serves 4

1 tablespoon extra-virgin olive oil
½ sweet onion, chopped
2 teaspoons minced garlic
1 cup chopped eggplant
1½ cups bulgur

4 cups low-sodium chicken broth
1 cup diced tomato
Sea salt and freshly ground black pepper, to taste
2 tablespoons chopped fresh basil

1. Place a large saucepan over medium-high heat. Add the oil and sauté the onion and garlic until softened and translucent, about 3 minutes.
2. Stir in the eggplant and sauté 4 minutes to soften.
3. Stir in the bulgur, broth, and tomatoes. Bring the mixture to a boil.
4. Reduce the heat to low, cover, and simmer until the water has been absorbed, about 25 minutes.
5. Season the pilaf with salt and pepper.
6. Garnish with the basil, and serve.

Per Serving
Calories: 300 | fat: 4.0g | protein: 14.0g | carbs: 54.0g | fiber: 12.0g | sugar: 7.0g | sodium: 358mg

Baby Spinach Walnut Salad

Prep time: 10 minutes | Cook time: 0 minutes | Serves 2

4 cups baby spinach
½ pear, cored, peeled, and chopped
¼ cup whole walnuts, chopped
2 tablespoons apple cider vinegar

2 tablespoons extra-virgin olive oil
1 teaspoon peeled and grated fresh ginger
½ teaspoon Dijon mustard
½ teaspoon sea salt

1. Layer the spinach on the bottom of two mason jars. Top with the pear and walnuts.
2. In a small bowl, whisk together the vinegar, oil, ginger, mustard, and salt. Put in another lidded container.
3. Shake the dressing before serving and add it to the mason jars. Close the jars and shake to distribute the dressing.

Per Serving
Calories: 254 | fat: 23g | protein: 4g | carbs: 10g | fiber: 4g | sugar: g | sodium: 340mg

Veggie Quinoa Zucchini Bowl

Prep time: 15 minutes | Cook time: 15 minutes | Serves 6

2 cups vegetable broth
1 cup quinoa, well rinsed and drained
1 teaspoon extra-virgin olive oil
½ sweet onion, chopped
2 teaspoons minced garlic
½ large green zucchini, halved lengthwise and

cut into half disks
1 red bell pepper, seeded and cut into thin strips
1 cup fresh or frozen corn kernels
1 teaspoon chopped fresh basil
Sea salt and freshly ground black pepper, to taste

1. Place a medium saucepan over medium heat and add the vegetable broth. Bring the broth to a boil and add the quinoa. Cover and reduce the heat to low.
2. Cook until the quinoa has absorbed all the broth, about 15 minutes. Remove from the heat and let it cool slightly.
3. While the quinoa is cooking, place a large skillet over medium-high heat and add the oil.
4. Sauté the onion and garlic until softened and translucent, about 3 minutes.
5. Add the zucchini, bell pepper, and corn, and sauté until the vegetables are tender-crisp, about 5 minutes.
6. Remove the skillet from the heat.
7. Add the cooked quinoa and the basil to the skillet, stirring to combine. Season with salt and pepper, and serve.

Per Serving
Calories: 159 | fat: 3.0g | protein: 7.1g | carbs: 26.1g | fiber: 2.9g | sugar: 3.0g | sodium: 300mg

Easy Cheesy Pan Cake with Bean Mixture

Prep time: 10 minutes | Cook time: 5 minutes | Serves 4

1 cup grated Parmesan cheese, divided
1 (15-ounce / 425-g) can low-sodium white beans, drained and rinsed
1 cucumber, peeled and finely diced
½ cup finely diced red onion
¼ cup thinly sliced

fresh basil
1 garlic clove, minced
½ jalapeño pepper, diced
1 tablespoon extra-virgin olive oil
1 tablespoon balsamic vinegar
¼ teaspoon salt
Freshly ground black pepper, to taste

1. Heat a medium nonstick skillet over medium heat. Sprinkle 2 tablespoons of cheese in a thin circle in the center of the pan, flattening it with a spatula.
2. When the cheese melts, use a spatula to flip the cheese and lightly brown the other side.
3. Remove the cheese "pancake" from the pan and place into the cup of a muffin tin, bending it gently with your hands to fit in the muffin cup.
4. Repeat with the remaining cheese until you have 8 cups.
5. In a mixing bowl, combine the beans, cucumber, onion, basil, garlic, jalapeño, olive oil, and vinegar, and season with the salt and pepper.
6. Fill each cup with the bean mixture just before serving.

Per Serving
Calories: 260 | fat: 12.1g | protein: 14.9 | carbs: 23.9g | fiber: 8.0g | sugar: 3.9g | sodium: 552mg

Veggie Pasta with Pesto & Parmesan

Prep time: 10 minutes | Cook time: 20 minutes | Serves 6

½ cup shredded kale
½ cup fresh basil
½ cup sun-dried tomatoes
¼ cup chopped almonds

2 tablespoons extra-virgin olive oil
8 ounces (227 g) dry whole-wheat linguine
½ cup grated Parmesan cheese

1. Place the kale, basil, sun-dried tomatoes, almonds, and olive oil in a food processor or blender, and pulse until a chunky paste forms, about 2 minutes. Scoop the pesto into a bowl and set it aside.
2. Place a large pot filled with water on high heat and bring to a boil.
3. Cook the pasta al dente, according to the package directions.
4. Drain the pasta and toss it with the pesto and the Parmesan cheese.
5. Serve immediately.

Per Serving
Calories: 218 | fat: 10.1g | protein: 9.1g | carbs: 25.1g | fiber: 1.1g | sugar: 2.9g | sodium: 195mg

Baked Navy Bean Oregano Mix

Prep time: 10 minutes | Cook time: 25 minutes | Serves 8

1 teaspoon extra-virgin olive oil
½ sweet onion, chopped
2 teaspoons minced garlic
2 sweet potatoes, peeled and diced
1 (28-ounce / 794-g) can low-sodium diced tomatoes
¼ cup sodium-free tomato paste

2 tablespoons granulated sweetener
2 tablespoons hot sauce
1 tablespoon Dijon mustard
3 (15-ounce / 425-g) cans sodium-free navy or white beans, drained
1 tablespoon chopped fresh oregano

1. Place a large saucepan over medium-high heat and add the oil.
2. Sauté the onion and garlic until translucent, about 3 minutes.
3. Stir in the sweet potatoes, diced tomatoes, tomato paste, sweetener, hot sauce, and mustard and bring to a boil.
4. Reduce the heat and simmer the tomato sauce for 10 minutes.
5. Stir in the beans and simmer for 10 minutes more.
6. Stir in the oregano and serve.

Per Serving
Calories: 256 | fat: 2.1g | protein: 15.1g | carbs: 48.1g | fiber: 11.9g | sugar: 8.1g | sodium: 150mg

Garlicky Bell Pepper Beans Chili Bowl

Prep time: 20 minutes | Cook time: 30 minutes | Serves 8

1 teaspoon extra-virgin olive oil
1 sweet onion, chopped
1 red bell pepper, seeded and diced
1 green bell pepper, seeded and diced
2 teaspoons minced garlic
1 (28-ounce / 794-g) can low-sodium diced tomatoes
1 (15-ounce / 425-g) can sodium-free black beans, rinsed and drained

1 (15-ounce / 425-g) can sodium-free red kidney beans, rinsed and drained
1 (15-ounce / 425-g) can sodium-free navy beans, rinsed and drained
2 tablespoons chili powder
2 teaspoons ground cumin
1 teaspoon ground coriander
¼ teaspoon red pepper flakes

1. Place a large saucepan over medium-high heat and add the oil.
2. Sauté the onion, red and green bell peppers, and garlic until the vegetables have softened, about 5 minutes.
3. Add the tomatoes, black beans, red kidney beans, navy beans, chili powder, cumin, coriander, and red pepper flakes to the pan.
4. Bring the chili to a boil, and then reduce the heat to low.
5. Simmer the chili, stirring occasionally, for at least 30 minutes.
6. Serve hot.

Per Serving
Calories: 480 | fat: 28.1g | protein: 15.1g | carbs: 45.1g | fiber: 16.9g | sugar: 4.0g | sodium: 16mg

Bell Pepper Black Olive Salad

Prep time: 10 minutes | Cook time: 0 minutes | Serves 2

2 cups chopped iceberg lettuce
10 cherry tomatoes, halved
1 cup pitted black olives, chopped
6 ounces ham, chopped
½ red onion, chopped
1 red bell pepper, seeded and chopped
10 basil leaves, torn
¼ cup Italian Vinaigrette

1. In a large bowl, combine the lettuce, tomatoes, olives, ham, onion, bell pepper, and basil leaves.
2. Toss with the vinaigrette just before serving.

Per Serving
Calories: 434 | fat: 31g | protein: 22g | carbs: 17g | fiber: 5g | sugar: 5.61g | sodium: 228mg

Spicy Cheesy Zucchini Macaroni Pie

Prep time: 15 minutes | Cook time: 30 minutes | Serves 6

1 pound (454-g) whole-wheat macaroni
2 celery stalks, thinly sliced
1 small yellow onion, chopped
2 garlic cloves, minced
Salt, to taste
¼ teaspoons freshly ground black pepper
2 tablespoons chickpea
flour
2 cups grated reduced-fat sharp Cheddar cheese
1 cup fat-free milk
2 large zucchini, finely grated and squeezed dry
2 roasted red peppers, chopped into ¼-inch pieces

1. Preheat the oven to 350ºF (180ºC).
2. Bring a pot of water to a boil, then add the macaroni and cook for 4 minutes or until al dente.
3. Drain the macaroni and transfer to a large bowl. Reserve 1 cup of the macaroni water.
4. Pour the macaroni water in an oven-safe skillet and heat over medium heat.
5. Add the celery, onion, garlic, salt, and black pepper to the skillet and sauté for 4 minutes or until tender.
6. Gently mix in the chickpea flour, and then fold in the cheese and milk. Keep stirring until the mixture is thick and smooth.

7. Add the cooked macaroni, zucchini, and red peppers. Stir to combine well.
8. Cover the skillet with aluminum foil and transfer it to the preheated oven.
9. Bake for 15 minutes or until the cheese melts, then remove the foil and bake for 5 more minutes or until lightly browned.
10. Remove the pie from the oven and serve immediately.

Per Serving
Calories: 378 | fat: 4.0g | protein: 24.0g | carbs: 67.0g | fiber: 8.0g | sugar: 6.0g | sodium: 332mg

Lemony Farro with Eggs and Avocado

Prep time: 5 minutes | Cook time: 25 minutes | Serves 4

3 cups water
1 cup uncooked farro
1 tablespoon extra-virgin olive oil
1 teaspoon ground cumin
½ teaspoon salt
½ teaspoons freshly
ground black pepper
4 hardboiled eggs, sliced
1 avocado, sliced
⅓ cup plain low-fat Greek yogurt
4 lemon wedges

1. In a medium saucepan, bring the water to a boil over high heat.
2. Pour the farro into the boiling water, and stir to submerge the grains. Reduce the heat to medium and cook for 20 minutes. Drain and set aside.
3. Heat a medium skillet over medium-low heat. When hot, pour in the oil, then add the cooked farro, cumin, salt, and pepper. Cook for 3 to 5 minutes, stirring occasionally.
4. Divide the farro into four equal portions, and top each with one-quarter of the eggs, avocado, and yogurt.
5. Add a squeeze of lemon over the top of each portion.

Per Serving
Calories: 333 | fat: 16.1g | protein: 15.1g | carbs: 31.9g | fiber: 7.9g | sugar: 2.0g | sodium: 360mg

Brown Rice Bowl with Egg and Avocado

Prep time: 15 minutes | Cook time: 15 minutes | Serves 8

2 teaspoons extra-virgin olive oil
½ sweet onion, chopped
1 teaspoon minced jalapeño pepper
1 teaspoon minced garlic
1 (15-ounce / 425-g) can sodium-free red kidney beans, rinsed
and drained
1 large tomato, chopped
1 teaspoon chopped fresh thyme
Sea salt and freshly ground black pepper, to taste
2 cups cooked brown rice

1. Place a large skillet over medium-high heat and add the olive oil.
2. Sauté the onion, jalapeño, and garlic until softened, about 3 minutes.
3. Stir in the beans, tomato, and thyme.
4. Cook until heated through, about 10 minutes. Season with salt and pepper.
5. Serve over the warm brown rice with Egg and Avocado.

Per Serving
Calories: 200 | fat: 2.1g | protein: 9.1g | carbs: 37.1g | fiber: 6.1g | sugar: 2.0g | sodium: 40mg

Thyme Pepper spiced Chicken Mushroom Rice

Prep time: 20 minutes | Cook time: 35 minutes | Serves 8

1 tablespoon extra-virgin olive oil
1 cup chopped button mushrooms
½ sweet onion, chopped
1 celery stalk, chopped
2 teaspoons minced garlic
2 cups brown basmati
rice
4 cups low-sodium chicken broth
1 teaspoon chopped fresh thyme
Sea salt and freshly ground black pepper, to taste
½ cup chopped hazelnuts

1. Place a large saucepan over medium-high heat and add the oil.
2. Sauté the mushrooms, onion, celery, and garlic until lightly browned, about 10 minutes.
3. Add the rice and sauté for an additional minute.
4. Add the chicken broth and bring to a boil.
5. Reduce the heat to low and cover the pot. Simmer until the liquid is absorbed and the rice is tender, about 20 minutes.
6. Stir in the thyme and season with salt and pepper.
7. Top with the hazelnuts, and serve.

Per Serving
Calories: 240 | fat: 6.1g | protein: 7.1g | carbs: 38.9g | fiber: 0.9g | sugar: 1.1g | sodium: 388mg

Wheat Couscous with Scallions & Pecans

Prep time: 10 minutes | Cook time: 5 minutes | Serves 6

Dressing:
¼ cup extra-virgin olive oil
2 tablespoons balsamic vinegar
1 teaspoon honey
Sea salt and freshly ground black pepper, to taste

Couscous:
1¼ cups whole-wheat couscous
Pinch sea salt
1 teaspoon butter
2 cups boiling water
1 scallion, white and green parts, chopped
½ cup chopped pecans
2 tablespoons chopped fresh parsley

Make Dressing:
1. Whisk together the oil, vinegar, and honey.
2. Season with salt and pepper and set it aside.

Make Couscous:
3. Put the couscous, salt, and butter in a large heat-proof bowl and pour the boiling water on top.
4. Stir and cover the bowl. Let it sit for 5 minutes. Uncover and fluff the couscous with a fork.
5. Stir in the dressing, scallion, pecans, and parsley. Serve warm.

Per Serving
Calories: 250 | fat: 12.9g | protein: 5.1g | carbs: 30.1g | fiber: 2.2g | sugar: 1.1g | sodium: 77mg

Lemony Black-Eyed Peas Dish

Prep time: 15 minutes | Cook time: 40 minutes | Serves 12

1 pound (454 g) dried black-eyed peas, rinsed and drained
4 cups vegetable broth
1 cup coconut water
1 cup chopped onion
4 large carrots, coarsely chopped
1½ tablespoons curry powder
1 tablespoon minced garlic
1 teaspoon peeled and minced fresh ginger
1 tablespoon extra-virgin olive oil
Kosher salt (optional)
Lime wedges, for serving

1. In the electric pressure cooker, combine the black-eyed peas, broth, coconut water, onion, carrots, curry powder, garlic, and ginger. Drizzle the olive oil over the top.
2. Close and lock the lid of the pressure cooker. Set the valve to sealing.
3. Cook on high pressure for 25 minutes.
4. When the cooking is complete, hit Cancel and allow the pressure to release naturally for 10 minutes, then quick release any remaining pressure.
5. Once the pin drops, unlock and remove the lid.
6. Season with salt (if using) and squeeze some fresh lime juice on each serving.

Per Serving
Calories: 113 | fat: 3.1g | protein: 10.1g | carbs: 30.9g | fiber: 6.1g | sugar: 6.0g | sodium: 672mg

Tomato Green chilies Soup with Lime Yogurt

Prep time: 8 hours 10 minutes | Cook time: 1 hour 33 minutes | Serves 8

2 tablespoons avocado oil
1 medium onion, chopped
1 (10-ounce / 284-g) can diced tomatoes and green chillies
1 pound (454 g) dried black beans, soaked in water for at least 8 hours, rinsed
1 teaspoon ground cumin
3 garlic cloves, minced
6 cup chicken bone broth, vegetable broth, or water
Kosher salt, to taste
1 tablespoon freshly squeezed lime juice
¼ cup Low-fat Greek yogurt

1. Heat the avocado oil in a nonstick skillet over medium heat until shimmering.
2. Add the onion and sauté for 3 minutes or until translucent.
3. Transfer the onion to a pot, then add the tomatoes and green chilies and their juices, black beans, cumin, garlic, broth, and salt. Stir to combine well.
4. Bring to a boil over medium-high heat, and then reduce the heat to low. Simmer for 1 hour and 30 minutes or until the beans are soft.
5. Meanwhile, combine the lime juice with Greek yogurt in a small bowl. Stir to mix well.
6. Pour the soup in a large serving bowl, and then drizzle with lime yogurt before serving.

Per Serving (1 Cup)
Calories: 285 | fat: 6.0g | protein: 19.0g | carbs: 42.0g | fiber: 10.0g | sugar: 3.0g | sodium: 174mg

Baked Margarine Cheesy Fish

Prep time: 10 minutes | Cook time: 20 minutes | Serves 4

1 pound (454 g) flounder
2 cups green beans
4 tablespoons margarine
8 basil leaves
1.75 ounces (50 g)
pork rinds
½ cup reduced fat Parmesan cheese
3 cloves garlic
Salt and ground black pepper, to taste
Nonstick cooking spray

1. Heat oven to 350ºF (180ºC). Spray a baking dish with cooking spray.
2. Steam green beans until they are almost tender, about 15 minutes, less if you use frozen or canned beans. Lay green beans in the prepared dish.
3. Place the fish filets over the green beans and season with salt and pepper.
4. Place the garlic, basil, pork rinds, and Parmesan in a food processor and pulse until mixture resembles crumbs. Sprinkle over fish. Cut margarine into small pieces and place on top.
5. Bake 15 to 20 minutes or until fish flakes easily with a fork. Serve.

Per Serving
Calories: 360 | fat: 20.0g | protein: 39.1g | carbs: 5.1g | fiber: 2.0g | sugar: 1.0g | sodium: 322mg

Veggie Salsa Fritters

Prep time: 10 minutes | Cook time: 25 minutes | Serves 20 Fritters

1¾ cups all-purpose flour
½ teaspoon cumin
2 teaspoons baking powder
2 teaspoons salt
½ teaspoon black pepper
4 egg whites, lightly

beaten
1 cup salsa
2 (16-ounce / 454-g) cans no-salt-added black beans, rinsed and drained
1 tablespoon canola oil, plus extra if needed

1. Combine the flour, cumin, baking powder, salt, and pepper in a large bowl, and then mix in the egg whites and salsa. Add the black beans and stir to mix well.
2. Heat the canola oil in a nonstick skillet over medium-high heat.
3. Spoon 1 teaspoon of the mixture into the skillet to make a fritter. Make more fritters to coat the bottom of the skillet.
4. Keep a little space between each two fritters. You may need to work in batches to avoid overcrowding.
5. Cook for 3 minutes or until the fritters are golden brown on both sides. Flip the fritters and flatten with a spatula halfway through the cooking time.
6. Repeat with the remaining mixture. Add more oil as needed.
7. Serve immediately.

Per Serving
Calories: 115 | fat: 1.0g | protein: 6.0g | carbs: 20.0g | fiber: 5.0g | sugar: 2.0g | sodium: 350mg

Classy Chicken Black Bean Soup

Prep time: 10 minutes | Cook time: 25 minutes | Serves 7

2 tablespoons olive oil
½ onion, diced
1 pound (454 g) boneless and skinless chicken breast, cut into ½-inch cubes
½ teaspoon Adobo seasoning, divided
¼ teaspoon black pepper
1 (15-ounce / 425-g) can no-salt-added

black beans, rinsed and drained
1 (14.5-ounce / 411-g) can fire-roasted tomatoes
½ cup frozen corn
½ teaspoon cumin
1 tablespoon chili powder
5 cups low-sodium chicken broth

1. Grease a stockpot with olive oil and heat over medium-high heat until shimmering.
2. Add the onion and sauté for 3 minutes or until translucent.
3. Add the chicken breast and sprinkle with Adobo seasoning and pepper. Put the lid on and cook for 6 minutes or until lightly browned. Shake the pot halfway through the cooking time.
4. Add the remaining ingredients. Reduce the heat to low and simmer for 15 minutes or until the black beans are soft.
5. Serve immediately.

Per Serving
Calories: 170 | fat: 3.5g | protein: 20.0g | carbs: 15.0g | fiber: 5.0g | sugar: 3.0g | sodium: 390mg

Fat free Sofrito Dumplings

Prep time: 20 minutes | Cook time: 15 minutes | Serves 8 to 10

4 cups water
4 cups low-sodium vegetable broth
1 cup cassava flour
1 cup gluten-free all-purpose flour

2 teaspoons baking powder
1 teaspoon salt
1 cup fat-free milk
2 tablespoons bottled chimichurri or sofrito

1. In a large pot, bring the water and the broth to a slow boil over medium-high heat.
2. In a large mixing bowl, whisk the cassava flour, all-purpose flour, baking powder, and salt together.
3. In a small bowl, whisk the milk and chimichurri together until combined.
4. Stir the wet ingredients into the dry ingredients a little at a time to create a firm dough.
5. With clean hands, pinch offs a small piece of dough. Roll into a ball, and gently flatten in the palm of your hand, forming a disk. Repeat until no dough remains.
6. Carefully drop the dumplings one at a time into the boiling liquid. Cover and simmer for 15 minutes, or until the dumplings are cooked through. You can test by inserting a fork into the dumpling; it should come out clean.
7. Serve warm.

Per Serving
Calories: 133 | fat: 1.1g | protein: 4.1g | carbs: 25.9g | fiber: 3.1g | sugar: 2.0g | sodium: 328mg

Chicken Rice with Almond Cranberry Salad

Prep time: 10 minutes | Cook time: 45 minutes | Serves 6 Cups

Rice:

2½ cups chicken bone broth, vegetable broth, or water

2 cups wild rice blend, rinsed

1 teaspoon kosher salt

Dressing:

Juice of 1 medium orange (about ¼ cup)

1½ teaspoons grated orange zest

¼ cup white wine

vinegar

1 teaspoon pure maple syrup

¼ cup extra-virgin olive oil

Salad:

½ cup sliced almonds, toasted

¾ cup unsweetened

dried cranberries

Freshly ground black pepper, to taste

Make the Rice:

1. Pour the broth in a pot, then add the rice and sprinkle with salt. Bring to a boil over medium-high heat.
2. Reduce the heat to low. Cover the pot, and then simmer for 45 minutes.
3. Turn off the heat and fluff the rice with a fork. Set aside until ready to use.

Make the Dressing:

4. When cooking the rice, make the dressing: Combine the ingredients for the dressing in a small bowl. Stir to combine well. Set aside until ready to use.

Make the Salad:

5. Put the cooked rice, almonds, and cranberries in a bowl, and then sprinkle with black pepper. Add the dressing, then toss to combine well.
6. Serve immediately.

Per Serving (¹/₃ Cup)

Calories: 126 | fat: 5.0g | protein: 3.0g | carbs: 18.0g | fiber: 2.0g | sugar: 2.0g | sodium: 120mg

Chickpea Wraps for Quesadillas

Prep time: 5 minutes | Cook time: 10 minutes | Serves 4

1 cup chickpea flour

1 cup water

¼ teaspoon salt

Nonstick cooking spray

1. In a large bowl, whisk all together until no lumps remain.
2. Spray a skillet with cooking spray and place over medium-high heat.
3. Pour batter in, ¼ cup at a time, and tilt pan to spread thinly.
4. Cook until golden brown on each side, about 2 minutes per side.
5. Use for taco shells, enchiladas, quesadillas or whatever you desire.

Per Serving

Calories: 90 | fat: 2.0g | protein: 5.1g | carbs: 13.1g | fiber: 3.0g | sugar: 3.0g | sodium: 161mg

Garlic Zucchini Chicken Soup

Prep time: 10 minutes | Cook time: 15 minutes | Serves 4

2 tablespoons extra-virgin olive oil

12 ounces (336 g) chicken breast, chopped

1 onion, chopped

2 carrots, chopped

2 celery stalks, chopped

2 garlic cloves

6 cups unsalted chicken broth

1 teaspoon dried thyme

1 teaspoon sea salt

2 medium zucchinis cut into noodles (or store-bought zucchini noodles)

1. In a large pot over medium-high heat, heat the olive oil until it shimmers.
2. Add the chicken and cook until it is opaque, about 5 minutes. With a slotted spoon, remove the chicken from the pot and set aside on a plate.
3. Add the onion, carrots, and celery to the pot. Cook, stirring occasionally, until the vegetables are soft, about 5 minutes.
4. Add the garlic and cook, stirring constantly, for 30 seconds. Add the chicken broth, thyme, and salt. Bring to a boil, and reduce the heat to medium.
5. Add the zucchini and return the chicken to the pan, adding any juices that have collected on the plate.
6. Cook, stirring occasionally, until the zucchini noodles are soft, 1 to 2 minutes more.

Per Serving

Calories: 236 | fat: 10g | protein: 27g | carbs: 11g | fiber: 3g | sugar: 17.3g | sodium: 201mg

Chapter 5: Meatless Mains and Seafood

Sodium Vegetable Callaloo

Prep time: 15 minutes | Cook time: 25 minutes | Serves 6

3 cups low-sodium vegetable broth
1 (13.5-ounce / 383-g) can light coconut milk
¼ cup coconut cream
1 tablespoon unsalted non-hydrogenated plant-based butter
12 ounces (340 g) okra, cut into 1-inch chunks
1 small onion, chopped
½ butternut squash, peeled, seeded, and cut into 4-inch chunks
1 bunch collard greens, stemmed and chopped
1 hot pepper (Scotch bonnet or habanero)

1. In an electric pressure cooker, combine the vegetable broth, coconut milk, coconut cream, and butter.
2. Layer the okra, onion, squash, collard greens, and whole hot pepper on top.
3. Close and lock the lid, and set the pressure valve to sealing.
4. Select the Manual/Pressure Cook setting, and cook for 20 minutes.
5. Once cooking is complete, quick-release the pressure. Carefully remove the lid.
6. Remove and discard the hot pepper. Carefully transfer the callaloo to a blender, and blend until smooth. Serve spooned over grits.

Per Serving

Calories: 174 | fat: 8.1g | protein: 4.1g | carbs: 24.9g | fiber: 5.1g | sugar: 10.0g | sodium: 126mg

Garlic Onion Egg Muffins

Prep time: 10 minutes | Cook time: 15 minutes | Serves 6

Nonstick cooking spray
2 tablespoons extra-virgin olive oil
1 onion, finely chopped
2 cups baby spinach
2 garlic cloves, minced
8 large eggs, beaten
¼ cup 1% or skim milk
½ teaspoon sea salt
¼ teaspoons freshly ground black pepper
1 cup shredded Swiss cheese

1. Preheat the oven to 375ºF (190ºC). Spray a 6-cup muffin tin with nonstick cooking spray.
2. In a large skillet over medium-high heat, heat the olive oil until it shimmers.
3. Add the onion and cook until soft, about 4 minutes. Add the spinach and cook, stirring, until the spinach softens, about 1 minute.
4. Add the garlic. Cook, stirring constantly, for 30 seconds. Remove from heat and let cool.
5. In a medium bowl, beat together the eggs, milk, salt, and pepper.
6. Fold the cooled vegetables and the cheese into the egg mixture. Spoon the mixture into the prepared muffin tins.
7. Bake until the eggs are set, about 15 minutes. Allow to rest for 5 minutes before serving.

Per Serving

Calories: 220 | fat: 17.1g | protein: 14.1g | carbs: 3.9g | fiber: 1.0g | sugar: 2.9g | sodium: 238mg

Delicious Dandelion Greens with Black Pepper

Prep time: 15 minutes | Cook time: 12 minutes | Serves 4

1 tablespoon extra-virgin olive oil
1 Vidalia onion, thinly sliced
2 garlic cloves, minced
2 bunches dandelion greens, roughly chopped
½ cup low-sodium vegetable broth
Freshly ground black pepper, to taste

1. Heat the olive oil in a large skillet over low heat.
2. Cook the onion and garlic for 2 to 3 minutes until tender, stirring occasionally.
3. Add the dandelion greens and broth and cook for 5 to 7 minutes, stirring frequently, or until the greens are wilted.
4. Transfer to a plate and season with black pepper. Serve warm.

Per Serving

Calories: 81 | fat: 3.8g | protein: 3.1g | carbs: 10.7g | fiber: 3.8g | sugar: 2.0g | sodium: 72mg

Ginger Garlic Lentil Tomatoes with Cilantro

Prep time: 10 minutes | Cook time: 25 minutes | Serves 6

1 tablespoon extra-virgin olive oil	Pinch cayenne pepper
1 sweet onion, chopped	2 cups cooked lentils
1 teaspoon minced garlic	1 (28-ounce / 794-g) can low-sodium diced tomatoes
1 tablespoon grated fresh ginger	1 (15-ounce / 425-g) can water-packed chickpeas, rinsed and drained
2 tablespoons red curry paste	¼ cup coconut milk
½ teaspoon turmeric	2 tablespoons chopped fresh cilantro
1 teaspoon ground cumin	

1. Heat the olive oil in a large saucepan over medium-high heat.
2. Add the onion, garlic, and ginger and sauté for about 3 minutes until tender, stirring occasionally.
3. Stir in the red curry paste, turmeric, cumin, and cayenne pepper and sauté for another 1 minute.
4. Add the cooked lentils, tomatoes, chickpeas, and coconut milk and stir to combine, and then bring the curry to a boil.
5. Once it starts to boil, reduce the heat to low and bring to a simmer for 20 minutes. Serve garnished with the cilantro.

Per Serving
Calories: 340 | fat: 8.2g | protein: 18.2g | carbs: 50.2g | fiber: 20.2g | sugar: 9.2g | sodium: 25mg

Mom's Special Sweet Potato Egg Bake

Prep time: 5 minutes | Cook time: 25 minutes | Serves 4

2 tablespoons extra-virgin olive oil	powder
1 red onion, chopped	½ teaspoon sea salt
1 green bell pepper, seeded and chopped	4 large eggs
1 sweet potato, cut into ½-inch pieces	½ cup shredded pepper Jack cheese
1 teaspoon chili	1 avocado, cut into cubes

1. Preheat the oven to 350ºF (180ºC).
2. In a large, ovenproof skillet over medium-high heat, heat the olive oil until it shimmers.
3. Add the onion, bell pepper, sweet potato, chili powder, and salt, and cook, stirring occasionally, until the vegetables start to brown, about 10 minutes.
4. Remove from heat. Arrange the vegetables in the pan to form 4 wells. Crack an egg into each well. Sprinkle the cheese on the vegetables, around the edges of the eggs.
5. Bake until the eggs set, about 10 minutes.
6. Top with avocado before serving.

Per Serving
Calories: 285 | fat: 21.1g | protein: 12.1g | carbs: 15.9g | fiber: 5.1g | sugar: 10.0g | sodium: 265mg

10 Ingredient Cheesy Butternut Noodles

Prep time: 10 minutes | Cook time: 15 minutes | Serves 4

¼ cup extra-virgin olive oil	3 garlic cloves, minced
½ red onion, finely chopped	½ cup dry white wine
1 pound (454 g) cremini mushrooms, sliced	Pinch red pepper flakes
1 teaspoon dried thyme	4 cups butternut noodles
½ teaspoon sea salt	4 ounces (113 g) Parmesan cheese, grated (optional)

1. Heat the olive oil in a large skillet over medium-high heat until shimmering.
2. Add the onion, mushrooms, thyme, and salt to the skillet. Sauté for 6 minutes, stirring occasionally, or until the mushrooms begin to brown.
3. Stir in the garlic and cook for 30 seconds until fragrant.
4. Fold in the wine and red pepper flakes and whisk to combine.
5. Add the butternut noodles to the skillet and continue cooking for 5 minutes, stirring occasionally, or until the noodles is softened.
6. Divide the mixture among four bowls. Sprinkle the grated Parmesan cheese on top, if desired.

Per Serving
Calories: 243 | fat: 14.2g | protein: 3.7g | carbs: 21.9g | fiber: 4.1g | sugar: 2.1g | sodium: 157mg

Cheddar Chili Mexican Bowl

Prep time: 5 minutes | Cook time: 35 minutes | Serves 8

3 eggs
1 cup Monterey jack pepper cheese, grated
¾ cup half-and-half
½ cup cheddar cheese, grated

2 (7-ounce / 198-g) cans whole green chilies, drain well
½ teaspoon salt
Nonstick cooking spray

1. Heat oven to 350ºF (180ºC). Spray a baking pan with cooking spray.
2. Slice each chili down one long side and lay flat.
3. Arrange half the chilies in the prepared baking pan, skin side down, in single layer.
4. Sprinkle with the pepper cheese and top with remaining chilies, skin side up.
5. In a small bowl, beat eggs, salt, and half-and-half. Pour over chilies. Top with cheddar cheese.
6. Bake 35 minutes, or until top is golden brown. Let rest 10 minutes before serving.

Per Serving
Calories: 296 | fat: 13.0g | protein: 13.1g | carbs: 36.1g | fiber: 14.0g | sugar: 21.0g | sodium: 463mg

Spicy Cheesy Quinoa with Zucchini and Pine nuts

Prep time: 20 minutes | Cook time: 30 minutes | Serves 4

1 teaspoon extra-virgin olive oil
½ sweet onion, chopped
2 teaspoons minced garlic
2 eggs, whisked
2 cups cooked quinoa
2 cups cherry tomatoes

½ cup low-fat ricotta cheese
Salt and ffreshly ground black pepper, to taste
1 zucchini, cut into thin ribbons
⅛ Cup toasted pine nuts

1. Preheat the oven to 350ºF (180ºC).
2. Heat the olive oil in a medium skillet over medium-high heat.
3. Sauté the onion and garlic for 3 minutes, stirring occasionally, or until softened.
4. Remove the skillet from the heat.
5. Add the whisked eggs, cooked quinoa, cherry tomatoes, and cheese and stir to incorporate. Sprinkle with salt and pepper.
6. Transfer the mixture to a baking dish.
7. Sprinkle the top with the zucchini ribbons and pine nuts.
8. Bake in the preheated oven for about 25 minutes, or until the casserole is heated through.
9. Cool for 5 to 10 minutes before serving.

Per Serving
Calories: 305 | fat: 9.3g | protein: 17.2g | carbs: 38.2g | fiber: 4.2g | sugar: 5.2g | sodium: 236mg

Cheesy Egg Broccoli Bake

Prep time: 10 minutes | Cook time: 1 hour | Serves 6

3 large eggs
2 cups broccoli florets, chopped
1 small onion, diced
1 cup cheddar cheese, grated
⅔ cup unsweetened almond milk

½ cup feta cheese, crumbled
1 tablespoon extra-virgin olive oil
½ teaspoon sea salt
¼ teaspoon black pepper
Nonstick cooking spray

1. Heat oven to 350ºF (180ºC). Spray a 9-inch baking dish with cooking spray.
2. Heat the oil in a large skillet over medium heat.
3. Add onion and cook 4 to 5 minutes, until onions are translucent.
4. Add broccoli and stir to combine. Cook until broccoli turns a bright green, about 2 minutes. Transfer to a bowl.
5. In a small bowl, whisk together almond milk, egg, salt, and pepper. Pour over the broccoli.
6. Add the cheddar cheese and stir it together. Pour into the prepared baking dish.
7. Sprinkle the feta cheese over the top and bake 35 minutes or until eggs are set in the middle and top is lightly browned. Serve.

Per Serving
Calories: 183 | fat: 14.0g | protein: 10.1g | carbs: 5.1g | fiber: 1.0g | sugar: 2.0g | sodium: 491mg

Cheesy Vegetables Topped with Yogurt

Prep time: 15 minutes | Cook time: 15 minutes | Serves 6

1 tablespoon extra-virgin olive oil
½ onion, chopped
3 garlic cloves, minced
½ green bell pepper, deseeded and chopped
½ red bell pepper, deseeded and chopped
2 small zucchinis, chopped
1 (10-ounce / 284-g) can low-sodium enchilada sauce
1 (15-ounce / 425-g) can low-sodium black beans, drained and
rinsed
1 teaspoon ground cumin
½ cup shredded cheddar cheese, divided
2 (6-inch) corn tortillas cut into strips
¼ teaspoon salt
¼ teaspoons freshly ground black pepper
Chopped fresh cilantro, for garnish
Plain yogurt, for serving

1. Preheat the broiler to high. Heat the olive oil in a large ovenproof skillet until it shimmers. Stir in the onion, garlic, bell peppers, and zucchinis and sauté for 3 to 5 minutes, or until the onion is translucent.
2. Add the enchilada sauce, black beans, cumin, and ¼ cup of cheese, tortilla strips, salt, and pepper and whisk to combine. Scatter the top with the remaining ¼ cup of cheese.
3. Place the skillet under the broiler and broil until the cheese melts, 5 to 8 minutes. Sprinkle the cilantro on top for garnish and serve topped with the yogurt.

Per Serving
Calories: 172 | fat: 7.2g | protein: 8.3g | carbs: 21.2g | fiber: 7.2g | sugar: 3.2g | sodium: 563mg

Instant Broiled Soy Salmon

Prep time: 5 minutes | Cook time: 4 minutes | Serves 4

⅓ Cup pineapple juice
⅓ Cup reduced-sodium soy sauce
¼ cup water
2 tablespoons rice vinegar
¼ tablespoon honey
1 garlic clove, minced
1 teaspoon peeled and grated fresh ginger
Pinch red pepper flakes
1 pound salmon fillet, cut into 4 pieces

1. Preheat the oven broiler on high.
2. In a small bowl, whisk together the pineapple juice, soy sauce, water, vinegar, honey, garlic, ginger, and red pepper flakes.
3. Place the salmon pieces flesh-side down in the mixture for 5 minutes.
4. Place the salmon on a rimmed baking sheet, flesh-side up. Gently brush with any leftover sauce.
5. Broil until the salmon is opaque, 3 to 5 minutes.

Per Serving
Calories: 202 | fat: 7g | protein: 24g | carbs: 9g | fiber: 1g | sugar: 19g | sodium: 752mg

Hot and Spicy Zoodles with Beet Mixture

Prep time: 20 minutes | Cook time: 40 minutes | Serves 2

1 medium red beet, peeled, chopped
½ cup walnut pieces, toasted
½ cup crumbled goat cheese
3 garlic cloves
2 tablespoons freshly
squeezed lemon juice
2 tablespoons plus 2 teaspoons extra-virgin olive oil, divided
¼ teaspoon salt
4 small zucchini, spiralizedd

1. Preheat the oven to 375ºF (190ºC).
2. Wrap the red beet in aluminium foil, making sure to seal the foil completely.
3. Roast in the preheated oven for 30 to 40 minutes until tender.
4. When ready, transfer the red beet to a food processor. Fold in the toasted walnut, goat cheese, garlic, and lemon juice, 2 tablespoons of olive oil, and salt and pulse until smooth. Transfer the beet mixture to a small bowl.
5. Heat the remaining 2 teaspoons of olive oil in a large skillet over medium heat. Add the zucchini, tossing to coat in the oil. Cook for 2 to 3 minutes, stirring constantly, or until the zucchini is softened.
6. Remove the zucchini from the heat to a plate and top with the beet mixture. Toss well and serve warm.

Per Serving
Calories: 424 | fat: 39.3g | protein: 8.1g | carbs: 17.2g | fiber: 6.2g | sugar: 10.1g | sodium: 340mg

Healthy Whole-Wheat Pita with Bulgur Mixture

Prep time: 20 minutes | Cook time: 0 minutes | Serves 4

1 cup cooked bulgur wheat
1 English cucumber, finely chopped
1 yellow bell pepper, deseeded and finely chopped
2 cups halved cherry tomatoes
½ cup fresh parsley, finely chopped
2 scallions, white and green parts, finely chopped
Juice of 1 lemon
2 tablespoons extra-virgin olive oil
Salt and freshly ground black pepper, to taste
4 whole-wheat pitas cut in half

1. Combine the bulgur wheat, cucumber, bell pepper, tomatoes, parsley, scallions, lemon juice, and olive oil in a large bowl and stir to mix well. Season with salt and pepper to taste.
2. Place the pita halves on a clean work surface. Evenly divide the bulgur mixture among pita halves and serve immediately.

Per Serving
Calories: 245 | fat: 8.2g | protein: 7.2g | carbs: 39.2g | fiber: 6.2g | sugar: 4.2g | sodium: 166mg

Spaghetti Eggplant-Zucchini with Cheese

Prep time: 10 minutes | Cook time: 2 hours | Serves 6

1 medium eggplant, peeled and cut into 1-inch cubes
1 medium zucchini, cut into 1-inch pieces
1 medium onion, cut into thin wedges
1 ½ cups purchased light spaghetti sauce
⅔ cup reduced fat Parmesan cheese, grated

1. Place the vegetables, spaghetti sauce and ⅓ cup Parmesan in the crock pot. Stir to combine. Cover and cook on high for 2 to 2 ½ hours, or on low 4 to 5 hours.
2. Sprinkle remaining Parmesan on top before serving.

Per Serving
Calories: 82 | fat: 2.0g | protein: 5.1g | carbs: 12.1g | fiber: 5.0g | sugar: 7.0g | sodium: 456mg

Egg Pea Salad fills in Kale Leaves

Prep time: 10 minutes | Cook time: 0 minutes | Serves 2

4 hard-boiled large eggs, chopped
1 cup fresh peas, shelled
2 tablespoons red onion, finely chopped
½ teaspoon sea salt
¼ teaspoon paprika
1 teaspoon Dijon mustard
1 tablespoon fresh dill, chopped
2 large kale leaves

1. Combine all the ingredients, except for the kale leaves, in a bowl. Stir to mix well.
2. Divide and spoon the mixture on the kale leaves, then roll up the leaves to wrap the mixture. Serve immediately.

Per Serving
Calories: 296 | fat: 18.2g | protein: 17.2g | carbs: 18.2g | fiber: 4.2g | sugar: 12.3 | sodium: 623mg

Healthy Pepper Egg Bowl

Prep time: 5 minutes | Cook time: 10 minutes | Serves 2

2 tablespoons extra-virgin olive oil
1 green bell pepper, deseeded and finely chopped
½ red onion, finely chopped
4 eggs whites
½ teaspoon sea salt
2 ounces (57 g) pepper Jack cheese, grated

1. Heat the olive oil in a nonstick skillet over medium-high heat..
2. Add the bell pepper and onion to the skillet and sauté for 5 minutes or until tender.
3. Sprinkle the egg white with salt in a bowl, and then pour the egg whites in the skillet. Cook for 3 minutes or until the egg whites are scrambled. Stir the egg whites halfway through.
4. Scatter with cheese and cook for an additional 1 minutes until the cheese melts.
5. Divide them onto two serving plates and serve warm.

Per Serving
Calories: 316 | fat: 23.3g | protein: 22.3g | carbs: 6.2g | fiber: 1.1g | sugar: 4.2g | sodium: 975mg

Pepper Mushroom Pesto Sandwich

Prep time: 5 minutes | Cook time: 13 to 17 minutes | Serves 2

1 teaspoon extra-virgin olive oil
½ red onion, sliced
½ cup sliced mushrooms
Salt and freshly ground black pepper,
to taste
¼ cup store-bought pesto sauce
2 whole-wheat flatbreads
¼ cup shredded Mozzarella cheese

1. Preheat the oven to 350ºF (180ºC).
2. Heat the olive oil in a small skillet over medium heat.
3. Add the onion slices and mushrooms to the skillet, and sauté for 3 to 5 minutes, stirring occasionally, or until they start to soften. Season with salt and pepper.
4. Meanwhile, spoon 2 tablespoons of pesto sauce onto each flatbread and spread it all over. Evenly divide the mushroom mixture between two flatbreads, and then scatter each top with 2 tablespoons of shredded cheese.
5. Transfer the flatbreads to a baking sheet and bake until the cheese melts and bubbles, about 10 to 12 minutes.
6. Let the flatbreads cool for 5 minutes and serve warm.

Per Serving
Calories: 346 | fat: 22.8g | protein: 14.2g | carbs: 27.6g | fiber: 7.3g | sugar: 4.0g | sodium: 790mg

Homely Rice Bowl with Radish and Avocado

Prep time: 15 minutes | Cook time: 12 minutes | Serves 4

2 cups sliced Brussels sprouts
2 teaspoons plus 2 tablespoons extra-virgin olive oil
1 teaspoon Dijon mustard
Juice of 1 lemon
1 garlic clove, minced
½ teaspoon salt
¼ teaspoons freshly ground black pepper
1 cup sliced radishes
1 cup cooked wild rice
1 avocado, sliced

1. Preheat the oven to 400ºF (205ºC). Line a baking sheet with parchment paper and set aside.
2. Add 2 teaspoons of olive oil and Brussels sprouts to a medium bowl, and toss to coat well.
3. Spread out the oiled Brussels sprouts on the prepared baking sheet. Roast in the preheated oven for 12 minutes, or until the Brussels sprouts are browned and crisp. Stir the Brussels sprouts once during cooking to ensure even cooking.
4. Meanwhile, make the dressing by whisking together the remaining olive oil, mustard, lemon juice, garlic, salt, and pepper in a small bowl. Remove the Brussels sprouts from the oven to a large bowl.
5. Add the radishes and cooked wild rice to the bowl. Drizzle with the prepared dressing and gently toss to coat everything evenly.
6. Divide the mixture into four bowls and scatter each bowl evenly with avocado slices. Serve immediately.

Per Serving
Calories: 177 | fat: 10.7g | protein: 2.3g | carbs: 17.6g | fiber: 5.1g | sugar: 2.0g | sodium: 297mg

My Favorite Veggie Broth with Tomato

Prep time: 10 minutes | Cook time: 20 minutes | Serves 4

1 cup low-sodium vegetable broth, divided
½ onion, thinly sliced
2 garlic cloves, thinly sliced
1 medium tomato, chopped
1 large bunch collard greens including stems, roughly chopped
1 teaspoon ground cumin
½ teaspoons freshly ground black pepper

1. Add ½ cup of vegetable broth to a Dutch oven over medium heat and bring to a simmer.
2. Stir in the onion and garlic and cook for about 4 minutes until tender.
3. Add the remaining broth, tomato, greens, cumin, and pepper, and gently stir to combine.
4. Reduce the heat to low and simmer uncovered for 15 minutes. Serve warm.

Per Serving
Calories: 68 | fat: 2.1g | protein: 4.8g | carbs: 13.8g | fiber: 7.1g | sugar: 2.0g | sodium: 67mg

Spicy Peppery Zucchini Tomato Bowl

Prep time: 10 minutes | Cook time: 10 minutes | Serves 4

1 tablespoon vegetable oil
1 sliced onion
2 pounds (907 g) zucchini, peeled and cut into 1-inch-thick slices
2 tomatoes, chopped
1 green bell pepper, chopped
Salt and freshly ground black pepper, to taste

1. Heat the vegetable oil in a nonstick skillet until it shimmers.
2. Sauté the onion slices in the oil for about 3 minutes until translucent, stirring occasionally.
3. Add the zucchini, tomatoes, bell pepper, salt, and pepper to the skillet and stir to combine.
4. Reduce the heat, cover, and continue cooking for about 5 minutes or until the veggies are tender.
5. Remove from the heat to a large plate and serve hot.

Per Serving
Calories: 110 | fat: 4.4g | protein: 6.9g | carbs: 10.7g | fiber: 3.4g | sugar: 2.2g | sodium: 11mg

Healthy Mushroom Whole Wheat Sandwich

Prep time: 5 minutes | Cook time: 10 minutes | Serves 2

2 large portabella mushroom caps
½ small zucchini, sliced
2 slices low fat cheese
2 whole wheat sandwiches thins
2 teaspoons roasted red bell peppers
2 teaspoons olive oil

1. Heat grill, or charcoal, to medium-high heat.
2. Lightly brush mushroom caps with olive oil. Grill mushroom caps and zucchini slices until tender, about 3 to 4 minutes per side.
3. Place on sandwich thin. Top with sliced cheese and roasted red bell pepper. Serve.

Per Serving
Calories: 178 | fat: 3.0g | protein: 15.1g | carbs: 26.1g | fiber: 8.0g | sugar: 3.0g | sodium: 520mg

Classic Italian Veggie Soup

Prep time: 10 minutes | Cook time: 20 minutes | Serves 2

2 tablespoons extra-virgin olive oil
1 onion, chopped
1 red bell pepper, seeded and chopped
2 garlic cloves, minced
2 cups green beans (fresh or frozen; halved if fresh)
1 cups low-sodium
vegetable broth
1 (14-ounce/397 g) can crushed tomatoes
1 tablespoon Italian seasoning
½ cup dried whole-wheat elbow macaroni
½ teaspoon sea salt
Pinch red pepper flakes (or to taste)

1. In a large pot over medium-high heat, heat the olive oil until it shimmers.
2. Add the onion and bell pepper and cook, stirring occasionally, until they soften, about 3 minutes.
3. Add the garlic and cook, stirring constantly, for 30 seconds.
4. Add the green beans, vegetable broth, tomatoes, and Italian seasoning and bring to a boil.
5. Add the elbow macaroni, salt, and red pepper flakes. Cook, stirring occasionally, until the macaroni is soft, about 8 minutes.

Per Serving
Calories: 200 | fat: 7g | protein: 5g | carbs: 29g | fiber: 7g | sugar: 29g | sodium: 477mg

Quick Zucchini Noodles with Pea Pesto

Prep time: 10 minutes | Cook time: 10 minutes | Serves 4

3 zucchinis
2 tablespoons extra-virgin olive oil
Pinch sea salt
3 tablespoon Pea Pesto

1. Using a vegetable peeler, cut the zucchini lengthwise into long strips. Use a knife to cut the strips into the desired width.
2. In a large skillet over medium-high heat, heat the olive oil until it shimmers.
3. Add the zucchini and cook until it starts to soften, about 3 minutes. Add the sea salt.
4. Toss the zucchini noodles with the pesto.

Per Serving
Calories: 348 | fat: 30g | protein: 10g | carbs: 13g | fiber: 1g | sugar: 0.14g | sodium: 343mg

Quick and Easy Peri Peri Shrimp

Prep time: 10 minutes | Cook time: 15 minutes | Serves 4

1 pound large shrimp, shelled and deveined
2 tablespoons extra-
virgin olive oil
Sea salt to taste
1 teaspoon Peri Peri

1. Preheat the oven broiler on high.
2. In a small pot, bring the Peri-Peri Sauce to a simmer.
3. Meanwhile, place the cleaned shrimp on a rimmed baking sheet, deveined-side down. Brush with the olive oil and sprinkle with the salt.
4. Broil until opaque, about 5 minutes.
5. Serve with the sauce on the side for dipping or spooned over the top of the shrimp.

Per Serving
Calories: 279 | fat: 16g | protein: 24g | carbs: 10g | fiber: 3g | sugar: 0g | sodium: 464mg

Broiled Cod with Salsa

Prep time: 10 minutes | Cook time: 10 minutes | Serves 4

1 pound (454 g) cod, cut into 4 fillets, pin bones removed
2 tablespoons extra-virgin olive oil
¾ teaspoon sea salt, divided
1 mango, pitted, peeled, and cut into
cubes
¼ cup chopped cilantro
½ red onion, finely chopped
1 jalapeño, seeded and finely chopped
1 garlic clove, minced
Juice of 1 lime

1. Preheat the oven broiler on high.
2. On a rimmed baking sheet, brush the cod with the olive oil and season with ½ teaspoon of the salt. Broil until the fish is opaque, 5 to 10 minutes.
3. Meanwhile, in a small bowl, combine the mango, cilantro, onion, jalapeño, garlic, lime juice, and remaining ¼ teaspoon of salt.
4. Serve the cod with the salsa spooned over the top.

Per Serving
Calories: 197 | fat: 8g | protein: 21g | carbs: 13g | fiber: 2g | sugar: 0.81g | sodium: 354mg

Delicious Peppery Tofu Curry

Prep time: 10 minutes | Cook time: 2 hours | Serves 4

2 cup green bell pepper, diced
1 cup firm tofu, cut into cubes
1 onion, peeled and diced
1 ½ cups canned coconut milk
1 cup tomato paste
2 cloves garlic, diced fine
2 tablespoons raw peanut butter
1 tablespoon garam masala
1 tablespoon curry powder
1 ½ teaspoons salt

1. Add all, except the tofu to a blender or food processor. Process until thoroughly combined.
2. Pour into a crock pot and add the tofu. Cover and cook on high 2 hours.
3. Stir well and serve over cauliflower rice.

Per Serving
Calories: 390 | fat: 28.0g | protein: 13.1g | carbs: 28.1g | fiber: 8.0g | sugar: 16.0g | sodium: 1004mg

Tofu Lettuce Leaf Wraps

Prep time: 15 minutes | Cook time: 20 minutes | Serves 4

1 package silken firm tofu, pressed
4 lettuce leaves
2 green onions, diced
¼ cup celery, diced
8 slices whole-wheat bread
2 tablespoons sweet
pickle relish
1 tablespoon Dijon mustard
¼ teaspoon turmeric
¼ teaspoon salt
⅛ teaspoon cayenne pepper

1. Press tofu between layers of paper towels for 15 minutes to remove excess moisture. Cut into small cubes.
2. In a medium bowl, stir together remaining. Fold in tofu. Spread over 4 slices of bread.
3. Top with a lettuce leaf and another slice of bread. Serve.

Per Serving
Calories: 380 | fat: 20.0g | protein: 24.1g | carbs: 15.1g | fiber: 2.0g | sugar: 2.0g | sodium: 575mg

Spicy Italian Spaghetti Pasta

Prep time: 20 minutes | Cook time: 35 minutes | Serves 6

1 tablespoon extra-virgin olive oil
3 teaspoons minced garlic
1 sweet onion, chopped
2 celery stalks, chopped
2 (28-ounce / 794-g) cans sodium-free diced tomatoes
1 tablespoon chopped fresh oregano
2 tablespoons chopped fresh basil
½ teaspoon red pepper flakes
½ cup quartered, pitted Kalamata olives
¼ cup freshly squeezed lemon juice
8 ounces (227 g) cooked whole-wheat spaghetti

1. Heat the olive oil in a large saucepan over medium-high heat.
2. Add the garlic, onion, and celery to the saucepan and sauté for about 3 minutes, stirring occasionally, or until softened.
3. Toss in the tomatoes, oregano, basil, and pepper flakes and stir to combine. Allow the sauce to boil, stirring often to prevent from sticking to the bottom of the pan.
4. Reduce the heat to low and bring the sauce to a simmer, stirring occasionally, about 20 minutes.
5. Add the olives and lemon juice to the sauce and mix well.
6. Remove from the heat and spoon the sauce over the spaghetti. Toss well and serve warm.

Per Serving
Calories: 199 | fat: 4.7g | protein: 7.2g | carbs: 34.9g | fiber: 3.9g | sugar: 8.1g | sodium: 89mg

The Best Veggie Chili Ever

Prep time: 10 minutes | Cook time: 15 minutes | Serves 4

2 tablespoons extra-virgin olive oil
1 onion, finely chopped
1 green bell pepper, deseeded and chopped
1 (14-ounce / 397-g) can kidney beans, drained and rinsed
2 (14-ounce / 397-g)
cans crushed tomatoes
2 cups veggie crumbles
1 teaspoon garlic powder
1 tablespoon chili powder
½ teaspoon sea salt

1. Heat the olive oil in a large skillet over medium-high heat until shimmering.
2. Add the onion and bell pepper and sauté for 5 minutes, stirring occasionally.
3. Fold in the beans, tomatoes, veggie crumbles, garlic powder, chili powder, and salt. Stir to incorporate and bring them to a simmer.
4. Reduce the heat and cook for an additional 5 minutes, stirring occasionally, or until the mixture is heated through.
5. Allow the mixture to cool for 5 minutes and serve warm.

Per Serving
Calories: 282 | fat: 10.1g | protein: 16.7g | carbs: 38.2g | fiber: 12.9g | sugar: 7.2g | sodium: 1128mg

Appetizing Cole slaw Bowl

Prep time: 10 minutes | Cook time: 20 minutes | Serves 4

1 large spaghetti squash, halved and seeds removed
3 stalks celery, sliced diagonally
1 onion, diced fine
2 cup Cole slaw mix
2 teaspoons fresh
ginger, grated
¼ cup Tamari
3 cloves garlic, diced fine
3-4 tablespoons water
2 tablespoons olive oil
1 tablespoon Splenda
¼ teaspoon pepper

1. Place squash, cut side down, in shallow glass dish and add water. Microwave on high 8 to 10 minutes, or until squash is soft. Use a fork to scoop out the squash into a bowl.
2. In a small bowl, whisk together Tamari, garlic, sugar, ginger and pepper.
3. Heat oil in large skillet over medium-high heat.
4. Add onion and celery and cook, stirring frequently, 3 to 4 minutes.
5. Add Cole slaw and cook until heated through, about 1 minute.
6. Add the squash and sauce mixture and stir well.
7. Cook 2 minutes, stirring frequently. Serve.

Per Serving
Calories: 130 | fat: 7.0g | protein: 3.1g | carbs: 13.1g | fiber: 2.0g | sugar: 6.0g | sodium: 1028mg

Cheesy Portobello Mushroom with Quinoa

Prep time: 15 minutes | Cook time: 27 to 30 minutes | Serves 8

1 tablespoon extra-virgin olive oil
1 Vidalia onion, thinly sliced
1 large Portobello mushroom, thinly sliced
6 yellow summer squash, thinly sliced
1 cup shredded

Parmesan cheese, divided
1 cup shredded Cheddar cheese
½ cup tri-color quinoa
½ cup whole-wheat bread crumbs
1 tablespoon Creole seasoning

1. Preheat the oven to 350ºF (180ºC).
2. Heat the olive oil in a large cast iron pan over medium heat.
3. Sauté the onion, mushroom, and squash in the oil for 7 to 10 minutes, stirring occasionally, or until the vegetables are softened.
4. Remove from the heat and add ½ cup of Parmesan cheese and the Cheddar cheese to the vegetables. Stir well.
5. Mix together the quinoa, bread crumbs, the remaining Parmesan cheese, Creole seasoning in a small bowl, then scatter the mixture over the vegetables.
6. Place the cast iron pan in the preheated oven and bake until browned and cooked through, about 20 minutes.
7. Cool for 10 minutes and serve on plates while warm.

Per Serving
Calories: 184 | fat: 8.9g | protein: 11.7g | carbs: 17.6g | fiber: 3.2g | sugar: 3.8g | sodium: 140mg

Scallion Tofu Vegetable Stir-Fry

Prep time: 10 minutes | Cook time: 20 minutes | Serves 4

3 tablespoons extra-virgin olive oil
4 scallions, sliced
12 ounces (340 g) firm tofu, cut into ½-inch pieces
4 cups broccoli, broken into florets
4 garlic cloves, minced

1 teaspoon peeled and grated fresh ginger
¼ cup vegetable broth
2 tablespoons soy sauce (use gluten-free soy sauce if necessary)
1 cup cooked brown rice

1. In a large skillet over medium-high heat, heat the olive oil until it shimmers.
2. Add the scallions, tofu, and broccoli and cook, stirring, until the vegetables begin to soften, about 6 minutes.
3. Add the garlic and ginger and cook, stirring constantly, for 30 seconds.
4. Add the broth, soy sauce, and rice. Cook, stirring, 1 to 2 minutes more to heat the rice through.

Per Serving
Calories: 235 | fat: 13.1g | protein: 11.1g | carbs: 20.9g | fiber: 4.1g | sugar: 12.3g | sodium: 362mg

One Pan Spicy Cauliflower Pepper

Prep time: 15 minutes | Cook time: 30 minutes | Serves 12

1 head cauliflower, grated
1 red bell pepper, diced fine
1 green bell pepper, diced fine
1 jalapeno pepper, seeded and diced fine
½ white onion, diced fine

1½ cups cheddar cheese, grated
1 teaspoon cilantro, diced fine
½ cup salsa
3 tablespoons water
1 teaspoon chili powder
Nonstick cooking spray

1. Heat oven to 350ºF (180ºC). Spray a 7x11x2-inch baking pan with cooking spray.
2. In a large skillet, over medium heat, cook onions and peppers until soft, about 5 minutes.
3. Add cilantro and chili powder and stir.
4. Place the cauliflower and water in a glass bowl and microwave on high for 3 minutes. Stir in 1 cup cheese and the salsa.
5. Stir the pepper mixture into the cauliflower and combine. Spread in prepared pan. Sprinkle the remaining cheese over the top and bake 30 to 35 minutes.
6. Let rest 5 minutes before cutting into 12 squares and serving.

Per Serving
Calories: 75 | fat: 5.0g | protein: 4.1g | carbs: 4.1g | fiber: 1.0g | sugar: 2.0g | sodium: 206mg

Healthy Whole-Wheat Elbow Macaroni Cheese Bowl

Prep time: 10 minutes | Cook time: 25 minutes | Serves 6

1 cup fat-free evaporated milk
½ cup skim milk
½ cup low-fat Cheddar cheese
½ cup low-fat cottage cheese
1 teaspoon nutmeg

Pinch cayenne pepper
Sea salt and freshly ground black pepper, to taste
6 cups cooked whole-wheat elbow macaroni
2 tablespoons grated Parmesan cheese

1. Preheat the oven to 350ºF (180ºC).
2. Heat the milk in a large saucepan over low heat until it steams.
3. Add the Cheddar cheese and cottage cheese to the milk, and keep whisking, or until the cheese is melted.
4. Add the nutmeg and cayenne pepper and stir well. Sprinkle the salt and pepper to season.
5. Remove from the heat. Add the cooked macaroni to the cheese mixture and stir until well combined. Transfer the macaroni and cheese to a large casserole dish and top with the grated Parmesan cheese.
6. Bake in the preheated oven for about 20 minutes, or until bubbly and lightly browned.
7. Divide the macaroni and cheese among six bowls and serve.

Per Serving
Calories: 245 | fat: 2.1g | protein: 15.7g | carbs: 43.8g | fiber: 3.8g | sugar: 6.8g | sodium: 186mg

Cauliflower Mushrooms Italian Dish

Prep time: 10 minutes | Cook time: 30 minutes | Serves 2

1 medium head cauliflower, grated
8 ounces (227 g) Porcini mushrooms, sliced
1 yellow onion, diced fine
2 cup low sodium

vegetable broth
2 teaspoons garlic, diced fine
2 teaspoons white wine vinegar
Salt and ground black pepper, to taste
Olive oil cooking spray

1. Heat oven to 350ºF (180ºC). Line a baking sheet with foil.
2. Place the mushrooms on the prepared pan and spray with cooking spray. Sprinkle with salt and toss to coat.
3. Bake 10 to 12 minutes, or until golden brown and the mushrooms start to crisp.
4. Spray a large skillet with cooking spray and place over medium-high heat. Add onion and cook, stirring frequently, until translucent, about 3 to 4 minutes.
5. Add garlic and cook 2 minutes, until golden.
6. Add the cauliflower and cook 1 minute, stirring.
7. Place the broth in a saucepan and bring to a simmer. Add to the skillet, ¼ cup at a time, mixing well after each addition.
8. Stir in vinegar. Reduce heat to low and let simmer, 4 to 5 minutes, or until most of the liquid has evaporated.
9. Spoon cauliflower mixture onto plates, or in bowls, and top with mushrooms. Serve.

Per Serving
Calories: 135 | fat: 0g | protein: 10.1g | carbs: 22.1g | fiber: 2.0g | sugar: 5.0g | sodium: 1105mg

Lettuce Wraps in Soy Sauce

Prep time: 5 minutes | Cook time: 5 minutes | Serves 2

1 package tempeh, crumbled
1 head butter-leaf lettuce
½ red bell pepper, diced
½ onion, diced
1 tablespoon garlic, diced fine

1 tablespoon olive oil
1 tablespoon low-sodium soy sauce
1 teaspoon ginger,
1 teaspoon onion powder
1 teaspoon garlic powder

1. Heat oil and garlic in a large skillet over medium heat.
2. Add onion, tempeh, and bell pepper and sauté for 3 minutes.
3. Add soy sauce and spices and cook for another 2 minutes.
4. Spoon mixture into lettuce leaves.

Per Serving
Calories: 131 | fat: 5.0g | protein: 8.1g | carbs: 14.1g | fiber: 4.0g | sugar: 2.0g | sodium: 268mg

a Patties with Tartar Sauce

Prep time: 5 minutes | Cook time: 10 minutes | Serves 4

1 pound canned tuna, drained	fresh dill
1 cup whole-wheat bread crumbs	Juice and zest of 1 lemon
2 large eggs, beaten	3 tablespoons extra-virgin olive oil
½ onion, grated	½ cup tartar sauce, for serving
1 tablespoon chopped	

1. In a large bowl, combine the tuna, bread crumbs, eggs, onion, dill, and lemon juice and zest. Form the mixture into 4 patties and chill for 10 minutes.
2. In a large non-stick skillet over medium-high heat, heat the olive oil until it shimmers.
3. Add the patties and cook until browned on both sides, 4 to 5 minutes per side.
4. Serve topped with the tartar sauce.

Per Serving

Calories: 530 | fat: 34g | protein: 35g | carbs: 18g | fiber: 2g | sugar: 8.8g | sodium: 674mg

Cheesed Tomato Garlic Pepper Soup

Prep time: 20minutes | Cook time: 35 minutes | Serves 6

2 tablespoons extra-virgin olive oil, plus more to oil the pan	4 garlic cloves, lightly crushed
16 tomatoes, cored, halved	Sea salt to taste
4 red bell peppers, seeded, halved	Freshly ground black pepper
4 celery stalks, coarsely chopped	6 cups low-sodium chicken broth
1 onion, cut into eighths	2 tablespoons chopped fresh basil
	2 ounces goat cheese

1. Preheat the oven to 400°F(204°C).
2. Lightly oil a large baking dish with olive oil.
3. Place the tomatoes cut-side down in the dish, and then scatter the bell peppers, celery, onion, and garlic on the tomatoes.
4. Drizzle the vegetables with 2 tablespoons of olive oil and lightly season with salt and pepper.
5. Roast the vegetables until they are soft and slightly charred, about 30 minutes.
6. Remove the vegetables from the oven and purée them in batches, with the chicken broth, in a food processor or blender until smooth.
7. Transfer the puréed soup to a medium saucepan over medium-high heat and bring the soup to a simmer.
8. Stir in the basil and goat cheese just before serving.

Per Serving

Calories: 188 | fat: 10g | protein: 8g | carbs: 21g | fiber: 6g | sugar: 30g | sodium: 826m

Cauliflower rice with Tofu

Prep time: 15 minutes | Cook time: 10 minutes | Serves 4

1 package extra firm tofu	sliced
1 red bell pepper, sliced	2 tablespoons low-sodium soy sauce
1 orange bell pepper, sliced	1 tablespoon olive oil
2 cup cauliflower rice, cooked	1 teaspoon ginger, 1 teaspoon garlic powder
2 cups broccoli, chopped	1 teaspoon onion powder
¼ cup green onion,	1 teaspoon chili paste

1. Remove tofu from package and press with paper towels to absorb all excess moisture, let set for 15 minutes.
2. Chop tofu into cubes. Add tofu and seasonings to a large Ziploc bag and shake to coat.
3. Heat oil in a large skillet over medium heat. Add tofu and vegetables and cook, stirring frequently, 5 to 8 minutes, until tofu is browned on all sides and vegetables are tender.
4. To serve, place ½ cup cauliflower rice on 4 plates and top evenly with tofu mixture.

Per Serving

Calories: 95 | fat: 3.0g | protein: 7.1g | carbs: 12.1g | fiber: 4.0g | sugar: 5.0g | sodium: 310mg

Cucumber Whole Wheat Pita

Prep time: 20 minutes | Cook time: 10 minutes | Serves 4

4 whole-wheat pitas
1 cup cooked bulgur wheat
1 English cucumber, finely chopped
2 cups halved cherry tomatoes
1 yellow bell pepper, seeded and finely chopped
2 scallions, white and green parts, finely chopped
½ cup finely chopped fresh parsley
2 tablespoons extra-virgin olive oil
Juice of 1 lemon
Sea salt to taste
Freshly ground black pepper

1. Cut the pitas in half and split them open. Set them aside.
2. In a large bowl, stir together the bulgur, cucumber, tomatoes, bell pepper, scallions, parsley, olive oil, and lemon juice.
3. Season the bulgur mixture with salt and pepper.
4. Spoon the bulgur mixture evenly into the pita halves and serve.

Per Serving
Calories: 242 | fat: 8g | protein: 7g | carbs: 39g | fiber: 6g | sugar: 4g | sodium: 164mg

Sweet Potato White Beans Bowl

Prep time: 10 minutes | Cook time: 25 minutes | Serves 8

1 teaspoon extra-virgin olive oil
½ sweet onion, chopped
2 teaspoons minced garlic
2 sweet potatoes, peeled and diced
1 (28-ounce/793.7 g) can low-sodium diced tomatoes
¼ cup sodium-free tomato paste
2 tablespoons granulated sweetener
2 tablespoons hot sauce
1 tablespoon Dijon mustard
3 (15-ounce/425.2 g) cans sodium-free navy or white beans, drained
1 tablespoon chopped fresh oregano

1. Place a large saucepan over medium-high heat and add the oil.
2. Sauté the onion and garlic until translucent, about 3 minutes.
3. Stir in the sweet potatoes, diced tomatoes, tomato paste, sweetener, hot sauce, and mustard and bring to a boil.
4. Reduce the heat and simmer the tomato sauce for 10 minutes.
5. Stir in the beans and simmer for 10 minutes more.
6. Stir in the oregano and serve.

Per Serving
Calories: 255 | fat: 2g | protein: 15g | carbs: 48g | fiber: 12g | sugar: 8g | sodium: 149mg

Hot Garlic Beans Veggie Chili

Prep time: 20 minutes | Cook time: 60 minutes | Serves 8

1 teaspoon extra-virgin olive oil
1 sweet onion, chopped
1 red bell pepper, seeded and diced
1 green bell pepper, seeded and diced
2 teaspoons minced garlic
1 (28-ounce/793.7 g) can low-sodium diced tomatoes
1 (15-ounce/425.2 g) can sodium-free black beans, rinsed and drained
1 (15-ounce/425.2 g) can sodium-free red kidney beans, rinsed and drained
1 (15-ounce/425.2 g) can sodium-free navy beans, rinsed and drained
2 tablespoons chili powder
2 teaspoons ground cumin
1 teaspoon ground coriander
¼ teaspoon red pepper flakes

1. Place a large saucepan over medium-high heat and add the oil.
2. Sauté the onion, red and green bell peppers, and garlic until the vegetables have softened, about 5 minutes.
3. Add the tomatoes, black beans, red kidney beans, navy beans, chili powder, cumin, coriander, and red pepper flakes to the pan.
4. Bring the chili to a boil, and then reduce the heat to low.
5. Simmer the chili, stirring occasionally, for at least 1 hour. Serve hot.

Per Serving
Calories: 479 | fat: 28g | protein: 15g | carbs: 45g | fiber: 17g | sugar: 4g | sodium: 15mg

Tomato Chickpea Curry

Prep time: 10 minutes | Cook time: 25 minutes | Serves 6

1 tablespoon extra-virgin olive oil
1 sweet onion, chopped
1 tablespoon grated fresh ginger
1 teaspoon minced garlic
2 tablespoons red curry paste
1 teaspoon ground cumin
½ teaspoon turmeric
Pinch cayenne pepper
1 (28-ounce/793.7 g) can sodium-free diced tomatoes
2 cups cooked lentils
1 (15-ounce/425.2 g) can water-packed chickpeas, rinsed and drained
¼ cup coconut milk
2 tablespoons chopped fresh cilantro

1. Place a large saucepan over medium-high heat and add the oil.
2. Sauté the onion, ginger, and garlic until softened, about 3 minutes.
3. Add the curry paste, cumin, turmeric, and cayenne and sauté 1 minute more.
4. Stir in the tomatoes, lentils, chickpeas, and coconut milk.
5. Bring the curry to a boil, and then reduce the heat to low and simmer for 20 minutes.
6. Remove the curry from the heat and garnish with the cilantro.

Per Serving
Calories: 338 | fat: 8g | protein: 18g | carbs: 50g | fiber: 20g | sugar: 9g | sodium: 22mg

Low Fat Ricotta Zucchini Bake

Prep time: 20 minutes | Cook time: 30 minutes | Serves 4

1 teaspoon extra-virgin olive oil
½ onion, chopped
2 teaspoons minced garlic
2 cups cooked quinoa
2 eggs
½ cup low-fat ricotta cheese
Sea salt to taste
Freshly ground black pepper
2 cups cherry tomatoes
1 zucchini, cut into thin ribbons
⅛ Cup pine nuts, toasted

1. Preheat the oven to 350°F (176.6°C).Place a medium skillet over medium-high heat and add the olive oil.
2. Sauté the onion and garlic until softened and translucent, about 3 minutes.
3. Remove the skillet from the heat and stir in the quinoa, eggs, and ricotta.
4. Season the mixture with salt and pepper.
5. Stir in the cherry tomatoes and spoon the casserole into an 8-by-8-inch baking dish.
6. Scatter the zucchini ribbons and pine nuts on top, and bake the casserole until it is heated through, about 25 minutes.

Per Serving
Calories: 302 | fat: 9g | protein: 17g | carbs: 38g | fiber: 4g | sugar: 5g | sodium: 234mg

Margarine Cauliflower Bake

Prep time: 5 minutes | Cook time: 50 minutes | Serves 6

1 small head cauliflower, separated into small florets
1½ cup reduced-fat sharp cheddar cheese, grated
1 cup low-fat milk
½ cup chopped onion
2 tablespoons margarine, divided
2 tablespoons whole wheat flour
2 tablespoons whole wheat bread crumbs
1 teaspoon olive oil
1 teaspoon yellow mustard
½ teaspoon garlic powder
¼ teaspoon salt
¼ teaspoon black pepper
Nonstick cooking spray

1. Heat oven to 400°F (205°C). Coat a baking sheet with cooking spray.
2. In a medium bowl, combine oil, salt, pepper, onion, and cauliflower. Toss until cauliflower is coated evenly. Spread on baking sheet and cook 25 to 30 minutes until lightly browned.
3. In a medium saucepan, over medium heat, melt 1½ tablespoons margarine. Whisk in flour until no lumps remain.
4. Add milk and continue whisking until sauce thickens. Stir in mustard, garlic powder, and cheese until melted and smooth.
5. Add cauliflower and mix well. Pour into a 1½-quart baking dish.
6. In a small glass bowl, melt remaining margarine in microwave. Stir in bread crumbs until moistened.
7. Sprinkle evenly over cauliflower. Bake 20 minutes until bubbling and golden brown on top.

Per Serving
Calories: 155 | fat: 8.0g | protein: 8.1g | carbs: 15.1g | fiber: 3.0g | sugar: 4.0g | sodium: 445mg

Homemade Low Sugar Italian Pasta

Prep time: 20 minutes | Cook time: 35 minutes | Serves 6

1 tablespoon extra-virgin olive oil
1 onion, chopped
2 celery stalks, chopped
3 teaspoons minced garlic
2 (28-ounce/793.7 g) cans sodium-free diced tomatoes
2 tablespoons chopped

fresh basil
1 tablespoon chopped fresh oregano
½ teaspoon red pepper flakes
½ cup quartered, pitted Kalamata olives
¼ cup freshly squeezed lemon juice
8 ounces (226.7 g) whole-wheat spaghetti

1. Place a large saucepan over medium-high heat and add the oil.
2. Sauté the onion, celery, and garlic until they are translucent, about 3 minutes.
3. Add the tomatoes, basil, oregano, and red pepper flakes, and bring the sauce to a boil, stirring occasionally.
4. Reduce the heat to low and simmer 20 minutes, stirring occasionally.
5. Stir in the olives and lemon juice and remove the saucepan from the heat.
6. Cook the pasta according to the package instructions.
7. Spoon the sauce over the pasta and serve.

Per Serving
Calories: 200 | fat: 5g | protein: 7g | carbs: 35g | fiber: 4g | sugar: 8g | sodium: 88mg

Homemade Carrot Celery Veggie Soup

Prep time: 10 minutes | Cook time: 55 minutes | Serves 4

1 teaspoon extra-virgin olive oil
1 onion, chopped
1 tablespoon minced garlic
4 celery stalks, with the greens, chopped
3 carrots, peeled and diced
3 cups red lentils, picked over, washed,

and drained
1 cups low-sodium vegetable broth
3 cups water
2 bay leaves
2 teaspoons chopped fresh thyme
Sea salt to taste
Freshly ground black pepper

1. Place a large stockpot on medium-high heat and add the oil.
2. Sauté the onion and garlic until translucent, about 3 minutes.
3. Stir in the celery and carrots and sauté 5 minutes.
4. Add the lentils, broth, water, and bay leaves, and bring the soup to a boil.
5. Reduce the heat to low and simmer until the lentils are soft and the soup is thick, about 45 minutes.
6. Remove the bay leaves and stir in the thyme.
7. Season with salt and pepper and serve.

Per Serving
Calories: 284 | fat: 2g | protein: 20g | carbs: 47g | fiber: 24g | sugar: 17g | sodium: 419mg

Creamy Cauliflower Veggie Casserole

Prep time: 10 minutes | Cook time: 35 minutes | Serves 8

2 cup cauliflower, grated
1 cup fat free sour cream
1 cup reduced fat cheddar cheese, grated
1 cup reduced fat Mexican cheese blend, grated
½ cup red onion, diced
1 (11-ounce / 312-g)

can Mexicorn, drain
10 ounces (283 g) tomatoes and green chilies
2.25 ounces (64 g) black olives, drain
1 cup black beans, rinsed
1 cup salsa
¼ teaspoon pepper
Nonstick cooking spray

1. Heat oven to 350ºF (180ºC). Spray a 2½-quart baking dish with cooking spray.
2. In a large bowl, combine beans, corn, tomatoes, salsa, sour cream, cheddar cheese, pepper, and cauliflower. Transfer to baking dish.
3. Sprinkle with onion and olives.
4. Bake 30 minutes. Sprinkle with Mexican blend cheese and bake another 5 to 10 minutes, or until cheese is melted and casserole is heated through. Let rest 10 minutes before serving.

Per Serving
Calories: 267 | fat: 8.0g | protein: 16.1g | carbs: 33.1g | fiber: 6.0g | sugar: 8.0g | sodium: 812mg

Tender Vegetables with Green onions & Sesame seeds

Prep time: 15 minutes | Cook time: 30 minutes | Serves 6

12 ounces (340 g) extra firm tofu organic, cut into 1-inch cubes	¼ cup lime juice
	2 cloves garlic, diced fine
2 zucchini, shredded into long zoodles	2 tablespoons reduced fat peanut butter
1 carrot, grated	2 tablespoons tamari
3 cups bean sprouts	1 tablespoon sesame seeds
2 Green onions sliced	
1 cup red cabbage, shredded	½ tablespoon sesame oil
¼ cup cilantro, chopped	2 teaspoons red chili flakes

1. Heat half the oil in a saucepan over medium heat.
2. Add tofu and cook until it starts to brown, about 5 minutes. Add garlic and stir until light brown.
3. Add zucchini, carrot, cabbage, lime juice, peanut butter, tamari, and chili flakes. Stir to combine all.
4. Cook, stirring frequently, until vegetables are tender, about 5 minutes. Add bean sprouts and remove from heat.
5. Serve topped with green onions, sesame seeds and cilantro.

Per Serving
Calories: 135 | fat: 6.0g | protein: 12.1g | carbs: 13.1g | fiber: 2.0g | sugar: 3.0g | sodium: 450mg

Grilled Tofu with Lettuce and Carrot

Prep time: 15 minutes | Cook time: 15 minutes | Serves 2

2 (3-ounce / 85-g) tofu portions, extra firm, pressed between paper towels 15 minutes	Butter leaf lettuce, for serving
	2 whole wheat sandwiches thins
¼ red onion, sliced	1 tablespoon teriyaki marinade
2 tablespoons carrot, grated	1 tablespoon Sriracha
1 teaspoon margarine	1 teaspoon red chili flakes

1. Heat grill, or charcoal, to a medium heat.

2. Marinate tofu in teriyaki marinade, red chili flakes and Sriracha.
3. Melt margarine in a small skillet over medium-high heat.
4. Add onions and cook until caramelized, about 5 minutes.
5. Grill tofu for 3 to 4 minutes per side.
6. To assemble, place tofu on bottom roll. Top with lettuce, carrot, and onion. Add top of the roll and serve.

Per Serving
Calories: 180 | fat: 5.0g | protein: 12.1g | carbs: 27.1g | fiber: 7.0g | sugar: 5.0g | sodium: 580mg

Scrambled Eggs with Veggies and Salsa

Prep time: 15 minutes | Cook time: 5 minutes | Serves 4

8 egg whites	chopped
4 egg yolks	2 tablespoons fresh lime juice
3 tomatoes cut in ½-inch pieces	
	12 tortilla chips, broken into small pieces
1 jalapeno pepper, slice thin	
½ avocado cut in ½-inch pieces	2 tablespoons water
	1 tablespoon olive oil
½ red onion, diced fine	¾ teaspoon pepper, divided
½ head Romaine lettuce, torn	½ teaspoon salt, divided
½ cup cilantro,	

1. In a medium bowl, combine tomatoes, avocado, onion, jalapeno, cilantro, lime juice, ¼ teaspoon salt, and ¼ teaspoon pepper.
2. In a large bowl, whisk egg whites, egg yolks, water, and remaining salt and pepper. Stir in tortilla chips.
3. Heat oil in a large skillet over medium heat. Add egg mixture and cook, stirring frequently, 3 to 5 minutes, or desired doneness.
4. To serve, divide lettuce leaves among 4 plates.
5. Add scrambled egg mixture and top with salsa.

Per Serving
Calories: 281 | fat: 21.0g | protein: 15.1g | carbs: 10.1g | fiber: 4.0g | sugar: 4.0g | sodium: 441mg

Cheesy Spinach Pizza

Prep time: 15 minutes | Cook time: 20 minutes | Serves 2

1¾ cup grated
Mozzarella cheese
½ cup frozen spinach,
thaw
1 egg
2 tablespoons reduced
fat Parmesan cheese,
grated
2 tablespoons cream

cheese, soft
¾ cup almond flour
¼ cup light Alfredo
sauce
½ teaspoon Italian
seasoning
¼ teaspoon red
pepper flakes
Pinch of salt

1. Heat oven to 400ºF (205ºC).
2. Squeeze all the excess water out of the spinach.
3. In a glass bowl, combine Mozzarella and almond flour. Stir in cream cheese. Microwave 1 minute on high, and then stir. If the mixture is not melted, microwave another 30 seconds.
4. Stir in the egg, seasoning, and salt. Mix well. Place dough on a piece of parchment paper and press into a 10-inch circle.
5. Place directly on the oven rack and bake 8 to 10 minutes or until lightly browned.
6. Remove the crust and spread with the Alfredo sauce, then add spinach, Parmesan and red pepper flakes evenly over top. Bake another 8 to 10 minutes. Slice and serve.

Per Serving
Calories: 442 | fat: 35.0g | protein: 24.1g | carbs: 14.1g | fiber: 5.0g | sugar: 4.0g | sodium: 1178mg

Creamy Mushroom Bowl with Parsley

Prep time: 10 minutes | Cook time: 120 minutes | Serves 2

8 cups mushrooms cut
into quarters
1 onion, halved and
sliced thin
4 tablespoons fresh
parsley, chopped
1½ tablespoons low fat
sour cream

1 cup low sodium
vegetable broth
3 cloves garlic, diced
fine
2 teaspoons smoked
paprika
Salt and ground black
pepper, to taste

1. Add all, except sour cream and parsley to crock pot.

2. Cover and cook on high 2 hours.
3. Stir in sour cream and serve garnished with parsley.

Per Serving
Calories: 113 | fat: 2.0g | protein: 10.1g | carbs: 18.1g | fiber: 4.0g | sugar: 8.0g | sodium: 595mg

Spicy Cauliflower Sauce with Scallions

Prep time: 15 minutes | Cook time: 45 minutes | Serves 4

1 large head
cauliflower, separated
in florets
3 scallions, sliced
1 onion, diced fine
1 (15-ounce / 425-g)
can petite tomatoes,
diced
4 cloves garlic, diced
fine
4 tablespoons olive oil,

divided
1 tablespoon red wine
vinegar
1 tablespoon balsamic
vinegar
3 teaspoons Splenda
1 teaspoon salt
1 teaspoon ground
black pepper
½ teaspoon chili
powder

1. Heat oven to 400ºF (205ºC).
2. Place cauliflower on a large baking sheet and drizzle with 2 tablespoons of oil. Sprinkle with salt and pepper, to taste. Use hands to rub oil and seasoning into florets then lay in single layer. Roast until fork tender.
3. Heat 1 tablespoon oil in a large skillet over medium-low heat. Add onion and cook until soft.
4. Stir in tomatoes, with juice, Splendid, both vinegars, and the teaspoon of salt.
5. Bring to a boil, reduce heat and simmer 20 to 25 minutes. For a smooth sauce, use an immersion blender to process until smooth, or leave it chunky.
6. In a separate skillet, heat remaining oil over medium-low heat and sauté garlic 1 to 2 minutes.
7. Stir in tomato sauce, and increase heat to medium. Cook, stirring frequently, 5 minutes.
8. Add chili powder and cauliflower and toss to coat. Serve garnished.

Per Serving
Calories: 108 | fat: 0g | protein: 6.1g | carbs: 23.1g | fiber: 7.0g | sugar: 12.0g | sodium: 751mg

Zucchini Tofu with Sesame seeds

Prep time: 15 minutes | Cook time: 15 minutes | Serves 6

1 block tofu
2 small zucchini, sliced
1 red bell pepper, cut into 1-inch cubes
1 yellow bell pepper, cut into 1-inch cubes
1 red onion, cut into 1-inch cubes
2 cups cherry tomatoes

2 tablespoons lite soy sauce
3 teaspoons barbecue sauce
2 teaspoons sesame seeds
Salt and ground black pepper, to taste
Nonstick cooking spray

1. Press tofu to extract liquid, for about half an hour. Then, cut tofu into cubes and marinate in soy sauce for at least 15 minutes.
2. Heat the grill to medium-high heat. Spray the grill rack with cooking spray.
3. Assemble skewers with tofu alternating with vegetables.
4. Grill for 2 to 3 minutes per side until vegetables start to soften, and tofu is golden brown. At the very end of cooking time, season with salt and pepper and brush with barbecue sauce.
5. Serve garnished with sesame seeds.

Per Serving
Calories: 65 | fat: 2.0g | protein: 5.1g | carbs: 10.1g | fiber: 3.0g | sugar: 6.0g | sodium: 237mg

Peppery Spinach Muffins

Prep time: 10 minutes | Cook time: 15 minutes | Serves 6

Non-stick cooking spray
2 tablespoons extra-virgin olive oil
1 onion, finely chopped
2 cups baby spinach
2 garlic cloves, minced

8 large eggs, beaten
¼ cup 1% or skim milk
½ teaspoon sea salt
¼ teaspoons freshly ground black pepper
1 cup shredded Swiss cheese

1. Preheat the oven to 375°F (190.5°C). Spray a 6-cup muffin tin with non-stick cooking spray.
2. In a large skillet over medium-high heat, heat the olive oil until it shimmers.

3. Add the onion and cook until soft, about 4 minutes. Add the spinach and cook, stirring, until the spinach softens, about 1 minute.
4. Add the garlic. Cook, stirring constantly, for 30 seconds. Remove from heat and let cool.
5. In a medium bowl, beat together the eggs, milk, salt, and pepper.
6. Fold the cooled vegetables and the cheese into the egg mixture. Spoon the mixture into the prepared muffin tins.
7. Bake until the eggs are set, about 15 minutes. Allow to rest for 5 minutes before serving.

Per Serving
Calories: 218 | fat: 17g | protein: 14g | carbs: 4g | fiber: 1g | sugar: 22g | sodium: 237 mg

Balsamic Mushrooms with Basil

Prep time: 5 minutes | Cook time: 10 minutes | Serves 4

8 Portobello mushrooms, stems removed
1 cup Mozzarella cheese, grated
1 cup cherry tomatoes, sliced
½ cup crushed tomatoes
½ cup fresh basil, chopped

2 tablespoons balsamic vinegar
1 tablespoon olive oil
1 tablespoon oregano
1 tablespoon red pepper flakes
½ tablespoon garlic powder
¼ teaspoon pepper
Pinch salt to taste

1. Heat oven to broil. Line a baking sheet with foil.
2. Place mushrooms, stem side down, on foil and drizzle with oil. Sprinkle with garlic powder, salt and pepper. Broil for 5 minutes.
3. Flip mushrooms over and top with crushed tomatoes, oregano, parsley, pepper flakes, cheese and sliced tomatoes. Broil another 5 minutes.
4. Top with basil and drizzle with balsamic. Serve.

Per Serving
Calories: 115 | fat: 5.0g | protein: 9.1g | carbs: 11.1g | fiber: 4.0g | sugar: 3.0g | sodium: 257mg

Sweet Potato Egg Bake with Avocado

Prep time: 5 minutes | Cook time: 25 minutes | Serves 4

2 tablespoons extra-virgin olive oil
1 red onion, chopped
1 green bell pepper, seeded and chopped
1 sweet potato, cut into ½-inch pieces
1 teaspoon chili powder
½ teaspoon sea salt
4 large eggs
½ cup shredded pepper Jack cheese
1 avocado, cut into cubes

1. Preheat the oven to 350°F (176.6°C). In a large, ovenproof skillet over medium-high heat, heat the olive oil until it shimmers.
2. Add the onion, bell pepper, sweet potato, chili powder, and salt, and cook, stirring occasionally, until the vegetables start to brown, about 10 minutes.
3. Remove from heat. Arrange the vegetables in the pan to form 4 wells. Crack an egg into each well.
4. Sprinkle the cheese on the vegetables, around the edges of the eggs.
5. Bake until the eggs set, about 10 minutes. Top with avocado before serving.

Per Serving
Calories: 284 | fat: 21g | protein: 12g | carbs: 16g | fiber: 5g | sugar: 9.1g | sodium: 264mg

Garlicky Mushroom Noodles with Parmesan

Prep time: 10 minutes | Cook time: 20 minutes | Serves 4

¼ cup extra-virgin olive oil
1 pound cremini mushrooms, sliced
½ red onion, finely chopped
1 teaspoon dried thyme
½ teaspoon sea salt
3 garlic cloves, minced
½ cup dry white wine
Pinch red pepper flakes
4 cups butternut noodles
4 ounces grated Parmesan cheese (optional, for serving)

1. In a large skillet over medium-high heat, heat the olive oil until it shimmers.
2. Add the mushrooms, onion, thyme, and salt. Cook, stirring occasionally, until the mushrooms start to brown, about 6 minutes.
3. Add the garlic and cook, stirring constantly, for 30 seconds. Add the white wine and red pepper flakes. Stir to combine.
4. Add the noodles. Cook, stirring occasionally, until the noodles are tender, about 5 minutes.
5. If desired, serve topped with grated Parmesan.

Per Serving
Calories: 244 | fat: 14g | protein: 4g | carbs: 22g | fiber: 4g | sugar: 12.7g | sodium: 159mg

Homemade Onion Shiitake Mushrooms Omelet

Prep time: 5 minutes | Cook time: 10 minutes | Serves 4

2 tablespoons extra-virgin olive oil
½ onion, finely chopped
1 cup broccoli florets
1 cup sliced shiitake mushrooms
1 garlic clove, minced
8 large eggs, beaten
½ teaspoon sea salt
½ cup grated Parmesan cheese

1. Preheat the oven broiler on high.
2. In a medium ovenproof skillet over medium-high heat, heat the olive oil until it shimmers.
3. Add the onion, broccoli, and mushrooms, and cook, stirring occasionally, until the vegetables start to brown, about 5 minutes.
4. Add the garlic and cook, stirring constantly, for 30 seconds. Arrange the vegetables in an even layer on the bottom of the pan.
5. While the vegetables cook, in a small bowl, whisk together the eggs and salt. Carefully pour the eggs over the vegetables.
6. Cook without stirring, allowing the eggs to set around the vegetables. As the eggs begin to set around the edges, use a spatula to pull the edges away from the sides of the pan.
7. Tilt the pan and allow the uncooked eggs to run into the spaces. Cook 1 to 2 minutes more, until it sets around the edges. The eggs will still be runny on top.
8. Sprinkle with the Parmesan and place the pan in the broiler. Broil until brown and puffy, about 3 minutes. Cut into wedges to serve.

Per Serving
Calories: 281 | fat: 21.1g | protein: 19.1g | carbs: 6.9g | fiber: 2.1g | sugar: 4.0g| sodium: 655mg

Tofu that Tastes Good Stir Fry

Prep time: 10 minutes | Cook time: 20 minutes | Serves 4

3 tablespoons extra-virgin olive oil
4 scallions, sliced
12 ounces firm tofu, cut into ½-inch pieces
4 cups broccoli, broken into florets
4 garlic cloves, minced

1 teaspoon peeled and grated fresh ginger
¼ cup vegetable broth
2 tablespoons soy sauce (use gluten-free soy sauce if necessary)
1 cup cooked brown rice

1.   In a large skillet over medium-high heat, heat the olive oil until it shimmers.
2.   Add the scallions, tofu, and broccoli and cook, stirring, until the vegetables begin to soften, about 6 minutes.
3.   Add the garlic and ginger and cook, stirring constantly, for 30 seconds.
4.   Add the broth, soy sauce, and rice. Cook, stirring, 1 to 2 minutes more to heat the rice through.

Per Serving
Calories: 236 | fat: 13g | protein: 11g | carbs: 21g | fiber: 4g | sugar: 8.8g | sodium: 361mg

Margarine Zucchini with Garlic Sauce

Prep time: 40 minutes | Cook time: 10 minutes | Serves 4

3 zucchinis, grated
2 eggs
1 onion, diced
¾ cups feta cheese, crumbled
¼ cup fresh dill, chopped
Garlic Dipping Sauce:
1 cup Greek yogurt
1 tablespoon fresh dill, diced fine

1 tablespoon margarine
½ cup flour
1 teaspoon salt
Pepper to taste
Oil for frying

2 cloves garlic, diced fine

1.   Combine the ingredients for the garlic dipping sauce in a small bowl. Stir to mix well. Reserve the bowl in the refrigerator until ready to serve.
2.   Place zucchini in a large colander and sprinkle with the salt. Toss with fingers and let sit 30 minutes. Squeeze with back of spoon to remove the excess water.
3.   Place the zucchini between paper towels and squeeze again. Place in large bowl and let dry.
4.   Melt margarine in a large skillet over medium-high heat. Add onion and cook until soft, about 5 minutes. Add to zucchini along with the feta and dill and mix well.
5.   In a small bowl, whisk together the flour and eggs. Pour over zucchini and mix well.
6.   Add oil to the skillet to equal ½-inch and heat over medium-high heat until very hot.
7.   Drop golf ball sized scoops of zucchini mixture into oil and flatten into a patty. Cook until golden brown on both sides. Transfer to paper towel line plate.
8.   Serve with the garlic dipping sauce.

Per Serving
Calories: 254 | fat: 15.0g | protein: 10.1g | carbs: 21.1g | fiber: 3.0g | sugar: 5.0g | sodium: 922mg

Homemade Spicy Veggie Bowl

Prep time: 10 minutes | Cook time: 15 minutes | Serves 4

2 tablespoons extra-virgin olive oil
1 onion, finely chopped
1 green bell pepper, seeded and chopped
2 (14-ounce/396 g) cans crushed tomatoes
1 (14-ounce/396g) can kidney beans, drained and rinsed

2 cups veggie crumbles (such as Morningstar Farms Grillers Crumbles)
1 tablespoon chili powder
1 teaspoon garlic powder
½ teaspoon sea salt

1.   In a large skillet over medium-high heat, heat the olive oil until it shimmers.
2.   Add the onion and bell pepper and cook, stirring occasionally, for 5 minutes.
3.   Add the tomatoes, beans, veggie crumbles, chili powder, garlic powder, and salt.
4.   Bring to a simmer, stirring. Reduce heat and cook for 5 minutes more, stirring occasionally.

Per Serving
Calories: 283 | fat: 1g | protein: 17g | carbs: 39g | fiber: 13g | sugar: 19g | sodium: 113mg

Scallops filled Lettuce with Remoulade

Prep time: 10minutes | Cook time: 10 minutes | Serves 4

1 cup whole-wheat bread crumbs
2 teaspoons sea salt
1 teaspoon dried oregano
¼ teaspoon cayenne (or to taste)
½ cup whole-wheat

flour
2 large eggs
1 pound sea scallops
4 large lettuce leaves, for serving
1 recipe Remoulade, for serving

1. Preheat the oven to 450°F (232°C)
2. In a medium bowl, whisk together the bread crumbs, salt, oregano, and cayenne until well combined. Put the flour in a separate bowl.
3. In a small bowl, beat the eggs well. Dip the scallops in the flour and pat off any excess. Dip them in the eggs, and then into the bread crumb mixture. Place on a rimmed baking sheet.
4. Bake until the breading is browned, 8 to 10 minutes.
5. Spoon the scallops into the lettuce leaves. Serve topped with the Remoulade.

Per Serving
Calories: 447 | fat: 20g | protein: 28g | carbs: 37g | fiber: 2g | sugar: 1.71g | sodium: 134mg

Low Fat Peppery Macaroni with Parmesan

Prep time: 10minutes | Cook time: 25 minutes | Serves 6

1 cup fat-free evaporated milk
½ cup skim milk
½ cup low-fat Cottage cheese
½ cup low-fat Cheddar cheese
1 teaspoon nutmeg

Pinch cayenne pepper
Sea salt to taste
Freshly ground black pepper
6 cups cooked whole-wheat elbow macaroni
2 tablespoons grated Parmesan cheese

1. Preheat the oven to 350°F (176.6°C). Place a large saucepan over low heat and add the evaporated milk and skim milk.
2. Heat the evaporated milk and skim milk until steaming, and then stir in the cottage cheese and Cheddar, stirring until they melt.

3. Stir in the nutmeg and cayenne.
4. Season the sauce with salt and black pepper and remove from the heat.
5. Stir the cooked pasta into the sauce, then spoon the mac and cheese into a large casserole dish.
6. Sprinkle the top with the Parmesan cheese, and bake until it is bubbly and lightly browned, about 20 minutes.

Per Serving
Calories: 246 | fat: 2g | protein: 16g | carbs: 44g | fiber: 4g | sugar: 7g | sodium: 187mg

15 Minute Bacon Pot Recipe

Prep time: 10 minutes | Cook time: 15 minutes | Serves 4

2 tablespoons extra-virgin olive oil
3 slices pepper bacon, chopped
1 onion, chopped
1 red bell pepper, seeded and chopped
1 fennel bulb, chopped

3 tablespoons flour
5 cups low-sodium or unsalted chicken broth
6 ounces chopped canned clams, undrained
½ teaspoon sea salt
½ cup milk

1. In a large pot over medium-high heat, heat the olive oil until it shimmers.
2. Add the bacon and cook, stirring, until browned, about 4 minutes. Remove the bacon from the fat with a slotted spoon, and set it aside on a plate.
3. Add the onion, bell pepper, and fennel to the fat in the pot. Cook, stirring occasionally, until the vegetables are soft, about 5 minutes. Add the flour and cook, stirring constantly, for 1 minute.
4.
5. Add the broth, clams, and salt. Bring to a simmer. Cook, stirring, until the soup thickens, about 5 minutes more.
6. Stir in the milk and return the bacon to the pot. Cook, stirring, 1 minute more.

Per Serving
Calories: 335 | fat: 20g | protein: 20g | carbs: 21g | fiber: 3g | sugar: 28g | sodium: 496mg

Chapter 6: Vegetable Sides

Spiced Avocado with Jicama Dip

Prep time: 5 minutes | Cook time: 0 minutes | Serves 4

1 avocado, cut into cubes
Juice of ½ limes
2 tablespoons finely chopped red onion
2 tablespoons chopped fresh cilantro
1 garlic clove, minced
¼ teaspoon sea salt
1 cup sliced jicama

1. In a small bowl, combine the avocado, lime juice, onion, cilantro, garlic, and salt. Mash lightly with a fork.
2. Serve with the jicama for dipping.

Per Serving
Calories: 74 | fat: 5.1g | protein: 1.1g | carbs: 7.9g | fiber: 4.9g | sugar: 3.0g | sodium: 80mg

Spicy Lemony Broccoli

Prep time: 10 minutes | Cook time: 25 minutes | Serves 8

2 large broccoli heads, cut into florets
2 tablespoons extra-virgin olive oil
3 garlic cloves, minced
¼ teaspoon salt
¼ teaspoon ground black pepper
2 tablespoons freshly squeezed lemon juice

1. Preheat the oven to 425ºF (220ºC) and line a large baking sheet with parchment paper.
2. In a large bowl, add the broccoli, olive oil, garlic, salt, and pepper. Toss well until the broccoli is coated completely. Transfer the broccoli to the prepared baking sheet.
3. Roast in the preheated oven for about 25 minutes, flipping the broccoli halfway through, or until the broccoli is browned and fork-tender.
4. Remove from the oven to a plate and let cool for 5 minutes. Serve drizzled with the lemon juice.

Per Serving
Calories: 33 | fat: 2.1g | protein: 1.2g | carbs: 3.1g | fiber: 1.1g | sugar: 1.1g | sodium: 85mg

Tahini Zucchini with Pepper Dip

Prep time: 10 minutes | Cook time: 0 minutes | Serves 4

2 zucchini, chopped
3 garlic cloves
2 tablespoons extra-virgin olive oil
2 tablespoons tahini
Juice of 1 lemon
½ teaspoon sea salt
1 red bell pepper, seeded and cut into sticks

1. In a blender or food processor, combine the zucchini, garlic, olive oil, tahini, lemon juice, and salt. Blend until smooth.
2. Serve with the red bell pepper for dipping.

Per Serving
Calories: 120 | fat: 11.1g | protein: 2.1g | carbs: 6.9g | fiber: 2.9g | sugar: 4.0g | sodium: 155mg

One Pan Garlic Onion Cucumber Pickle

Prep time: 15 minutes | Cook time: 5 minutes | Serves 10

2 cucumbers cut into ¼-inch slices
½ onion, sliced thin
1½ cups vinegar
2 tablespoons stevia
1 tablespoon dill
2 cloves garlic, sliced thin
1 teaspoon peppercorns
1 teaspoon coriander seeds
½ teaspoon salt
¼ teaspoon red pepper flakes

1. In a medium saucepan, combine vinegar and spices. Bring to a boil over high heat. Set aside.
2. Place the cucumbers, onions, and garlic into a quart-sized jar, or plastic container, with an air tight lid. Pour hot liquid over the vegetables, making sure they are completely covered.
3. Add the lid and chill at least a day before serving.

Per Serving
Calories: 35 | fat: 0g | protein: 0g | carbs: 6.1g | fiber: 0g | sugar: 4.0g | sodium: 124mg

One Pot Hot Corn

Prep time: 10 minutes | Cook time: 20 minutes | Serves 12

6 ears corn

1. Remove the husks and silk from the corn. Cut or break each ear in half.
2. Pour 1 cup of water into the bottom of the electric pressure cooker. Insert a wire rack or trivet.
3. Place the corn upright on the rack, cut-side down. Close and lock the lid of the pressure cooker. Set the valve to sealing.
4. Cook on high pressure for 5 minutes.
5. When the cooking is complete, hit Cancel and quick release the pressure.
6. Once the pin drops, unlock and remove the lid.
7. Use tongs to remove the corn from the pot. Season as desired and serve immediately.

Per Serving
Calories: 64 | fat: 1.1g | protein: 2.1g | carbs: 13.9g | fiber: 0.9g | sugar: 5.0g | sodium: 12mg

Cheese Stuffed Mushroom Caps

Prep time: 5 minutes | Cook time: 20 minutes | Serves 4

12 cremini mushrooms, stems removed	cheese, grated
	⅓ cup reduced fat Parmesan cheese
4 ounces (113 g) low fat cream cheese, soft	6 tablespoons basil pesto
½ cup Mozzarella	Nonstick cooking spray

1. Heat oven to 375ºF (190ºC). Line a square baking dish with foil and spray with cooking spray. Arrange the mushrooms in the baking pan. Set aside.
2. In a medium bowl, beat cream cheese, pesto and Parmesan until smooth and creamy. Spoon mixture into mushroom caps.
3. Top with a heaping teaspoon of Mozzarella.
4. Bake 20 to 23 minutes or until cheese is melted and golden brown. Let cook 5 to 10 minutes before serving.

Per Serving
Calories: 77 | fat: 3.0g | protein: 8.2g | carbs: 4.1g | fiber: 0g | sugar: 1.0g | sodium: 541mg

Spicy Asparagus Cashews Bake

Prep time: 10 minutes | Cook time: 15 to 20 minutes | Serves 4

2 pounds (907 g) asparagus, woody ends trimmed	ground black pepper, to taste
1 tablespoon extra-virgin olive oil	½ cup chopped cashews
Sea salt and freshly	Zest and juice of 1 lime

1. Preheat the oven to 400ºF (205ºC). Line a baking sheet with aluminum foil.
2. Toss the asparagus with the olive oil in a medium bowl. Sprinkle the salt and pepper to season.
3. Arrange the asparagus on the baking sheet and bake for 15 to 20 minutes, or until lightly browned and tender.
4. Remove the asparagus from the oven to a serving bowl.
5. Add the cashews, lime zest and juice, and toss to coat well. Serve immediately.

Per Serving
Calories: 173 | fat: 11.8g | protein: 8.0g | carbs: 43.7g | fiber: 4.9g | sugar: 5.0g | sodium: 65mg

Browny Cauliflower Bowl

Prep time: 5 minutes | Cook time: 20 minutes | Serves 4

1 head cauliflower, separated into bite-sized florets	¼ teaspoon salt
	⅛ Teaspoon black pepper
¼ teaspoon garlic powder	Butter-flavored cooking spray

1. Heat oven to 400ºF (205ºC).
2. Place cauliflower in a large bowl and spray with cooking spray, making sure to coat all sides. Sprinkle with seasonings and toss to coat.
3. Place in a single layer on a cookie sheet.
4. Bake for 20 to 25 minutes or until cauliflower starts to brown. Serve warm.

Per Serving
Calories: 55 | fat: 0g | protein: 4.2g | carbs: 11.1g | fiber: 5.0g | sugar: 5.0g | sodium: 165mg

Asparagus with Bell Peppers with Italian Dressing

Prep time: 5 minutes | Cook time: 15 minutes | Serves 4

1 pound (454 g) asparagus, woody ends trimmed, cut into 2-inch segments
2 red bell peppers, seeded, cut into 1-inch pieces
1 small onion, quartered
2 tablespoons Italian dressing

1. Preheat the oven to 400ºF (205ºC). Line a baking sheet with parchment paper and set aside.
2. Combine the asparagus with the peppers, onion, and dressing in a large bowl, and toss well.
3. Arrange the vegetables on the baking sheet and roast for about 15 minutes until softened. Flip the vegetables with a spatula once during cooking.
4. Transfer to a large platter and serve.

Per Serving
Calories: 92 | fat: 4.8g | protein: 2.9g | carbs: 10.7g | fiber: 4.0g | sugar: 5.7g | sodium: 31mg

Citrusy Wax Beans Bowl

Prep time: 5 minutes | Cook time: 15 minutes | Serves 4

2 pounds (907 g) wax beans
2 tablespoons extra-virgin olive oil
Sea salt to taste
Freshly ground black pepper
Juice of ½ lemon

1. Preheat the oven to 400ºF (204ºC). Line a baking sheet with aluminium foil.
2. In a large bowl, toss the beans and olive oil. Season lightly with salt and pepper.
3. Transfer the beans to the baking sheet and spread them out.
4. Roast the beans until caramelized and tender, about 10 to 12 minutes.
5. Transfer the beans to a serving platter and sprinkle with the lemon juice.

Per Serving
Calories: 100 | fat: 7g | protein: 2g | carbs: 8g | fiber: 4g | sugar: 4g | sodium: 813mg

Butter Sautéed Green Beans

Prep time: 15 minutes | Cook time: 5 minutes | Serves 4

1 tablespoon butter
1½ pounds (680 g) green beans, trimmed
1 teaspoon ground nutmeg
Sea salt, to taste

1. Melt the butter in a large skillet over medium heat.
2. Sauté the green beans in the melted butter for 5 minutes until tender but still crisp, stirring frequently.
3. Season with nutmeg and salt and mix well.
4. Remove from the heat and cool for a few minutes before serving.

Per Serving
Calories: 83 | fat: 3.2g | protein: 3.2g | carbs: 12.2g | fiber: 6.1g | sugar: 3.2g | sodium: 90mg

Oven Baked Lemony Cauliflower

Prep time: 5 minutes | Cook time: 25 minutes | Serves 4

1 cauliflower head, broken into small florets
2 tablespoons extra-virgin olive oil
½ teaspoon salt, or more to taste
½ teaspoon ground chipotle chili powder
Juice of 1 lime

1. Preheat the oven to 450ºF (235ºC) and line a large baking sheet with parchment paper. Set aside.
2. Toss the cauliflower florets in the olive oil in a large bowl. Season with salt and chipotle chili powder.
3. Arrange the cauliflower florets on the baking sheet.
4. Roast in the preheated oven for 15 minutes until lightly browned. Flip the cauliflower and continue to roast until crisp and tender, about 10 minutes.
5. Remove from the oven and season as needed with salt.
6. Cool for 6 minutes and drizzle with the lime juice, then serve.

Per Serving
Calories: 100 | fat: 7.1g | protein: 3.2g | carbs: 8.1g | fiber: 3.2g | sugar: 3.2g | sodium: 285mg

One Plate Egg Spinach Quiches

Prep time: 10 minutes | Cook time: 15 minutes | Serves 6

2 tablespoons olive oil, divided
1 onion, finely chopped
2 garlic cloves, minced
2 cups baby spinach
8 large eggs
¼ cup 1% or skim milk
½ teaspoon sea salt
¼ teaspoons freshly ground black pepper
1 cup Swiss cheese, shredded

Special Equipment:
A 6-cup muffin tin

1. Preheat the oven to 375ºF (190ºC). Grease a 6-cup muffin tin with 1 tablespoon olive oil.
2. Heat the olive oil in a nonstick skillet over medium-high heat. Add the onion and garlic to the skillet and sauté for 4 minutes until translucent.
3. Add the spinach to the skillet and sauté for 1 minute until tender. Transfer them to a plate and set aside.
4. Whisk together the eggs, milk, salt, and black pepper in a bowl. Dunk the cooked vegetables in the bowl of egg mixture, and then scatter with the cheese.
5. Divide the mixture among the muffin cups. Bake in the preheated oven for 15 minutes until puffed and the edges are golden brown. Transfer the quiches to six small plates and serve warm.

Per Serving
Calories: 220 | fat: 17.2g | protein: 14.3g | carbs: 4.2g | fiber: 0.8g | sugar: 27g | sodium: 235mg

Garlic and Soy Sauce Sautéed Cabbage

Prep time: 10 minutes | Cook time: 10 minutes | Serves 8

2 tablespoons extra-virgin olive oil
1 collard greens bunch, stemmed and thinly sliced
½ small green cabbage, thinly sliced
6 garlic cloves, minced
1 tablespoon low-sodium soy sauce

1. Heat the olive oil in a large skillet over medium-high heat.
2. Sauté the collard greens in the oil for about 2 minutes, or until the greens start to wilt.
3. Toss in the cabbage and mix well. Reduce the heat to medium-low, cover, and cook for 5 to 7 minutes, stirring occasionally, or until the greens are softened.
4. Fold in the garlic and soy sauce and stir to combine. Cook for about 30 seconds more until fragrant.
5. Remove from the heat to a plate and serve.

Per Serving
Calories: 73 | fat: 4.1g | protein: 3.2g | carbs: 5.9g | fiber: 2.9g | sugar: 0g | sodium: 128mg

Cheesy Spinach Portobello Mushrooms Mix

Prep time: 5 minutes | Cook time: 20 minutes | Serves 4

8 large Portobello mushrooms
3 teaspoons extra-virgin olive oil, divided
4 cups fresh spinach
1 medium red bell pepper, diced
¼ cup feta cheese, crumbled

1. Preheat the oven to 450ºF (235ºC).
2. On your cutting board, remove the mushroom stems. Scoop out the gills with a spoon and discard. Grease the mushrooms with 2 tablespoons olive oil.
3. Arrange the mushrooms, cap-side down, on a baking sheet. Roast in the preheated oven for 20 minutes until browned on top.
4. Meanwhile, in a skillet, heat the remaining olive oil over medium heat until shimmering.
5. Add the spinach and red bell pepper to the skillet and sauté for 8 minutes until the vegetables are tender, stirring occasionally. Remove from the heat to a bowl.
6. Remove the mushrooms from the oven to a plate. Using a spoon to stuff the mushrooms with the vegetables and sprinkle with the feta cheese. Serve warm.

Per Serving
Calories: 118 | fat: 6.3g | protein: 7.2g | carbs: 12.2g | fiber: 4.1g | sugar: 6.1g | sodium: 128mg

Simple Veggie Eggs Bake

Prep time: 5 minutes | Cook time: 25 minutes | Serves 4

2 tablespoons extra-virgin olive oil
1 red onion, chopped
1 sweet potato, cut into ½-inch pieces
1 green bell pepper, seeded and chopped
½ teaspoon sea salt
1 teaspoon chili powder
4 large eggs
½ cup shredded pepper Jack cheese
1 avocado, cut into cubes

1. Preheat the oven to 350°F (180°C).
2. Heat the olive oil in a large skillet over medium-high heat until shimmering.
3. Add the onion, sweet potato, bell pepper, salt, and chili powder. Cook for about 10 minutes, stirring constantly, or until the vegetables are lightly browned.
4. Remove from the heat. With the back of a spoon, make 4 wells in the vegetables, then crack an egg into each well. Scatter the shredded cheese over the vegetables.
5. Bake in the preheated oven for about 10 minutes until the cheese is melted and eggs are set.
6. Remove from the heat and sprinkle the avocado on top before serving.

Per Serving
Calories: 286 | fat: 21.3g | protein: 12.3g | carbs: 16.2g | fiber: 5.2g | sugar: 9.1 g | sodium: 266mg

Sundried Tomato with Brussels sprouts Roast

Prep time: 15 minutes | Cook time: 20 minutes | Serves 4

1 pound (454 g) Brussels sprouts, trimmed and halved
1 tablespoon extra-virgin olive oil
Sea salt and freshly ground black pepper,
to taste
½ cup sun-dried tomatoes, chopped
2 tablespoons freshly squeezed lemon juice
1 teaspoon lemon zest

1. Preheat the oven to 400°F (205°C). Line a large baking sheet with aluminum foil.
2. Toss the Brussels sprouts in the olive oil in a large bowl until well coated. Sprinkle with salt and pepper.
3. Spread out the seasoned Brussels sprouts on the prepared baking sheet in a single layer.
4. Roast in the preheated oven for 20 minutes, shaking the pan halfway through, or until the Brussels sprouts are crispy and browned on the outside.
5. Remove from the oven to a serving bowl.
6. Add the tomatoes, lemon juice, and lemon zest, and stir to incorporate. Serve immediately.

Per Serving
Calories: 111 | fat: 5.8g | protein: 5.0g | carbs: 13.7g | fiber: 4.9g | sugar: 2.7g | sodium: 103mg

Simple Acorn Squash with Parmesan

Prep time: 10 minutes | Cook time: 20 minutes | Serves 4

1 acorn squash (about 1 pound / 454 g)
1 tablespoon extra-virgin olive oil
1 teaspoon dried sage leaves, crumbled
¼ teaspoon freshly grated nutmeg
⅛ Teaspoon kosher salt
⅛ Teaspoon freshly ground black pepper
2 tablespoons freshly grated Parmesan cheese

1. Cut the acorn squash in half lengthwise and remove the seeds. Cut each half in half for a total of 4 wedges. Snap off the stem if it's easy to do.
2. In a small bowl, combine the olive oil, sage, nutmeg, salt, and pepper. Brush the cut sides of the squash with the olive oil mixture.
3. Pour 1 cup of water into the electric pressure cooker and insert a wire rack or trivet.
4. Place the squash on the trivet in a single layer, skin-side down.
5. Close and lock the lid of the pressure cooker. Set the valve to sealing. Cook on high pressure for 20 minutes.
6. When the cooking is complete, hit Cancel and quick release the pressure. Once the pin drops, unlock and remove the lid.
7. Carefully remove the squash from the pot, sprinkle with the Parmesan, and serve.

Per Serving
Calories: 86 | fat: 4.1g | protein: 2.1g | carbs: 11.9g | fiber: 2.1g | sugar: 0g | sodium: 283mg

Garlic Veggie Broth Onion Bowl

Prep time: 10 minutes | Cook time: 20 minutes | Serves 2

2 tablespoons extra-virgin olive oil
1 chopped onion
1 red bell pepper, seeded and chopped
2 minced garlic cloves
1 (14-ounce / 397-g) can crushed tomatoes
2 cups green beans (fresh or frozen;
halved if fresh)
3 cups low-sodium vegetable broth
1 tablespoon Italian seasoning
½ cup dried whole-wheat elbow macaroni
Pinch red pepper flakes (or to taste)
½ teaspoon sea salt

1. Heat the olive oil in a large saucepan over medium-high heat until shimmering.
2. Sauté the onion and bell pepper for about 3 minutes, stirring frequently, or until they start to soften.
3. Add the garlic and cook for 30 seconds until fragrant, stirring occasionally.
4. Stir in the tomatoes, green beans, vegetable broth, and Italian seasoning, and then bring the mixture to a boil.
5. Add the elbow macaroni, red pepper flakes, and salt. Continue to cook for 8 minutes, stirring occasionally, or until the macaroni is cooked through.
6. Remove from the heat to a large bowl and cool for 6 minutes before serving.

Per Serving
Calories: 202 | fat: 7.2g | protein: 5.2g | carbs: 29.2g | fiber: 7.2g | sugar: 29g | sodium: 479mg

Brown rice with Tofu Broccoli Stir fry

Prep time: 10 minutes | Cook time: 10 minutes | Serves 4

3 tablespoons extra-virgin olive oil
12 ounces (340 g) firm tofu, cut into ½-inch pieces
4 cups broccoli, broken into florets
4 scallions, sliced
1 teaspoon peeled and
grated fresh ginger
4 garlic cloves, minced
2 tablespoons soy sauce (use gluten-free soy sauce if necessary)
¼ cup vegetable broth
1 cup cooked brown rice

1. Heat the olive oil in a large skillet over medium-high heat until simmering.
2. Add the tofu, broccoli, and scallions and stir fry for 6 minutes, or until the vegetables start to become tender.
3. Add the ginger and garlic and cook for about 30 seconds, stirring constantly.
4. Fold in the soy sauce, vegetable broth, and brown rice. Stir to combine and cook for an additional 1 to 2 minutes until the rice is heated through.
5. Let it cool for 5 minutes before serving.

Per Serving
Calories: 238 | fat: 13.2g | protein: 11.1g | carbs: 21.2g | fiber: 4.2g | sugar: 8.8g | sodium: 360 mg

Sweet and Creamy Pumpkin Seeds

Prep time: 10 minutes | Cook time: 30 minutes | Serves 8

2 cup raw fresh pumpkin seeds wash and pat dry
1 tablespoon butter
1 tablespoon honey
1 tablespoon coconut oil
1 teaspoon cinnamon

1. Heat oven to 275ºF (135ºC). Line a baking sheet with parchment paper, making sure it hangs over both ends.
2. Place the pumpkin seeds in a medium bowl.
3. In a small microwave safe bowl, add butter, coconut oil, and honey. Microwave until the butter melts and the honey is runny.
4. Pour the honey mixture over the pumpkin seeds and stir. Add the cinnamon and stir again.
5. Dump the pumpkin seeds into the middle of the paper and place it in the oven.
6. Bake for 30 to 40 minutes until the seeds and honey are a deep golden brown, stirring every 10 minutes.
7. When the seeds are roasted, remove from the oven and stir again.
8. Stir a few times as they cool to keep them from sticking in one big lump.
9. Enjoy the seeds once they are cool enough to eat. Store uncovered for up to one week. Serving size is ¼ cup.

Per Serving
Calories: 270 | fat: 22.0g | protein: 8.2g | carbs: 13.1g | fiber: 1.0g | sugar: 7.0g | sodium: 87mg

My Favorite Egg Zucchini

Prep time: 10 minutes | Cook time: 10 minutes | Serves 4

3 zucchini, slice ¼- to ⅛-inch thick
2 eggs
½ cup sunflower oil

⅓ cup coconut flour
¼ cup reduced fat Parmesan cheese
1 tablespoon water

1. Heat oil in a large skillet over medium heat.
2. In a shallow bowl whisk the egg and water together.
3. In another shallow bowl, stir flour and Parmesan together.
4. Coat zucchini in the egg then flour mixture. Add, in a single layer, to the skillet.
5. Cook 2 minutes per side until golden brown. Transfer to paper towel lined plate. Repeat.
6. Serve immediately with your favorite dipping sauce.

Per Serving
Calories: 140 | fat: 11.0g | protein: 6.2g | carbs: 6.1g | fiber: 2.0g | sugar: 3.0g | sodium: 139mg

Grandma's Citrusy Broccoli Tofu

Prep time: 15 minutes | Cook time: 2 hours | Serves 4

1 package extra firm tofu, pressed for at least 15 minutes, cut into cubes
2 cups broccoli florets, fresh
1 tablespoon

margarine
¼ cup orange juice
¼ cup reduced sodium soy sauce
¼ cup honey
2 cloves garlic, diced fine

1. Melt butter in a medium skillet, over medium high heat. Add tofu and garlic and cook, stirring occasionally until tofu starts to brown, about 5 to 10 minutes. Transfer to crock pot.
2. Whisk the wet together in a small bowl. Pour over tofu and add the broccoli.
3. Cover and cook on high 90 minutes, or on low 2 hours.
4. Serve warm.

Per Serving
Calories: 138 | fat: 4.0g | protein: 4.1g | carbs: 24.1g | fiber: 2.0g | sugar: 20.0g | sodium: 592mg

Peppery Egg Butternut Fritters

Prep time: 15 minutes | Cook time: 15 minutes | Serves 6

5 cup butternut squash, grated
2 large eggs
1 tablespoon fresh sage, diced fine

⅔ cup flour
2 tablespoons olive oil
Salt and pepper, to taste

1. Heat oil in a large skillet over medium-high heat.
2. In a large bowl, combine squash, eggs, sage and salt and pepper to taste. Fold in flour.
3. Drop ¼ cup mixture into skillet, keeping fritters at least 1 inch apart. Cook till golden brown on both sides, about 2 minutes per side.
4. Transfer to paper towel lined plate. Repeat. Serve immediately with your favorite dipping sauce.

Per Serving
Calories: 165 | fat: 6.0g | protein: 4.1g | carbs: 24.1g | fiber: 3.0g | sugar: 3.0g | sodium: 55mg

One Pan Spiced Tofu with Spinach

Prep time: 15 minutes | Cook time: 1 hour 25 minutes | Serves 4

1 package extra firm tofu, pressed 15 minutes and cut into cubes
1 package fresh baby spinach
2 limes
1 tablespoon margarine

½ cup raw peanut butter
2 tablespoons lite soy sauce
3 cloves garlic, chopped fine
½ teaspoon ginger
¼ teaspoon red pepper flakes

1. Melt margarine in a large saucepan. Add tofu and garlic and cook, stirring occasionally, 5 to 10 minutes, or until tofu starts to brown.
2. Add remaining, except spinach and bring to simmer. Reduce heat, cover and cook, stirring occasionally 30 to 35 minutes.
3. Stir in the spinach and cook 15 minutes more. Serve.

Per Serving
Calories: 326 | fat: 24.0g | protein: 18.1g | carbs: 15.1g | fiber: 5.0g | sugar: 5.0g | sodium: 635mg

Oven Baked Squash with Black Pepper

Prep time: 10 minutes | Cook time: 20 minutes | Serves 4

1 (1- to 1½-pound/454-680 g) delicate squash, halved, seeded, and cut into ½-inch-thick strips
1 tablespoon extra-virgin olive oil
½ teaspoon dried thyme
¼ teaspoon salt
¼ teaspoons freshly ground black pepper

1. Preheat the oven to 400ºF (205ºC). Line a baking sheet with parchment paper and set aside.
2. Add the squash strips, olive oil, thyme, salt, and pepper in a large bowl, and toss until the squash strips are fully coated.
3. Place the squash strips on the prepared baking sheet in a single layer. Roast for about 20 minutes until lightly browned, flipping the strips halfway through.
4. Remove from the oven and serve on plates.

Per Serving
Calories: 78 | fat: 4.2g | protein: 1.1g | carbs: 11.8g | fiber: 2.1g | sugar: 2.9g | sodium: 122mg

Delicious Golden Onion Rings

Prep time: 5 minutes | Cook time: 15 minutes | Serves 4

1 large onion, slice ½-inch thick
1 egg
¼ cup sunflower oil
2 tablespoons coconut flour
2 tablespoons reduced fat Parmesan cheese
¼ teaspoon parsley flakes
⅛ teaspoon garlic powder
⅛ teaspoon cayenne pepper
Salt, to taste
Ketchup, for serving

1. Heat oil in a large skillet over medium-high heat.
2. In a shallow bowl, combine flour, Parmesan, and seasonings.
3. Beat the egg.
4. Separate onion slices into individual rings and place in large bowl, adds beaten egg and toss to coat well. Let rest 1 to 2 minutes.
5. In small batches, coat onion in flour mixture and add to skillet. Cook 1 to 2 minutes per side, or until golden brown. Transfer to paper towel lined cookie sheet.
6. Serve with ketchup.

Per Serving
Calories: 185 | fat: 16.0g | protein: 3.2g | carbs: 8.1g | fiber: 3.0g | sugar: 2.0g | sodium: 95mg

Homemade Veggie Fajitas with Guacamole

Prep time: 10 minutes | Cook time: 15 minutes | Serves 4

Guacamole:
2 small avocados, pitted and peeled
1 teaspoon freshly squeezed lime juice
¼ teaspoon salt
9 halved cherry tomatoes

Fajitas:
1 red bell pepper, cut into into ½-inch slices
1 green bell pepper, cut into into ½-inch slices
1 small white onion, cut into into ½-inch slices
1 cup canned low-sodium black beans, drained and rinsed
¼ teaspoon garlic powder
¼ teaspoon chili powder
½ teaspoon ground cumin
4 (6-inch) yellow corn tortillas
Avocado oil cooking spray

1. In a bowl, add the avocados and lime juice. Using a fork to mash until a uniform consistency is achieved. Season with salt and fold in the cherry tomatoes. Stir well and set aside.
2. Heat a large skillet over medium heat until hot. Cover the bottom with cooking spray.
3. Add the bell peppers, white onion, black beans, garlic powder, chili powder, and cumin to the skillet. Stir and cook for about 15 minutes until the beans are tender.
4. Remove from the heat to a plate. Arrange the corn tortillas on a clean work surface and evenly divide the fajita mixture among the tortillas. Serve topped with the guacamole.

Per Serving
Calories: 273 | fat: 15.2g | protein: 8.1g | carbs: 30.1g | fiber: 11.2g | sugar: 5.2g | sodium: 176mg

Peppery Bok Choy with Toasted Sliced Almonds

Prep time: 15 minutes | Cook time: 7 minutes | Serves 4

2 teaspoons sesame oil
2 pounds (907 g) bok choy, cleaned and quartered
2 teaspoons low-

sodium soy sauce
Pinch red pepper flakes
½ cup toasted sliced almonds

1. Heat the sesame oil in a large skillet over medium heat until hot.
2. Sauté the bok choy in the hot oil for about 5 minutes, stirring occasionally, or until tender but still crisp.
3. Add the soy sauce and red pepper flakes and stir to combine. Continue sautéing for 2 minutes.
4. Transfer to a plate and serve topped with sliced almonds.

Per Serving
Calories: 118 | fat: 7.8g | protein: 6.2g | carbs: 7.9g | fiber: 4.1g | sugar: 3.0g | sodium: 293mg

Low Sugar Bok Choy Bowl

Prep time: 15 minutes | Cook time: 7 minutes | Serves 4

2 teaspoons sesame oil
2 pounds (907 g) bok choy, cleaned and quartered
2 teaspoons low-

sodium soy sauce
Pinch red pepper flakes
½ cup toasted sliced almonds

1. Place a large skillet over medium heat and add the oil.
2. When the oil is hot, sauté the bok choy until tender-crisp, about 5 minutes.
3. Stir in the soy sauce and red pepper flakes and sauté 2 minutes more.
4. Remove the bok choy to a serving bowl and top with the sliced almonds.

Per Serving
Calories: 119 | fat: 8g | protein: 6g | carbs: 8g | fiber: 4g | sugar: 3g | sodium: 294mg

Broiled Peppery Spinach Bowl

Prep time: 5 minutes | Cook time: 4 minutes | Serves 4

8 cups spinach, thoroughly washed and spun dry
1 tablespoon extra-virgin olive oil

¼ teaspoon ground cumin
Sea salt to taste
Freshly ground black pepper to taste

1. Preheat the broiler. Put an oven rack in the upper third of the oven.
2. Set a wire rack on a large baking sheet.
3. In a large bowl, massage the spinach, oil, and cumin together until all the leaves are well coated.
4. Spread half the spinach out on the rack, with as little overlap as possible. Season the greens lightly with salt and pepper.
5. Broil the spinach until the edges are crispy, about 2 minutes.
6. Remove the baking sheet from the oven and transfer the spinach to a large serving bowl.
7. Repeat with the remaining spinach. Serve immediately.

Per Serving
Calories: 40 | fat: 4g | protein: 2g | carbs: 2g | fiber: 1g | sugar: 0g | sodium: 106mg

Sautéed Peppery Mushrooms

Prep time: 10 minutes | Cook time: 12 minutes | Serves 4

1 tablespoon butter
2 teaspoons extra-virgin olive oil
2 pounds button mushrooms, halved
2 teaspoons minced

fresh garlic
1 teaspoon chopped fresh thyme
Sea salt to taste
Freshly ground black pepper

1. Place a large skillet over medium-high heat and add the butter and olive oil.
2. Sauté the mushrooms, stirring occasionally, until they are lightly caramelized and tender, about 10 minutes.
3. Add the garlic and thyme and sauté for 2 more minutes.
4. Season the mushrooms with salt and pepper before serving.

Per Serving
Calories: 97 | fat: 6g | protein: 7g | carbs: 8g | fiber: 2g | sugar: 4g | sodium: 92mg

Cardamom spiced Kale and Chard

Prep time: 10 minutes | Cook time: 10 minutes | Serves 4

2 tablespoons extra-virgin olive oil
1 pound (454 g) kale, coarse stems removed and leaves chopped
1 pound (454 g) Swiss chard, coarse stems removed and leaves

chopped
1 tablespoon freshly squeezed lemon juice
½ teaspoon ground cardamom
Sea salt to taste
Freshly ground black pepper

1. Place a large skillet over medium-high heat and add the olive oil.
2. Add the kale, chard, lemon juice, and cardamom to the skillet. Use tongs to toss the greens continuously until they are wilted, about 10 minutes or less.
3. Season the greens with salt and pepper. Serve immediately.

Per Serving
Calories: 140 | fat: 7g | protein: 6g | carbs: 16g | fiber: 4g | sugar: 1g | sodium: 351mg

Classic Chicken Brussels sprouts

Prep time: 10 minutes | Cook time: 20 minutes | Serves 4

1 pound (454 g) Brussels sprouts
2 tablespoons avocado oil, divided
1 cup chicken bone broth
1 tablespoon minced garlic

½ teaspoon kosher salt
Freshly ground black pepper, to taste
½ medium lemons
½ tablespoon poppy seeds

1. Trim the Brussels sprouts by cutting off the stem ends and removing any loose outer leaves. Cut each in half lengthwise (through the stem).
2. Set the electric pressure cooker to the Sauté/More setting. When the pot is hot, pour in 1 tablespoon of the avocado oil.
3. Add half of the Brussels sprouts to the pot, cut-side down, and let them brown for 3 to 5 minutes without disturbing.
4. Transfer to a bowl and add the remaining tablespoon of avocado oil and the remaining Brussels sprouts to the pot. Hit Cancel and return all of the Brussels sprouts to the pot.
5. Add the broth, garlic, salt, and a few grinds of pepper. Stir to distribute the seasonings.

6. Close and lock the lid of the pressure cooker. Set the valve to sealing. Cook on high pressure for 2 minutes.
7. While the Brussels sprouts are cooking, zest the lemon, then cut it into quarters.
8. When the cooking is complete, hit Cancel and quick release the pressure. Once the pin drops, unlock and remove the lid.
9. Using a slotted spoon, transfer the Brussels sprouts to a serving bowl.
10. Toss with the lemon zest, a squeeze of lemon juice, and the poppy seeds. Serve immediately.

Per Serving
Calories: 126 | fat: 8.1g | protein: 4.1g | carbs: 12.9g | fiber: 4.9g | sugar: 3.0g | sodium: 500mg

Citrusy Butter Yams

Prep time: 7 minutes | Cook time: 45 minutes | Serves 8 (½ cup each)

2 medium jewel yams cut into 2-inch dices
2 tablespoons unsalted butter
Juice of 1 large orange
1½ teaspoons ground cinnamon

¼ teaspoon ground ginger
¾ teaspoon ground nutmeg
⅛ Teaspoon ground cloves

1. Preheat the oven to 350ºF (180ºC).
2. Arrange the yam dices on a rimmed baking sheet in a single layer. Set aside.
3. Add the butter, orange juice, cinnamon, ginger, nutmeg, and garlic cloves to a medium saucepan over medium-low heat. Cook for 3 to 5 minutes, stirring continuously, or until the sauce begins to thicken and bubble.
4. Spoon the sauce over the yams and toss to coat well.
5. Bake in the preheated oven for 40 minutes until tender.
6. Let the yams cool for 8 minutes in the baking sheet before removing and serving.

Per Serving
Calories: 129 | fat: 2.8g | protein: 2.1g | carbs: 24.7g | fiber: 5.0g | sugar: 2.9g | sodium: 28mg

Gingery Eggplant with Green Onions

Prep time: 10 minutes | Cook time: 40 minutes | Serves 4

1 large eggplant, sliced into fourths
3 green onions, diced, green tips only
1 teaspoon fresh ginger, peeled and diced fine
¼ cup plus 1 teaspoon cornstarch
1½ tablespoons soy

sauce
1½ tablespoons sesame oil
1 tablespoon vegetable oil
1 tablespoon fish sauce
2 teaspoons Splenda
¼ teaspoon salt

1. Place eggplant on paper towels and sprinkle both sides with salt. Let for 1 hour to remove excess moisture. Pat dry with more paper towels.
2. In a small bowl, whisk together soy sauce, sesame oil, fish sauce, Splenda, and 1 teaspoon cornstarch.
3. Coat both sides of the eggplant with the ¼ cup cornstarch, use more if needed.
4. Heat oil in a large skillet, over medium-high heat.
5. Add ½ the ginger and 1 green onion, then lay 2 slices of eggplant on top. Use ½ the sauce mixture to lightly coat both sides of the eggplant. Cook 8 to 10 minutes per side. Repeat.
6. Serve garnished with remaining green onions.

Per Serving
Calories: 156 | fat: 9.0g | protein: 2.1g | carbs: 18.1g | fiber: 5.0g | sugar: 6.0g | sodium: 719mg

Cheese Coated Egg Muffins

Prep time: 10 minutes | Cook time: 20 minutes | Serves 4

4 egg whites
½ teaspoon fresh parsley, diced fine
3 tablespoons reduced fat Parmesan cheese,

divided
2 teaspoons water
½ teaspoon salt
Truffle oil to taste
Nonstick cooking spray

1. Heat oven to 400ºF (205ºC). Spray two muffin pans with cooking spray.
2. In a small bowl, whisk together egg whites, water, and salt until combined.
3. Spoon just enough egg white mixture into each muffin cup to barely cover the bottom. Sprinkle a small pinch of Parmesan on each egg white.
4. Bake 10 to 15 minutes or until the edges are dark brown, be careful not to burn them.
5. Let cool in the pans 3 to 4 minutes then transfer to a small bowl and drizzle lightly with truffle oil.
6. Add parsley and ½ tablespoon Parmesan and toss to coat. Serve.

Per Serving
Calories: 47 | fat: 3.0g | protein: 4.1g | carbs: 0g | fiber: 0g | sugar: 0g | sodium: 671mg

Tender Veggie Spring Peas

Prep time: 10 minutes | Cook time: 12 minutes | Serves 6 (½ cup each)

1 tablespoon unsalted butter
½ Vidalia onion, thinly sliced
1 cup low-sodium

vegetable broth
3 cups fresh shelled peas
1 tablespoon minced fresh tarragon

1. Melt the butter in a skillet over medium heat.
2. Sauté the onion in the melted butter for about 3 minutes until translucent stirs occasionally.
3. Pour in the vegetable broth and whisk well. Add the peas and tarragon to the skillet and stir to combine.
4. Reduce the heat to low, cover, and cook for about 8 minutes more, or until the peas are tender.
5. Let the peas cool for 5 minutes and serve warm.

Per Serving
Calories: 82 | fat: 2.1g | protein: 4.2g | carbs: 12.0g | fiber: 3.8g | sugar: 4.9g | sodium: 48mg

Aromatic Thyme Spiced Button Mushrooms

Prep time: 10 minutes | Cook time: 12 minutes | Serves 4

1 tablespoon butter
2 teaspoons extra-virgin olive oil
2 pounds (907 g) button mushrooms, halved
2 teaspoons minced

fresh garlic
1 teaspoon chopped fresh thyme
Sea salt and freshly ground black pepper, to taste

1. Heat the butter and olive oil in a large skillet over medium-high heat.
2. Add the mushrooms and sauté for 10 minutes, stirring occasionally, or until the mushrooms are lightly browned and cooked though.
3. Stir in the garlic and thyme and cook for an additional 2 minutes.
4. Season with salt and pepper and serve on a plate.

Per Serving
Calories: 96 | fat: 6.1g | protein: 6.9g | carbs: 8.2g | fiber: 1.7g | sugar: 3.9g | sodium: 91mg

Cardamom Spiced Swiss chard

Prep time: 10 minutes | Cook time: 10 minutes | Serves 4

2 tablespoons extra-virgin olive oil
1 pound (454 g) Swiss chard, coarse stems removed and leaves chopped
1 pound (454 g) kale, coarse stems removed

and leaves chopped
½ teaspoon ground cardamom
1 tablespoon freshly squeezed lemon juice
Sea salt and freshly ground black pepper, to taste

1. Heat the olive oil in a large skillet over medium-high heat.
2. Add the Swiss chard, kale, cardamom, and lemon juice to the skillet, and stir to combine. Cook for about 10 minutes, stirring continuously, or until the greens are wilted.

3. Sprinkle with the salt and pepper and stir well.
4. Serve the greens on a plate while warm.

Per Serving
Calories: 139 | fat: 6.8g | protein: 5.9g | carbs: 15.8g | fiber: 3.9g | sugar: 1.0g | sodium: 350mg

Chicken Broth Cauliflower Soup

Prep time: 10 minutes | Cook time: 15 minutes | Serves 6

2½ pounds (1.1 kg) cauliflower florets
½ leek, white and pale green part, halved
4 tablespoons butter
2 teaspoons fresh parsley, diced
2 tablespoons low

sodium chicken broth
2 teaspoons extra virgin olive oil
4 cloves garlic, diced fine
¼ teaspoon salt
¼ teaspoon pepper

1. Place the cauliflower in a steamer basket over boiling water. Cover and steam 10 to 15 minutes or until fork tender.
2. Rinse the leek under water and pat dry. Chop into thin slices.
3. Heat oil in a large skillet over medium-low heat. Add the leek and cook 2 to 3 minutes, or until soft. Add the garlic and cook 1 minute more.
4. Add all to a food processor and pulse until almost smooth. Serve warm, or refrigerate for a later use.

Per Serving
Calories: 147 | fat: 9.0g | protein: 5.1g | carbs: 14.1g | fiber: 6.0g | sugar: 6.0g | sodium: 218mg

Chapter 7: Fish and Seafood

Caramelized Sprouts with Sun dried Tomato

Prep time: 15 minutes | Cook time: 20 minutes | Serves 4

1 pound (454 g) Brussels sprouts, trimmed and halved
1 tablespoon extra-virgin olive oil
Sea salt to taste
Freshly ground black
pepper
½ cup sun-dried tomatoes, chopped
2 tablespoons freshly squeezed lemon juice
1 teaspoon lemon zest

1. Preheat the oven to 400°F (204°C). Line a large baking sheet with aluminium foil.
2. In a large bowl, toss the Brussels sprouts with oil and season with salt and pepper.
3. Spread the Brussels sprouts on the baking sheet in a single layer.
4. Roast the sprouts until they are caramelized, about 20 minutes.
5. Transfer the sprouts to a serving bowl. Mix in the sun-dried tomatoes, lemon juice, and lemon zest.
6. Stir to combine, and serve.

Per Serving
Calories: 110 | fat: 6g | protein: 5g | carbs: 14g | fiber: 5g | sugar: 3g| sodium: 105mg

Navy Beans & Scallions Bowl

Prep time: 20 minutes | Cook time: 20 minutes | Serves 4

2½ cups cooked navy beans
1 tomato, diced
½ red bell pepper, seeded and chopped
¼ jalapeño pepper, chopped
1 scallion, white and
green parts, chopped
1 teaspoon minced garlic
1 teaspoon ground cumin
½ teaspoon ground coriander

1. Put the beans, tomato, bell pepper, jalapeño, scallion, garlic, cumin, and coriander in a medium bowl and stir until well mixed.
2. Serve.

Per Serving
Calories: 224 | fat: 4g | protein: 14g | carbs: 34g | fiber: 13g | sugar: 164g| sodium: 164mg

One Pan Chicken Broth and Chickpeas

Prep time: 10 minutes | Cook time: 20 minutes | Serves 6

1 tablespoon extra-virgin olive oil
1 small fennel bulb, trimmed and cut into ¼-inch-thick slices
1 sweet onion, thinly sliced
1 (15½-ounce/439 g) can sodium-free chickpeas, rinsed and
drained
1 cup low-sodium chicken broth
2 teaspoons chopped fresh thyme
¼ teaspoon sea salt
¼ teaspoons freshly ground black pepper
¼ tablespoon butter

1. Place a large saucepan over medium-high heat and add the oil.
2. Sauté the fennel and onion until tender and lightly browned, about 10 minutes.
3. Add the chickpeas, broth, thyme, salt, and pepper.
4. Cover and cook, stirring occasionally, for 10 minutes, until the liquid has reduced by about half.
5. Remove the pan from the heat and stir in the butter. Serve hot.

Per Serving
Calories: 215 | fat: 5g | protein: 12g | carbs: 32g | fiber: 15g | sugar: 2g | sodium: 253mg

Basil Tuna Steaks Bowl

Prep time: 5 minutes | Cook time: 10 minutes | Serves 6

6 (6-ounce / 170-g) tuna steaks
3 tablespoons fresh basil, diced
4½ teaspoon olive oil
¾ teaspoon salt
¼ teaspoon pepper
Nonstick cooking spray

1. Heat grill to medium heat. Spray rack with cooking spray.
2. Drizzle both sides of the tuna with oil. Sprinkle with basil, salt and pepper.
3. Place on grill and cook 5 minutes per side, tuna should be slightly pink in the center. Serve.

Per Serving
Calories: 344 | fat: 14.0g | protein: 51.2g | carbs: 0g | fiber: 0g | sugar: 0g | sodium: 367mg

Cheesy Shrimp with Pasta

Prep time: 10 minutes | Cook time: 30 minutes | Serves 4

½ pound (227 g) shrimp, peeled and deveined
4 ounces (113 g) sun-dried tomatoes
1 cup half-and-half
1 cup reduced fat Parmesan cheese
4 cloves garlic, diced fine
2 tablespoons olive oil
1 teaspoon dried basil
¼ teaspoon salt
¼ teaspoon paprika
¼ teaspoon crushed red pepper
1 cup corn pasta, cooked and drained

1. Heat oil in a large skillet over medium heat. Add garlic and tomatoes and cook 1 minute.
2. Add shrimp, sprinkle with salt and paprika, and cook about 2 minutes.
3. Add half-and-half, basil, and crushed red pepper and bring to boil. Reduce heat to simmer. Whisk the Parmesan cheese into the hot cream and stir to melt cheese, on low heat.
4. Remove from heat. Add pasta and stir to coat. Serve.

Per Serving
Calories: 354 | fat: 22.0g | protein: 37.2g | carbs: 23.1g | fiber: 3.0g | sugar: 3.0g | sodium: 724mg

Cayenne pepper Catfish Fillets

Prep time: 5 minutes | Cook time: 15 minutes | Serves 4

4 (8-ounce / 227-g) catfish fillets
2 tablespoons olive oil
2 teaspoons garlic salt
2 teaspoons thyme
2 teaspoons paprika
½ teaspoon cayenne
pepper
½ teaspoon red hot sauce
¼ teaspoon black pepper
Nonstick cooking spray

1. Heat oven to 450ºF (235ºC). Spray a baking dish with cooking spray.
2. In a small bowl whisk together everything but catfish. Brush both sides of fillets, using all the spice mix.
3. Bake 10 to 13 minutes or until fish flakes easily with a fork. Serve.

Per Serving
Calories: 367 | fat: 24.0g | protein: 35.2g | carbs: 0g | fiber: 0g | sugar: 0g | sodium: 70mg

Spicy Tomatoes Flounder Mix

Prep time: 10 minutes | Cook time: 15 minutes | Serves 4

4 flounder fillets
2½ cups tomatoes, diced
¾ cup onion, diced
¾ cup green bell pepper, diced
2 cloves garlic, diced fine
1 tablespoon Cajun seasoning
1 teaspoon olive oil

1. Heat oil in a large skillet over medium-high heat. Add onion and garlic and cook 2 minutes, or until soft.
2. Add tomatoes, peppers and spices, and cook 2 to 3 minutes until tomatoes soften.
3. Lay fish over top. Cover, reduce heat to medium and cook, 5 to 8 minutes, or until fish flakes easily with a fork.
4. Transfer fish to serving plates and top with sauce.

Per Serving
Calories: 195 | fat: 3.0g | protein: 32.2g | carbs: 8.1g | fiber: 2.0g | sugar: 5.0g | sodium: 1278mg

Lemony Shrimp with Cilantro

Prep time: 5 minutes | Cook time: 5 minutes | Serves 4

1½ pounds (680 g) shrimp, peel and devein
4 lime wedges
4 tablespoons cilantro, chopped
4 cloves garlic, diced
1 tablespoon chili powder
1 tablespoon paprika
1 tablespoon olive oil
2 teaspoons honey
1 teaspoon cumin
1 teaspoon oregano
1 teaspoon garlic powder
1 teaspoon salt
½ teaspoon pepper

1. In a small bowl combine seasonings and honey.
2. Heat oil in a skillet over medium-high heat. Add shrimp, in a single layer, and cook 1 to 2 minutes per side.
3. Add seasonings, and cook, stirring, 30 seconds. Serve garnished with cilantro and a lime wedge.

Per Serving
Calories: 253 | fat: 7.0g | protein: 39.2g | carbs: 7.1g | fiber: 1.0g | sugar: 2.0g | sodium: 846mg

Oysters with Low-sodium Ketchup and Lime

Prep time: 20 minutes | Cook time: 10 minutes | Serves 2

1 dozen fresh oysters, shucked and left on the half shell
3 slices thick cut bacon, cut into thin strips
Juice of ½ lemons
⅓ cup low-sodium ketchup
¼ cup Worcestershire sauce
1 teaspoon horseradish
Dash of hot sauce
Lime wedges, for garnish
Rock salt, to taste

1. Heat oven to broil. Line a shallow baking dish with rock salt. Place the oysters snugly into the salt.
2. In a large bowl, combine remaining and mix well.
3. Add a dash of Worcestershire to each oyster then top with bacon mixture.
4. Cook 10 minutes, or until bacon is crisp. Serve with lime wedges.

Per Serving
Calories: 235 | fat: 13.0g | protein: 13.2g | carbs: 10.1g | fiber: 0g | sugar: 9.0g | sodium: 1310mg

Ginger Cod Chard Bake

Prep time: 10 minutes | Cook time: 15 minutes | Serves 4

1 chard bunch, stemmed, leaves and stems cut into thin strips
1 red bell pepper, seeded and cut into strips
1 pound (454 g) cod fillets cut into 4 pieces
1 tablespoon grated fresh ginger
3 garlic cloves, minced
2 tablespoons white wine vinegar
2 tablespoons low-sodium tamari or gluten-free soy sauce
½ tablespoon honey

1. Preheat the oven to 425ºF (220ºC).
2. Cut four pieces of parchment paper, each about 16 inches wide. Lay the four pieces out on a large workspace.
3. On each piece of paper, arrange a small pile of chard leaves and stems, topped by several strips of bell pepper. Top with a piece of cod.

4. In a small bowl, mix the ginger, garlic, vinegar, tamari, and honey. Top each piece of fish with one-fourth of the mixture.
5. Fold the parchment paper over so the edges overlap. Fold the edges over several times to secure the fish in the packets. Carefully place the packets on a large baking sheet.
6. Bake for 12 minutes. Carefully open the packets, allowing steam to escape, and serve.

Per Serving
Calories: 120 | fat: 1.0g | protein: 19.1g | carbs: 8.9g | fiber: 1.1g | sugar: 6.1g | sodium: 716mg

Peppery Halibut Fillet with Beans

Prep time: 10 minutes | Cook time: 15 minutes | Serves 4

1 pound (454 g) green beans, trimmed
2 red bell peppers, seeded and cut into strips
1 onion, sliced
Zest and juice of 2 lemons
3 garlic cloves, minced
2 tablespoons extra-
virgin olive oil
1 teaspoon dried dill
1 teaspoon dried oregano
4 (4-ounce / 113-g) halibut fillets
½ teaspoon salt
¼ teaspoons freshly ground black pepper

1. Preheat the oven to 400ºF (205ºC). Line a baking sheet with parchment paper.
2. In a large bowl, toss the green beans, bell peppers, onion, lemon zest and juice, garlic, olive oil, dill, and oregano.
3. Use a slotted spoon to transfer the vegetables to the prepared baking sheet in a single layer, leaving the juice behind in the bowl.
4. Gently place the halibut fillets in the bowl, and coat in the juice.
5. Transfer the fillets to the baking sheet, nestled between the vegetables, and drizzle them with any juice left in the bowl.
6. Sprinkle the vegetables and halibut with the salt and pepper.
7. Bake for 15 to 20 minutes until the vegetables are just tender and the fish flakes apart easily.

Per Serving
Calories: 235 | fat: 9.1g | protein: 23.9g | carbs: 16.1g | fiber: 4.9g | sugar: 8.1g | sodium: 350mg

Lemony Chick Pea Egg Bake

Prep time: 15 minutes | Cook time: 20 minutes | Serves 4

4 medium egg whites
½ cup fat-free milk
1 cup chickpea crumbs
¼ teaspoons freshly ground black pepper
½ teaspoon ground cumin
3 cups frozen chopped scallops, thawed

1 small onion, finely chopped
1 small green bell pepper, finely chopped
2 celery stalks, finely chopped
2 garlic cloves, minced
Juice of 2 limes

1. Preheat the oven to 350ºF (180ºC).
2. In a large bowl, combine the egg whites, milk, and chickpea crumbs.
3. Add the black pepper and cumin and mix well.
4. Add the scallops, onion, bell pepper, celery, and garlic.
5. Form golf ball–size patties and place on a rimmed baking sheet 1 inch apart.
6. Transfer the baking sheet to the oven and cook for 5 to 7 minutes, or until golden brown.
7. Flip the patties, return to the oven, and bake for 5 to 7 minutes, or until golden brown.
8. Top with the lime juice, and serve.

Per Serving
Calories: 338 | fat: 0g | protein: 50.1g | carbs: 24.1g | fiber: 5.9g | sugar: 4.0g | sodium: 465mg

Fruity Cod with Salsa

Prep time: 10 minutes | Cook time: 10 minutes | Serves 4

1 pound (454 g) cod, cut into 4 fillets, pin bones removed
2 tablespoons extra-virgin olive oil
¾ teaspoon sea salt, divided
1 mango, pitted, peeled, and cut into

cubes
¼ cup chopped cilantro
½ red onion, finely chopped
1 jalapeño, seeded and finely chopped
1 garlic clove, minced
Juice of 1 lime

1. Preheat the oven broiler on high.
2. On a rimmed baking sheet, brush the cod with the olive oil and season with ½ teaspoon of the salt. Broil until the fish is opaque, 5 to 10 minutes.
3. Meanwhile, in a small bowl, combine the mango, cilantro, onion, jalapeño, garlic, lime juice, and remaining ¼ teaspoon of salt.
4. Serve the cod with the salsa spooned over the top.

Per Serving
Calories: 200 | fat: 8.0g | protein: 21.1g | carbs: 12.9g | fiber: 1.9g | sugar: 7.6g | sodium: 355mg

Butter Sautéed Scallops with Asparagus

Prep time: 10 minutes | Cook time: 15 minutes | Serves 4

3 teaspoons extra-virgin olive oil, divided
1 pound (454 g) asparagus, trimmed and cut into 2-inch segments
1 tablespoon butter

1 pound (454 g) sea scallops
¼ cup dry white wine
Juice of 1 lemon
2 garlic cloves, minced
¼ teaspoons freshly ground black pepper.

1. In a large skillet, heat 1½ teaspoons of oil over medium heat.
2. Add the asparagus and sauté for 5 to 6 minutes until just tender, stirring regularly. Remove from the skillet and cover with aluminum foil to keep warm.
3. Add the remaining 1½ teaspoons of oil and the butter to the skillet. When the butter is melted and sizzling, place the scallops in a single layer in the skillet.
4. Cook for about 3 minutes on one side until nicely browned. Use tongs to gently loosen and flip the scallops, and cook on the other side for another 3 minutes until browned and cooked through. Remove and cover with foil to keep warm.
5. In the same skillet, combine the wine, lemon juice, garlic, and pepper. Bring to a simmer for 1 to 2 minutes, stirring to mix in any browned pieces left in the pan.
6. Return the asparagus and the cooked scallops to the skillet to coat with the sauce. Serve warm.

Per Serving
Calories: 253 | fat: 7.1g | protein: 26.1g | carbs: 14.9g | fiber: 2.1g | sugar: 3.1g | sodium: 494mg

Low-sodium Chicken Broth Sole Fillets

Prep time: 10 minutes | Cook time: 20 minutes | Serves 4

1 teaspoon extra-virgin olive oil
4 (5-ounce / 142-g) sole fillets, patted dry
3 tablespoons butter
2 teaspoons minced garlic
2 tablespoons all-purpose flour
2 cups low-sodium chicken broth
Juice and zest of ½ lemons
2 tablespoons capers

1. Heat the olive oil in a large skillet over medium heat.
2. Add the sole fillets to the skillet and sear each side for about 4 minutes or until the fish is opaque and flakes easily.
3. Remove from the heat to a plate and set aside.
4. Melt the butter in the skillet and sauté the garlic for 3 minutes until fragrant.
5. Add the flour and cook for about 2 minutes, stirring frequently, or until the mixture is bubbly and foamy. It should look like a thick paste.
6. Stir in the chicken broth, lemon juice and zest and cook for 4 minutes, whisking constantly, or until the sauce is thickened.
7. Scatter with the capers and spoon the sauce over the fish. Serve immediately.

Per Serving
Calories: 273 | fat: 13.3g | protein: 30.3g | carbs: 7.1g | fiber: 0g | sugar: 2.2g | sodium: 414mg

Peppery Haddock with Yogurt Cucumber Sauce

Prep time: 10 minutes | Cook time: 10 minutes | Serves 4

Cucumber Sauce:
½ English cucumber, grated and liquid squeezed out
¼ cup Low-fat Greek yogurt
½ scallions, white and
green parts, finely chopped
2 teaspoons chopped fresh mint
1 teaspoon honey
A pinch of salt
Fish:
4 (5-ounce / 142-g) haddock fillets, patted dry
Sea salt and ffreshly
ground black pepper, to taste
Non-stick cooking spray

1. Whisk together all the ingredients for the cucumber sauce in a small bowl and set aside.
2. On a clean work surface, lightly season the haddock fillets with salt and pepper.
3. Heat a large skillet over medium-high heat and spritz with nonstick cooking spray.
4. Cook the haddock fillets for 10 minutes, flipping them halfway through, or until the fish is lightly browned and cooked through.
5. Divide the haddock fillets among four plates and top with the cucumber sauce. Serve warm.

Per Serving
Calories: 165 | fat: 2.2g | protein: 27.3g | carbs: 4.2g | fiber: 0g | sugar: 3.2g | sodium: 105mg

Spicy Flounder Fillets

Prep time: 5 minutes | Cook time: 12 minutes | Serves 4

2 cups low-fat buttermilk
½ teaspoon onion powder
½ teaspoon garlic powder
4 (4-ounce / 113-g) flounder fillets
½ cup chickpea flour
½ cup plain yellow cornmeal
¼ teaspoon cayenne pepper
Freshly ground black pepper, to taste

1. Whisk together the buttermilk, onion powder, and garlic powder in a large bowl.
2. Add the flounder fillets, coating well on both sides. Let the fish marinate for 20 minutes.
3. Thoroughly combine the chickpea flour, cornmeal, cayenne pepper, and pepper in a shallow bowl.
4. Dredge each fillet in the flour mixture until they are completely coated.
5. Preheat the air fryer to 380ºF (190ºC).
6. Arrange the fish in the air fryer basket and bake for 12 minutes, flipping the fish halfway through, or until the fish is cooked through.
7. Serve warm.

Per Serving
Calories: 231 | fat: 6.2g | protein: 28.2g | carbs: 16.2g | fiber: 2.2g | sugar: 7.1g | sodium: 240mg

Broiled Cod Fillets with Garlic Mango Salsa

Prep time: 10 minutes | Cook time: 5 to 10 minutes | Serves 4

Cod:

1 pound (454 g) cod, cut into 4 fillets, pin bones removed

2 tablespoons extra-

virgin olive oil

¾ teaspoon sea salt, divided

Mango Salsa:

1 mango, pitted, peeled, and cut into cubes

¼ cup chopped cilantro

1 jalapeño, deseeded

and finely chopped

½ red onion, finely chopped

Juice of 1 lime

1 garlic clove, minced

1. Preheat the broiler to high. Place the cod fillets on a rimmed baking sheet. Brush both sides of the fillets with the olive oil. Sprinkle with ½ teaspoon of the salt.
2. Broil in the preheated broiler for 5 to 10 minutes until the flesh flakes easily with a fork.
3. Meanwhile, make the mango salsa by stirring together the mango, cilantro, jalapeño, red onion, lime juice, garlic, and remaining salt in a small bowl.
4. Serve the cod warm topped with the mango salsa.

Per Serving

Calories: 198 | fat: 8.1g | protein: 21.2g | carbs: 13.2g | fiber: 2.2g | saturated fat: 1g | sodium: 355mg

Mango Shrimp Fruit Bowl

Prep time: 15 minutes | Cook time: 3 minutes | Serves 4

1 pound (454 g) medium shrimp, peeled and deveined

1 cup diced mango

2 ripe avocados, diced

¼ cup finely diced red onion

2 Roma tomatoes, diced

¼ cup chopped fresh cilantro

2 tablespoons low-carb tomato ketchup

Juice of 1 lime

Juice of 1 orange

1 tablespoon extra-virgin olive oil

1 jalapeño pepper, seeded and minced

Lime wedges, for serving

1. Fill a large pot about halfway with water and bring to a boil. Meanwhile, fill a large bowl ⅔ of the way with ice and about 1 cup of cold water.
2. Add the shrimp to the boiling water and cook for 3 minutes until they are opaque and firm. Drain and quickly transfer to the ice water bath for 3 minutes to stop the cooking and cool them. Drain and pat the shrimp dry with a clean paper towel.
3. In a large bowl, mix together the shrimp, mango, avocado, red onion, tomatoes, and cilantro.
4. In a small bowl, combine the ketchup, lime juice, orange juice, oil, and jalapeño. Mix well and gently fold the sauce into the shrimp mixture.
5. Divide among 4 glasses or small dishes, with a lime wedge on the rim of each.

Per Serving

Calories: 278 | fat: 16.1g | protein: 17.9g | carbs: 20.1g | fiber: 6.1g | sugar: 9.9g | sodium: 675mg

Butter Cod with Lemony Asparagus

Prep time: 5 minutes | Cook time: 10 minutes | Serves 4

4 (4-ounce / 113-g) cod fillets

¼ teaspoon garlic powder

¼ teaspoon salt

¼ teaspoons freshly ground black pepper

2 tablespoons unsalted

butter

24 asparagus spears, woody ends trimmed

½ cup brown rice, cooked

1 tablespoon freshly squeezed lemon juice

1. In a large bowl, sseason the cod fillets with the garlic powder, salt, and pepper. Set aside.
2. Melt the butter in a skillet over medium-low heat.
3. Place the cod fillets and asparagus in the skillet in a single layer. Cook covered for 8 minutes, or until the cod is cooked through.
4. Divide the cooked brown rice, cod fillets, and asparagus among four plates. Serve drizzled with the lemon juice.

Per Serving

Calories: 233 | fat: 8.2g | protein: 22.1g | carbs: 20.1g | fiber: 5.2g | sugar: 2.2g | sodium: 275mg

Lemony Salmon Fillets

Prep time: 10 minutes | Cook time: 30 minutes | Serves 4

1 teaspoon extra-virgin olive oil
½ sweet onion, finely chopped
1 teaspoon minced garlic
3 cups baby spinach
1 cup kale, tough stems removed, torn

into 3-inch pieces
Sea salt and freshly ground black pepper, to taste
4 (5-ounce / 142-g) salmon fillets
Lemon wedges, for serving

1. Preheat the oven to 350°F (180°C).
2. Place a large skillet over medium-high heat and add the oil.
3. Sauté the onion and garlic until softened and translucent, about 3 minutes.
4. Add the spinach and kale and sauté until the greens wilt, about 5 minutes.
5. Remove the skillet from the heat and season the greens with salt and pepper.
6. Place the salmon fillets so they are nestled in the greens and partially covered by them. Bake the salmon until it is opaque, about 20 minutes.
7. Serve immediately with a squeeze of fresh lemon.

Per Serving
Calories: 282 | fat: 15.9g | protein: 28.9g | carbs: 4.1g | fiber: 1.1g | sugar: 0.9g | sodium: 92mg

Delicious Tacos with Greek Yogurt Sauce

Prep time: 5 minutes | Cook time: 10 minutes | Serves 4

Yogurt Sauce:
½ cup plain low-fat Greek yogurt
½ teaspoon ground

cumin
½ teaspoon garlic powder

Tacos:
2 tablespoons extra-virgin olive oil
4 (6-ounce / 170-g) cod fillets
8 (10-inch) yellow corn tortillas

2 cups packaged shredded cabbage
¼ cup chopped fresh cilantro
4 lime wedges

1. Whisk together all the ingredients for the yogurt sauce in a small bowl. Set aside.

2. Make the tacos: Heat the olive oil in a medium skillet over medium-low heat.
3. Add the fish and cook each side for 4 minutes until flaky.
4. Arrange the tortillas on a clean work surface. Top each tortilla evenly with the shredded cabbage, cooked fish, and cilantro, yogurt sauce, finished by a squeeze of lime. Serve immediately.

Per Serving
Calories: 375 | fat: 13.2g | protein: 36.2g | carbs: 30.2g | fiber: 4.2g | sugar: 4.1g | sodium: 340mg

Cod Fillet Quinoa Asparagus Bowl

Prep time: 5 minutes | Cook time: 15 minutes | Serves 4

½ cup uncooked quinoa
4 (4-ounce / 113-g) cod fillets
½ teaspoon garlic powder, divided
¼ teaspoon salt
¼ teaspoons freshly

ground black pepper
24 asparagus spears cut the bottom 1½ inches off
1 tablespoon avocado oil
1 cup half-and-half

1. Put the quinoa in a pot of salted water. Bring to a boil. Reduce the heat to low and simmer for 15 minutes or until the quinoa is soft and has a white "tail". Cover and turn off the heat. Let sit for 5 minutes.
2. On a clean work surface, rub the cod fillets with ¼ teaspoon of garlic powder, salt, and pepper.
3. Heat the avocado oil in a non-stick skillet over medium-low heat.
4. Add the cod fillets and asparagus in the skillet and cook for 8 minutes or until they are tender. Flip the cod and shake the skillet halfway through the cooking time.
5. Pour the half-and-half in the skillet, and sprinkle with remaining garlic powder. Turn up the heat to high and simmer for 2 minutes until creamy.
6. Divide the quinoa, cod fillets, and asparagus in four bowls and serve warm.

Per Serving
Calories: 258 | fat: 7.9g | protein: 25.2g | carbs: 22.7g | fiber: 5.2g | sugar: 3.8g | sodium: 410mg

Breadcrumbs Tuna Flat Cake

Prep time: 5 minutes | Cook time: 8 to 10 minutes | Serves 4

1 pound (454 g) canned tuna, drained
1 cup whole-wheat bread crumbs
2 large eggs, lightly beaten
Juice and zest of 1 lemon
½ onion, grated
1 tablespoon chopped fresh dill
3 tablespoons extra-virgin olive oil
½ cup tartar sauce, for topping

1. Mix together the tuna with the bread crumbs, beaten eggs, lemon juice and zest, onion, and dill in a large bowl, and stir until well incorporated.
2. Scoop out the tuna mixture and shape into 4 equal-sized patties with your hands.
3. Transfer the patties to a plate and chill in the refrigerator for 10 minutes.
4. Once chilled, heat the olive oil in a large nonstick skillet over medium-high heat.
5. Add the patties to the skillet and cook each side for 4 to 5 minutes, or until nicely browned on both sides.
6. Remove the patties from the heat and top with the tartar sauce.

Per Serving
Calories: 529 | fat: 33.6g | protein: 34.9g | carbs: 18.3g | fiber: 2.1g | sugar: 3.8g | sodium: 673mg

Grilled Shrimp Yogurt and Chili Sauce

Prep time: 10 minutes | Cook time: 12 minutes | Serves 4

1 pound (454 g) shrimp, shelled and deveined
½ cup Low-fat Greek yogurt
½ tablespoon chili
paste
½ tablespoon lime juice
Chopped green onions, for garnish

Special Equipment:
Wooden skewers, soaked in water for at least 30 minutes

1. Thread the shrimp onto skewers, piercing once near the tail and once near the head. You can place about 5 shrimps on each skewer.

2. Preheat the grill to medium.
3. Place the shrimp skewers on the grill and cook for about 6 minutes, flipping the shrimp halfway through, or until the shrimp are totally pink and opaque.
4. Meanwhile, make the yogurt and chili sauce: In a small bowl, stir together the yogurt, chili paste, and lime juice.
5. Transfer the shrimp skewers to a large plate. Scatter the green onions on top for garnish and serve with the yogurt and chili sauce on the side.

Per Serving
Calories: 122 | fat: 0.8g | protein: 26.1g | carbs: 2.9g | fiber: 0.5g | sugar: 1.3g | sodium: 175mg

Peppery White Fish Fillets with Parsley Mixture

Prep time: 10minutes | Cook time: 10 minutes | Serves 4

4 (6-ounce / 170-g) lean white fish fillets, rinsed and patted dry
Cooking spray
Paprika, to taste
Salt and pepper, to taste
2 tablespoons parsley,
finely chopped
½ teaspoon lemon zest
¼ cup extra virgin olive oil
¼ teaspoon dried dill
1 medium lemon, halved

1. Preheat the oven to 400ºF (205ºC). Line a baking sheet with aluminum foil and spray with cooking spray.
2. Place the fillets on the foil and scatter with the paprika. Season as desired with salt and pepper.
3. Bake in the preheated oven for 10 minutes or until the flesh flakes easily with a fork.
4. Meanwhile, stir together the parsley, lemon zest, olive oil, and dill in a small bowl.
5. Remove the fish from the oven to four plates. Squeeze the lemon juice over the fish and serve topped with the parsley mixture.

Per Serving
Calories: 283 | fat: 17.2g | protein: 33.3g | carbs: 1.0g | fiber: 0g | sugar: 0g | sodium: 74mg

Onion Garlic Scallop Balls

Prep time: 15 minutes | Cook time: 10 to 14 minutes | Serves 4

4 medium egg whites
1 cup chickpea crumbs
½ cup fat-free milk
½ teaspoon ground cumin
¼ teaspoons freshly ground black pepper
3 cups frozen chopped scallops, thawed
1 small onion, finely chopped
2 garlic cloves, minced
2 celery stalks, finely chopped
1 small green bell pepper, finely chopped
Juice of 2 limes

1. Preheat the oven to 350ºF (180ºC). Whisk together the egg whites, chickpea crumbs, milk, cumin, and black pepper in a large bowl until well combined.
2. Stir in the scallops, onion, garlic, celery, and bell pepper. Shape the mixture into golf ball-sized balls and flatten them into patties with your hands.
3. Arrange the patties on a rimmed baking sheet, spacing them 1 inch apart.
4. Bake in the preheated oven for 10 to 14 minutes until golden brown. Flip the patties halfway through the cooking time.
5. Serve drizzled with the lime juice.

Per Serving
Calories: 338 | fat: 0g | protein: 50.2g | carbs: 24.2g | fiber: 6.2g | sugar: 4.2g | sodium: 465mg

Lemony Asparagus spears with Cod Fillets

Prep time: 5 minutes | Cook time: 9 to 12 minutes | Serves 4

1 pound (454 g) asparagus spears, ends trimmed
Cooking spray
4 (4-ounce / 113-g) cod fillets, rinsed and patted dry
¼ teaspoon black
pepper (optional)
¼ cup light butter with canola oil
Juice and zest of 1 medium lemon
¼ teaspoon salt (optional)

1. Heat a grill pan over medium-high heat.
2. Spray the asparagus spears with cooking spray. Cook the asparagus for 6 to 8 minutes until fork-tender, flipping occasionally.
3. Transfer to a large platter and keep warm.
4. Spray both sides of fillets with cooking spray. Season with ¼ teaspoon black pepper, if needed.
5. Add the fillets to the pan and sear each side for 3 minutes until opaque.
6. Meantime, in a small bowl, whisk together the light butter, lemon zest, and ¼ teaspoon salts (if desired).
7. Spoon and spread the mixture all over the asparagus. Place the fish on top and squeeze the lemon juice over the fish. Serve immediately.

Per Serving
Calories: 158 | fat: 6.4g | protein: 23.0g | carbs: 6.1g | fiber: 3.0g | sugar: 2.8g | sodium: 212mg

Peppery Trout and Italian Salsa and Lemon

Prep time: 5 minutes | Cook time: 10 minutes | Serves 6

6 (6-ounce / 170-g) trout filets
6 lemon slices
Italian Salsa:
4 plum tomatoes, diced
½ red onion, diced fine
2 tablespoons fresh parsley, diced
12 Kalamata olives, pitted and chopped
2 cloves garlic, diced
4 tablespoons olive oil
¾ teaspoon salt
½ teaspoon pepper

fine
1 tablespoon balsamic vinegar
1 tablespoon olive oil
2 teaspoons capers, drained
¼ teaspoon salt
¼ teaspoon pepper

1. Sprinkle filets with salt and pepper.
2. Heat oil in a large nonstick skillet over medium-high heat. Cook trout, 3 filets at a time, 2 to 3 minutes per side, or fish flakes easily with a fork. Repeat with remaining filets.
3. Meanwhile, combine the ingredients for the salsa in a small bowl.
4. Serve the trout topped with salsa and a slice of lemon.

Per Serving
Calories: 321 | fat: 21.0g | protein: 30.2g | carbs: 2.1g | fiber: 0g | sugar: 1.0g | sodium: 634mg

Sea Scallops with Thyme & Orange Sauce

Prep time: 10 minutes | Cook time: 10 minutes | Serves 4

2 pounds (907 g) sea scallops, patted dry
Sea salt and freshly ground black pepper, to taste
2 tablespoons extra-virgin olive oil
1 tablespoon minced

garlic
¼ cup freshly squeezed orange juice
1 teaspoon orange zest
2 teaspoons chopped fresh thyme, for garnish

1. In a bowl, season the scallops with salt and pepper. Set aside.
2. Heat the olive oil in a large skillet over medium-high heat until shimmering.
3. Add the garlic and sauté for about 3 minutes, stirring occasionally, or until the garlic is softened.
4. Add the scallops and cook each side for about 4 minutes or until the scallops is lightly browned and firm.
5. Remove the scallops from the heat to a plate and cover with foil to keep warm. Set aside.
6. Pour the orange juice and zest into the skillet and stir, scraping up any cooked bits.
7. Drizzle the scallops with the orange sauce and sprinkle the thyme on top for garnish before serving.

Per Serving
Calories: 268 | fat: 8.2g | protein: 38.2g | carbs: 8.3g | fiber: 0g | sugar: 1.1g | sodium: 360mg

Pineapple flavoured Salmon

Prep time: 5 minutes | Cook time: 3 to 5 minutes | Serves 4

⅓ cup low-sodium soy sauce
⅓ cup pineapple juice
¼ cup water
2 tablespoons rice vinegar
1 garlic clove, minced
1 tablespoon honey

1 teaspoon peeled and grated fresh ginger
Pinch red pepper flakes
1 pound (454 g) salmon fillet, cut into 4 pieces

1. Preheat the oven broiler on high. Stir together the soy sauce, pineapple juice, water, vinegar, garlic, honey, ginger, and red pepper flakes in a small bowl.
2. Marinate the fillets (flesh-side down) in the sauce for about 5 minutes.
3. Transfer the fillets (flesh-side up) to a rimmed baking sheet and brush them generously with any leftover sauce.
4. Broil the fish until it flakes apart easily and reaches an internal temperature of 145ºF (63ºC), about 3 to 5 minutes.
5. Let the fish cool for 5 minutes before serving.

Per Serving
Calories: 201 | fat: 6.8g | protein: 23.7g | carbs: 8.9g | fiber: 1.0g | sugar: 10.2g | sodium: 750mg

Shrimp & Cod with Italian Seasoning

Prep time: 10 minutes | Cook time: 15 minutes | Serves 4

2 tablespoons extra-virgin olive oil
1 onion, chopped finely
1 garlic clove, minced
½ cup dry white wine
1 (14-ounce / 397-g) can tomato sauce
8 ounces (227 g) shrimp, peeled and deveined

8 ounces (227 g) cod, pin bones removed and cut into 1-inch pieces
1 tablespoon Italian seasoning
½ teaspoon sea salt
Pinch red pepper flakes

1. Heat the olive oil in a large skillet over medium-high heat until it shimmers.
2. Toss in the onion and cook for 3 minutes, stirring occasionally, or until the onion is translucent. Stir in the garlic and cook for 30 seconds until fragrant.
3. Add the wine and cook for 1 minute, stirring continuously.
4. Stir in the tomato sauce and bring the mixture to a simmer.
5. Add the shrimp and cod, Italian seasoning, salt, and red pepper flakes, and whisk to combine. Continue simmering for about 5 minutes or until the fish is cooked through.
6. Remove from the heat and serve on plates.

Per Serving
Calories: 242 | fat: 7.8g | protein: 23.2g | carbs: 10.7g | fiber: 2.1g | sugar: 7.7g | sodium: 270mg

Classic Ginger Chili Marinated Salmon

Prep time: 10 minutes | Cook time: 8 to 12 minutes | Serves 4

1 tablespoon olive oil
1 tablespoon grated fresh ginger
1 small hot chili pepper
1 tablespoon lemongrass, minced
2 tablespoons low-sodium soy sauce
1 tablespoon Splenda
4 (4-ounce / 113-g) skinless salmon fillets

1. Except for the salmon, stir together all the ingredients in a medium bowl.
2. Brush the salmon fillets generously with the marinade and place in the fridge to marinate for 30 minutes.
3. Preheat the grill to medium heat.
4. Discard the marinade and transfer the salmon to the preheated grill.
5. Grill each side for 4 to 6 minutes, or until the fish is almost completely cooked through at the thickest part. Serve hot.

Per Serving
Calories: 223 | fat: 12.2g | protein: 25.7g | carbs: 2.0g | fiber: 0g | sugar: 2.9g | sodium: 203mg

Buttery Oysters with Scallions

Prep time: 30 minutes | Cook time: 15 minutes | Serves 2

2 cups coarse salt, for holding the oysters
1 dozen fresh oysters, scrubbed
1 tablespoon butter
½ cup artichoke hearts, finely chopped
¼ cup red bell pepper, finely chopped
¼ cup finely chopped
scallions, both white and green parts
1 tablespoon fresh parsley, finely chopped
Zest and juice of ½ lemons
1 garlic clove, minced
Salt and freshly ground black pepper, to taste

1. Spread the coarse salt in the bottom of a baking dish.
2. Shuck the oyster with a shucking knife, then discard the empty half and loose the oyster with the knife.
3. Arrange the oyster on the shells with juices, then place them on the coarse salt in the baking dish. Set aside.
4. Preheat the oven to 425ºF (220ºC).

5. Put the butter in a nonstick skillet, and melt over medium heat.
6. Add the artichokes hearts, bell pepper, and scallions to the skillet and sauté for 6 minutes or until soft.
7. Add the garlic to the skillet and sauté for 1 minute more until fragrant.
8. Remove them from the skillet in a large bowl, then spread the parsley and lemon zest on top, and drizzle with lemon juice, and then sprinkle with salt and black pepper.
9. Spoon the vegetable mixture in each oyster. Bake in the preheated oven for 12 minutes or until the vegetables are lightly wilted.
10. Remove them from the oven and serve warm.

Per Serving
Calories: 136 | fat: 6.9g | protein: 6.1g | carbs: 10.8g | fiber: 2.1g | sugar: 6.7g | sodium: 276mg

Peppery Trout Fillets

Prep time: 5 minutes | Cook time: 7 to 8 minutes | Serves 2

4 to 6 fresh rosemary sprigs
8 ounces (227 g) trout fillets, about ¼ inch thick; rinsed and patted dry
½ teaspoon olive oil
⅛ teaspoon salt
⅛ teaspoon pepper
1 teaspoon fresh lemon juice

1. Preheat the oven to 350ºF (180ºC).
2. Put the rosemary sprigs in a small baking pan in a single row. Spread the fillets on the top of the rosemary sprigs.
3. Brush both sides of each piece of fish with the olive oil. Sprinkle with the salt, pepper, and lemon juice.
4. Bake in the preheated oven for 7 to 8 minutes, or until the fish is opaque and flakes easily.
5. Divide the fillets between two plates and serve hot.

Per Serving
Calories: 180 | fat: 9.1g | protein: 23.8g | carbs: 0g | fiber: 0g | sugar: 0g | sodium: 210mg

Garlicky Cod Fillet Quinoa Bowl

Prep time: 5 minutes | Cook time: 15 minutes | Serves 4

½ cup uncooked quinoa	ground black pepper
4 (4-ounce / 113-g) cod fillets	24 asparagus spears cut the bottom 1½ inches off
½ teaspoon garlic powder, divided	1 tablespoon avocado oil
¼ teaspoon salt	1 cup half-and-half
¼ teaspoons freshly	

1. Put the quinoa in a pot of salted water. Bring to a boil. Reduce the heat to low and simmer for 15 minutes or until the quinoa is soft and has a white "tail". Cover and turn off the heat. Let sit for 5 minutes.
2. On a clean work surface, rub the cod fillets with ¼ teaspoon of garlic powder, salt, and pepper.
3. Heat the avocado oil in a non-stick skillet over medium-low heat.
4. Add the cod fillets and asparagus in the skillet and cook for 8 minutes or until they are tender.
5. Flip the cod and shake the skillet halfway through the cooking time.
6. Pour the half-and-half in the skillet, and sprinkle with remaining garlic powder. Turn up the heat to high and simmer for 2 minutes until creamy.
7. Divide the quinoa, cod fillets, and asparagus in four bowls and serve warm.

Per Serving
Calories: 258 | fat: 7.9g | protein: 25.2g | carbs: 22.7g | fiber: 5.2g | sugar: 3.8g | sodium: 410mg

Honey Soy Shrimp Veggie Stir-Fry

Prep time: 5 minutes | Cook time: 15 minutes | Serves 4

Sauce:

½ cup water	¼ teaspoon garlic powder
2½ tablespoons low-sodium soy sauce	Pinch ground ginger
½ tablespoon honey	1 tablespoon corn-starch
1 tablespoon rice vinegar	

Stir-Fry:

8 cups frozen vegetable stir-fry mix	40 medium fresh shrimp, peeled and deveined
2 tablespoons sesame oil	

1. Mix together the water, soy sauce, honey, vinegar, garlic powder, and ginger in a small saucepan and stir to combine. Fold in the corn starch and whisk constantly until everything is incorporated.
2. Let the sauce boil over medium heat for 1 minute. Remove from the heat and set aside in a bowl.
3. Heat a large saucepan over medium-high heat until hot. Add the vegetable stir-fry mix and cook for 8 to 10 minutes, stirring occasionally, or until the water has evaporated.
4. Reduce the heat, pour in the sesame oil and add the shrimp. Stir well and cook for 3 minutes, stirring occasionally, or until the shrimp are pink and cooked through.
5. Stir in the prepared sauce and cook for another 2 minutes.
6. Remove from the heat and let cool for 5 minutes before serving.

Per Serving
Calories: 299 | fat: 17.3g | protein: 24.3g | carbs: 14.2g | fiber: 2.2g | sugar: 9.1g | sodium: 453mg

Baked Salmon with Tomato

Prep time: 10 minutes | Cook time: 20 minutes | Serves 6

2½ pound (1.1 kg) salmon filet	½ cup margarine
2 tomatoes, sliced	½ cup basil pesto

1. Heat the oven to 400ºF (205ºC). Line a baking sheet with foil, making sure it covers the sides.
2. Place another large piece of foil onto the baking sheet and place the salmon filet on top of it.
3. Place the pesto and margarine in blender or food processor and pulse until smooth. Spread evenly over salmon. Place tomato slices on top.
4. Wrap the foil around the salmon, tenting around the top to prevent foil from touching the salmon as much as possible.
5. Bake 15 to 25 minutes, or salmon flakes easily with a fork. Serve.

Per Serving
Calories: 445 | fat: 24.0g | protein: 55.2g | carbs: 2.1g | fiber: 0g | sugar: 1.0g | sodium: 288mg

Citrus Shrimp with Tomatoes and Feta

Prep time: 10 minutes | Cook time: 30 minutes | Serves 4

3 tomatoes, coarsely chopped
½ cup chopped sun-dried tomatoes
2 teaspoons minced garlic
2 teaspoons extra-virgin olive oil
1 teaspoon chopped fresh oregano

Freshly ground black pepper
1½ pounds (16–20 count) shrimp, peeled, deveined, tails removed
4 teaspoons freshly squeezed lemon juice
½ cup low-sodium feta cheese, crumbled

1. Heat the oven to 450°F (232°C). In a medium bowl, toss the tomatoes, sun-dried tomatoes, garlic, oil, and oregano until well combined.
2. Season the mixture lightly with pepper.
3. Transfer the tomato mixture to a 9-by-13-inch glass baking dish.
4. Bake until softened, about 15 minutes.
5. Stir the shrimp and lemon juice into the hot tomato mixture and top evenly with the feta.
6. Bake until the shrimp are cooked through, about 15 minutes more.

Per Serving
Calories: 306 | fat: 11g | protein: 39g | carbs: 12g | fiber: 3g | sugar: 5g| sodium: 502mg

Simple Garlic Pepper Shrimp

Prep time: 15 minutes | Cook time: 8 minutes | Serves 4

1 teaspoon extra virgin olive oil
½ teaspoon garlic clove, minced
1 pound (454 g) large shrimp, peeled and deveined
¼ cup chopped fresh

cilantro, or more to taste
1 lime, zested and juiced
¼ teaspoon salt
⅛ teaspoon black pepper

1. In a large heavy skillet, heat the olive oil over medium-high heat.
2. Add the minced garlic and cook for 30 seconds until fragrant.
3. Toss in the shrimp and cook for about 5 to 6 minutes, stirring occasionally, or until they turn pink and opaque.
4. Remove from the heat to a bowl. Add the cilantro, lime zest and juice, salt, and pepper to the shrimp, and toss to combine. Serve immediately.

Per Serving
Calories: 133 | fat: 3.5g | protein: 24.3g | carbs: 1.0g | fiber: 0g | sugar: 0g | sodium: 258mg

Tuna Onion Broccoli Casserole

Prep time: 10 minutes | Cook time: 40 minutes | Serves 4

1 tablespoon avocado oil
1 medium yellow onion, diced
2 tablespoons whole-wheat flour
2 cups low-sodium chicken broth
1 cup unsweetened almond milk
1 (10-ounce / 284-

g) package zucchini noodles
1 cup fresh or frozen broccoli, cut into florets
2 (5-ounce / 142-g) cans chunk-light tuna, drained
1 cup Cheddar cheese, shredded

1. Preheat the oven to 375°F (190ºC). Heat the avocado oil in a nonstick skillet over medium heat until shimmering.
2. Add the onion to the skillet and cook for 3 minutes or until translucent.
3. Add the flour to the skillet and cook for 2 minutes. Stir constantly.
4. Gently fold in the chicken broth and almond milk, then turn up the heat to high and bring the mixture to a boil.
5. Add the zucchini noodles and broccoli to the skillet. Reduce the heat to medium and cook for 6 minutes until the mixture is lightly thickened. Add the tuna to the skillet.
6. Pour the mixture in a casserole dish, and spread the cheese on top. Cover the casserole dish with aluminum foil.
7. Bake in the preheated oven for 20 minutes or until the tuna is opaque. Remove the aluminum foil and broil for an additional 2 minutes.
8. Remove the casserole from the oven. Allow to cool for a few minutes and serve warm.

Per Serving
Calories: 273 | fat: 11.8g | protein: 29.1g | carbs: 11.1g | fiber: 3.2g | sugar: 2.8g | sodium: 349mg

Garlicky Veggie broth Pumpkin Shrimp

Prep time: 5 minutes | Cook time: 15 minutes | Serves 3

½ pound (227 g) raw shrimp, peel and deveined	vegetable broth
	¼ cup pumpkin purée
2 cups cauliflower, grated	¼ cup reduced fat Parmesan cheese
¼ cup half-and-half	2 cloves garlic, diced fine
2 tablespoons margarine	¼ teaspoon sage
½ cup low sodium	¼ teaspoon salt
	¼ teaspoon pepper

1. Melt margarine in a large skillet over medium-high heat. Add garlic and cook 1 to 2 minutes.
2. Add the broth, pumpkin, and half-and-half and whisk until smooth.
3. Add cauliflower and Parmesan and cook 5 minutes, or until cauliflower is tender.
4. Stir in shrimp and cook until they turn pink. Season with salt and pepper and serve.

Per Serving
Calories: 237 | fat: 13.0g | protein: 21.2g | carbs: 9.1g | fiber: 2.0g | sugar: 3.0g | sodium: 618mg

One Pan Citrus Roughly Filets

Prep time: 5 minutes | Cook time: 15 minutes | Serves 4

4 orange roughy filets	1 tablespoon Splenda
¼ cup fresh lemon juice	½ teaspoon ginger
¼ cup reduced sodium soy sauce	½ teaspoon lemon pepper
	Nonstick cooking spray

1. In a large Ziploc bag combine lemon juice, soy sauce, Splenda, and ginger. Add fish, seal, and turn to coat. Refrigerate 30 minutes.
2. Heat oven to 350ºF (180ºC). Spray a large baking sheet with cooking spray.
3. Place filets on prepared pan and sprinkle with lemon pepper.
4. Bake 12 to 15 minutes, or until fish flakes easily with fork.

Per Serving
Calories: 238 | fat: 12.0g | protein: 25.2g | carbs: 4.1g | fiber: 1.0g | sugar: 4.0g | sodium: 656mg

Delicious Citrus Wax Beans

Prep time: 5 minutes | Cook time: 15 minutes| Serves 4

2 pounds wax beans	Freshly ground black pepper
2 tablespoons extra-virgin olive oil	Juice of ½ lemon
Sea salt to taste	

1. Preheat the oven to 400°F (204°C).
2. Line a baking sheet with aluminium foil.
3. In a large bowl, toss the beans and olive oil. Season lightly with salt and pepper.
4. Transfer the beans to the baking sheet and spread them out.
5. Roast the beans until caramelized and tender, about 10 to 12 minutes.
6. Transfer the beans to a serving platter and sprinkle with the lemon juice.

Per Serving
Calories: 100 | fat: 7g | protein: 2g | carbs: 8g | fiber: 4g | sugar: 4g| sodium: 813mg

Quick and Healthy Spinach Bowl

Prep time: 5 minutes | Cook time: 4 minutes | Serves 4

8 cups spinach, thoroughly washed and spun dry	¼ teaspoon ground cumin
1 tablespoon extra-virgin olive oil	Sea salt to taste
	Freshly ground black pepper

1. Preheat the broiler. Put an oven rack in the upper third of the oven.
2. Set a wire rack on a large baking sheet.
3. In a large bowl, massage the spinach, oil, and cumin together until all the leaves are well coated.
4. Spread half the spinach out on the rack, with as little overlap as possible. Season the greens lightly with salt and pepper.
5. Broil the spinach until the edges are crispy, about 2 minutes.
6. Remove the baking sheet from the oven and transfer the spinach to a large serving bowl.
7. Repeat with the remaining spinach. Serve immediately.

Per Serving
Calories: 40 | fat: 4g | protein: 2g | carbs: 2g | fiber: 1g | sugar: 0g| sodium: 106mg

Cardamom spiced Kale and Chard

Prep time: 10 minutes | Cook time: 10 minutes | Serves 4

2 tablespoons extra-virgin olive oil
1 pound (454 g) kale, coarse stems removed and leaves chopped
1 pound (454 g) Swiss chard, coarse stems removed and leaves

chopped
1 tablespoon freshly squeezed lemon juice
½ teaspoon ground cardamom
Sea salt to taste
Freshly ground black pepper

1. Place a large skillet over medium-high heat and add the olive oil.
2. Add the kale, chard, lemon juice, and cardamom to the skillet. Use tongs to toss the greens continuously until they are wilted, about 10 minutes or less.
3. Season the greens with salt and pepper.
4. Serve immediately.

Per Serving
Calories: 140 | fat: 7g | protein: 6g | carbs: 16g | fiber: 4g | sugar: 1g| sodium: 351mg

Thyme Herbed Button Mushrooms

Prep time: 10 minutes | Cook time: 12 minutes | Serves 4

1 teaspoon butter
2 teaspoons extra-virgin olive oil
2 pounds (907 g) button mushrooms, halved
2 teaspoons minced

fresh garlic
1 teaspoon chopped fresh thyme
Sea salt to taste
Freshly ground black pepper to taste

1. Place a large skillet over medium-high heat and add the butter and olive oil.
2. Sauté the mushrooms, stirring occasionally, until they are lightly caramelized and tender, about 10 minutes.
3. Add the garlic and thyme and sauté for 2 more minutes.
4. Season the mushrooms with salt and pepper before serving.

Per Serving
Calories: 97 | fat: 6g | protein: 7g | carbs: 8g | fiber: 2g | sugar: 4g| sodium: 92mg

Low Sodium Soy Bok Choy with Almonds

Prep time: 15 minutes | Cook time: 7 minutes | Serves 4

2 teaspoons sesame oil
2 pounds (907 g) bok choy, cleaned and quartered
2 teaspoons low-

sodium soy sauce
Pinch red pepper flakes
½ cup toasted sliced almonds

1. Place a large skillet over medium heat and add the oil.
2. When the oil is hot, sauté the bok choy until tender-crisp, about 5 minutes.
3. Stir in the soy sauce and red pepper flakes and sauté 2 minutes more.
4. Remove the bok choy to a serving bowl and top with the sliced almonds.

Per Serving
Calories: 119 | fat: 8g | protein: 6g | carbs: 8g | fiber: 4g | sugar: 3g| sodium: 294mg

Peppery Asparagus with Citrus Cashews

Prep time: 10 minutes | Cook time: 20 minutes | Serves 4

2 pounds (907 g) asparagus, woody ends trimmed
1 tablespoon extra-virgin olive oil
Sea salt to taste

Freshly ground black pepper
½ cup chopped cashews
Zest and juice of 1 lime

1. Preheat the oven to 400°F (204°C) and line a baking sheet with aluminium foil.
2. In a large bowl, toss the asparagus with the oil and lightly season with salt and pepper.
3. Transfer the asparagus to the baking sheet and bake until tender and lightly browned, 15 to 20 minutes.
4. Transfer the asparagus to a serving bowl and toss them with the chopped cashews, lime zest, and lime juice.

Per Serving
Calories: 174 | fat: 12g | protein: 8g | carbs: 14g | fiber: 5g | sugar: 5g| sodium: 66mg

Sautéed Asparagus with Scallop

Prep time: 10 minutes | Cook time: 15 minutes | Serves 4

3 teaspoons extra-virgin olive oil, divided
1 pound (454 g) asparagus, trimmed and cut into 2-inch segments
1 tablespoon butter
1 pound (454 g) sea scallops
¼ cup dry white wine
2 garlic cloves, minced
Juice of 1 lemon
¼ teaspoons freshly ground black pepper

1. Heat half of olive oil in a nonstick skillet over medium heat until shimmering.
2. Add the asparagus to the skillet and sauté for 6 minutes until soft. Transfer the cooked asparagus to a large plate and cover with aluminum foil.
3. Heat the remaining half of olive oil and butter in the skillet until the butter is melted.
4. Add the scallops to the skillet and cook for 6 minutes or until opaque and browned. Flip the scallops with tongs halfway through the cooking time. Transfer the scallops to the plate and cover with aluminum foil.
5. Combine the wine, garlic, lemon juice, and black pepper in the skillet. Simmer over medium-low heat for 2 minutes. Keep stirring during the simmering.
6. Pour the sauce over the asparagus and scallops to coat well, then serve warm.

Per Serving
Calories: 256 | fat: 6.9g | protein: 26.1g | carbs: 14.9g | fiber: 2.1g | sugar: 2.9g | sodium: 491mg

Coriander spiced Coconut Shrimp

Prep time: 12 minutes | Cook time: 6 to 8 minutes | Serves 4

2 egg whites
1 tablespoon water
½ cup whole-wheat panko bread crumbs
¼ cup unsweetened coconut flakes
½ teaspoon turmeric
½ teaspoon ground coriander
½ teaspoon ground cumin
⅛ teaspoon salt
1 pound large raw shrimp, peeled, deveined, and patted dry
Nonstick cooking spray

1. Preheat the air fry to 400ºF (205ºC).
2. In a shallow dish, beat the egg whites and water until slightly foamy. Set aside.
3. In a separate shallow dish, mix the bread crumbs, coconut flakes, turmeric, coriander, cumin, and salt, and stir until well combined.
4. Dredge the shrimp in the egg mixture, shaking off any excess, then coat them in the crumb-coconut mixture.
5. Spritz the air fryer basket with nonstick cooking spray and arrange the coated shrimp in the basket.
6. Air fry for 6 to 8 minutes, flipping the shrimp once during cooking, or until the shrimp are golden brown and cooked through.
7. Let the shrimp cool for 5 minutes before serving.

Per Serving
Calories: 181 | fat: 4.2g | protein: 27.8g | carbs: 9.0g | fiber: 2.3g | sugar: 0.8g | sodium: 227mg

Easy Garlic Orange Scallops

Prep time: 10 minutes | Cook time: 10 minutes| Serves 4

2 pounds sea scallops
Sea salt to taste
Freshly ground black pepper
2 tablespoons extra-virgin olive oil
1 tablespoon minced garlic
¼ cup freshly squeezed orange juice
1 teaspoon orange zest
2 teaspoons chopped fresh thyme, for garnish

1. Clean the scallops and pat them dry with paper towels, then season them lightly with salt and pepper.
2. Place a large skillet over medium-high heat and add the olive oil.
3. Sauté the garlic until it is softened and translucent, about 3 minutes.
4. Add the scallops to the skillet and cook until they are lightly seared and just cooked through, turning once, about 4 minutes per side.
5. Transfer the scallops to a plate, cover to keep warm, and set them aside.
6. Add the orange juice and zest to the skillet and stir to scrape up any cooked bits.
7. Spoon the sauce over the scallops and serve, garnished with the thyme.

Per Serving
Calories: 267 | fat: 8g | protein: 3g | carbs: 8g | fiber: 0g | sugar: 1g| sodium: 361mg

Creamy Chicken Sole Piccata

Prep time: 10 minutes | Cook time: 20 minutes| Serves 4

1 teaspoon extra-virgin olive oil
4 (5-ounce/142 g) sole fillets, patted dry
3 tablespoons butter
2 teaspoons minced garlic

2 tablespoons all-purpose flour
2 cups low-sodium chicken broth
Juice and zest of ½ lemons
2 tablespoons capers

1. Place a large skillet over medium-high heat and add the olive oil.
2. Pat the sole fillets dry with paper towels then pan-sear them until the fish flakes easily when tested with a fork, about 4 minutes on each side. Transfer the fish to a plate and set it aside.
3. Return the skillet to the stove and add the butter.
4. Sauté the garlic until translucent, about 3 minutes.
5. Whisk in the flour to make a thick paste and cook, stirring constantly, until the mixture is golden brown, about 2 minutes.
6. Whisk in the chicken broth, lemon juice, and lemon zest.
7. Cook until the sauce has thickened, about 4 minutes.
8. Stir in the capers and serve the sauce over the fish.

Per Serving
Calories: 271 fat: 13g | protein: 30g | carbs: 7g | fiber: 0g | sugar: 2g| sodium: 413mg

Chili Garlic Spiced Sole

Prep time: 10 minutes | Cook time 10 minutes | Serves 4

1 teaspoon chili powder
1 teaspoon garlic powder
½ teaspoon lime zest
½ teaspoon lemon zest
¼ teaspoons freshly ground black pepper

¼ teaspoon smoked paprika
Pinch sea salt
4 (6-ounce) sole fillets, patted dry
1 tablespoon extra-virgin olive oil
2 teaspoons freshly squeezed lime juice

1. Preheat the oven to 450°F(232°C).
2. Line a baking sheet with aluminium foil and set it aside.

3. In a small bowl, stir together the chili powder, garlic powder, lime zest, lemon zest, pepper, paprika, and salt until well mixed.
4. Pat the fish fillets dry with paper towels, places them on the baking sheet, and rub them lightly all over with the spice mixture.
5. Drizzle the olive oil and lime juice on the top of the fish.
6. Bake until the fish flakes when pressed lightly with a fork, about 8 minutes. Serve immediately.

Per Serving
Calories: 184 | fat: 5g | protein: 32g | carbs: 0g | fiber: 0g | sugar: 0g| sodium: 137mg

Haddock Fillets with Cucumber Sauce

Prep time: 10 minutes | Cook time: 10 minutes | Serves 4

¼ cup 2 per cent Low-fat Greek yogurt
½ English cucumbers, grated, liquid squeezed out
½ scallions, white and green parts, finely chopped
2 teaspoons chopped fresh mint

½ teaspoon honey
Sea salt to taste
4 (5-ounce/142 g) haddock fillets
Freshly ground black pepper
Non-stick cooking spray

1. In a small bowl, stir together the yogurt, cucumber, scallion, mint, honey, and a pinch of salt. Set it aside.
2. Pat the fish fillets dry with paper towels and season them lightly with salt and pepper.
3. Place a large skillet over medium-high heat and spray lightly with cooking spray.
4. Cook the haddock, turning once, until it is just cooked through, about 5 minutes per side.
5. Remove the fish from the heat and transfer to plates. Serve topped with the cucumber sauce.

Per Serving
Calories: 164 | fat: 2g | protein: 27g | carbs: 4g | fiber: 0g | sugar: 3g| sodium: 104mg

Hot and Thyme Herbed Halibut

Prep time: 10 minutes | Cook time: 20 minutes | Serves 4

4 (5-ounce/142 g) halibut fillets
Extra-virgin olive oil, for brushing
½ cup coarsely ground unsalted pistachios
1 tablespoon chopped fresh parsley

1 teaspoon chopped fresh thyme
1 teaspoon chopped fresh basil
Pinch sea salt
Pinch freshly ground black pepper

1. Preheat the oven to 350°F (177°C).
2. Line a baking sheet with parchment paper.
3. Pat the halibut fillets dry with a paper towel and place them on the baking sheet.
4. Brush the halibut generously with olive oil.
5. In a small bowl, stir together the pistachios, parsley, thyme, basil, salt, and pepper.
6. Spoon the nut and herb mixture evenly on the fish, spreading it out so the tops of the fillets are covered.
7. Bake the halibut until it flakes when pressed with a fork, about 20 minutes. Serve immediately.

Per Serving
Calories: 262 | fat: 11g | protein: 32g | carbs: 4g | fiber: 2g | sugar: 1g| sodium: 77mg

Baked Citrus Salmon with Baby Spinach

Prep time: 10 minutes | Cook time: 30 minutes | Serves 4

1 teaspoon extra-virgin olive oil
½ sweet onion, finely chopped
1 teaspoon minced garlic
3 cups baby spinach
1 cup kale, tough stems removed, torn

into 3-inch pieces
Sea salt to taste
Freshly ground black pepper
4 (5-ounce) salmon fillets
Lemon wedges, for serving

1. Preheat the oven to 350°F(177°C)
2. Place a large skillet over medium-high heat and add the oil.
3. Sauté the onion and garlic until softened and translucent, about 3 minutes.
4. Add the spinach and kale and sauté until the greens wilt, about 5 minutes.

5. Remove the skillet from the heat and season the greens with salt and pepper.
6. Place the salmon fillets so they are nestled in the greens and partially covered by them. Bake the salmon until it is opaque, about 20 minutes.
7. Serve immediately with a squeeze of fresh lemon.

Per Serving
Calories: 281 | fat: 16g | protein: 29g | carbs: 4g | fiber: 1g | sugar: 1g| sodium: 91mg

Baked Citrus Veggie Salmon with Sauce

Prep time: 10 minutes | Cook time: 15 minutes | Serves 4

4 (5-ounce/142 g) salmon fillets
Sea salt to taste
Freshly ground black pepper
1 tablespoon extra-virgin olive oil
½ cup low-sodium vegetable broth

Juice and zest of 1 lemon
1 teaspoon chopped fresh thyme
½ cup fat-free sour cream
1 teaspoon honey
1 tablespoon chopped fresh chives

1. Preheat the oven to 400°F (204°C).
2. Season the salmon lightly on both sides with salt and pepper.
3. Place a large ovenproof skillet over medium-high heat and add the olive oil.
4. Sear the salmon fillets on both sides until golden, about 3 minutes per side.
5. Transfer the salmon to a baking dish and bake until it is just cooked through, about 10 minutes.
6. While the salmon is baking, whisk together the vegetable broth, lemon juice, zest, and thyme in a small saucepan over medium-high heat until the liquid reduces by about one-quarter, about 5 minutes.
7. Whisk in the sour cream and honey.
8. Stir in the chives and serve the sauce over the salmon.

Per Serving
Calories: 310 | fat: 18g | protein: 29g | carbs: 6g | fiber: 0g | sugar: 2g| sodium: 129mg

Quick Buttery Nutmeg Green Beans

Prep time: 15 minutes | Cook time: 5 minutes | Serves 4

1 tablespoon butter	1 teaspoon ground
1½ pounds (680 g)	nutmeg
green beans, trimmed	Sea salt to taste

1. Place a large skillet over medium heat and melt the butter.
2. Add the green beans and sauté, stirring often, until the beans are tender-crisp, about 5 minutes.
3. Stir in the nutmeg and season with salt.
4. Serve immediately.

Per Serving
Calories: 81 | fat: g | protein: 3g | carbs: 12g | fiber: 6g | sugar: 3g| sodium: 89mg

Delicious & Easy Fish Stew

Prep time: 20 minutes | Cook time: 30 minutes| Serves 6

1 tablespoon extra-virgin olive oil	2 teaspoons chopped fresh basil
1 sweet onion, chopped	2 teaspoons chopped fresh oregano
2 teaspoons minced garlic	2 (4-ounce/113 g) haddock fillets, cut into 1-inch chunks
3 celery stalks, chopped	1 pound mussels, scrubbed
2 carrots, peeled and chopped	8 ounces (16–20 count) shrimp, peeled, deveined, quartered
1 (28-ounce/794 g) can sodium-free diced tomatoes, undrained	Sea salt to taste
3 cups low-sodium chicken broth	Freshly ground black pepper to taste
½ cup clam juice	2 tablespoons chopped fresh parsley
¼ cup dry white wine	

1. Place a large saucepan over medium-high heat and add the olive oil.
2. Sauté the onion and garlic until softened and translucent, about 3 minutes.
3. Stir in the celery and carrots and sauté for 4 minutes.
4. Stir in the tomatoes, chicken broth, clam juice, white wine, basil, and oregano.
5. Bring the sauce to a boil, and then reduce the heat to low. Simmer for 15 minutes.

6. Add the fish and mussels, cover, and cook until the mussels open, about 5 minutes.
7. Discard any unopened mussels. Add the shrimp to the pan and cook until the shrimp are opaque, about 2 minutes.
8. Season with salt and pepper. Serve garnished with the chopped parsley.

Per Serving
Calories: 248 | fat: 7g | protein: 28g | carbs: 19g | fiber: 2g | sugar: 7g| sodium: 577mg

Coconut Shrimp with Tomato

Prep time: 10 minutes | Cook time: 25 minutes | Serves 4

1 pound (454 g) extra-large shrimp, peel and devein	fine
	1 tablespoon coconut oil
1 onion, diced fine	2 teaspoons coriander
1¾ cup coconut milk, unsweetened	1 teaspoon curry powder
2 tablespoons fresh lemon juice	1 teaspoon salt, or to taste
1 tablespoon fresh ginger, grated	½ teaspoon turmeric
1 (14½-ounce / 411-g) can tomatoes, diced	¾ teaspoon black pepper
3 cloves garlic, diced	¼ teaspoon cayenne

1. In a medium bowl combine lemon juice, ¼ teaspoon salt, ¼ teaspoon pepper and the cayenne pepper.
2. Add shrimp and toss to coat. Cover and refrigerate at least 10 minutes.
3. Heat the oil in a large, deep, skillet over medium-high heat.
4. Add onion and cook until it starts to soften, about 2 to 3 minutes. Add remaining seasonings and cook 1 minute more.
5. Add tomatoes with juices and coconut milk, stir and bring to boil. Cook, stirring occasionally, 5 minutes.
6. Add shrimp and marinade and cook till shrimp turn pink about 2 to 3 minutes. Serve.

Per Serving
Calories: 450 | fat: 30.0g | protein: 29.2g | carbs: 12.1g | fiber: 3.0g | sugar: 5.0g | sodium: 865mg

Milky Mashed Cauliflower with Chopped Chives

Prep time: 5 minutes | Cook time: 10 minutes | Serves 4

1 large head cauliflower (about 3 pounds/1.3 k g), cut into small florets
½ cup skim milk

2 tablespoons prepared horseradish
¼ teaspoon sea salt
2 teaspoons chopped fresh chives

1. Place a large pot of water on high heat and bring it to a boil.
2. Blanch the cauliflower until it is tender, about 5 minutes.
3. Drain the cauliflower completely and transfer it to a food processor.
4. Add the milk and horseradish to the cauliflower and purée until it is smooth and thick, about 2 minutes. Or mash it by hand with a potato masher.
5. Transfer the mashed cauliflower to a bowl and season with salt.
6. Serve immediately, topped with the chopped chives.

Per Serving
Calories: 100 | fat: 0g | protein: 8g | carbs: 20g | fiber: 9g | sugar: 10g| sodium: 259mg

Garlicky Broccoli Cauliflower Bake

Prep time: 15 minutes | Cook time: 40 minutes | Serves 4 to 6

½ cup ground almonds
¼ cup grated Parmesan cheese
1 tablespoon butter, melted, plus 2 tablespoons butter
Pinch freshly ground black pepper
1 head broccoli, cut into small florets
1 head cauliflower, cut into small florets

1 sweet onion, chopped
1 teaspoon minced garlic
2 tablespoons all-purpose flour
1 cup skim milk
2 ounces (28 g) goat cheese
¼ teaspoon ground nutmeg

1. Preheat the oven to 350°F (177°C). In a small bowl, mix together the almonds, Parmesan cheese, melted butter, and pepper. Set it aside.
2. Place a large pot full of water over high heat and bring to a boil.
3. Blanch the broccoli and cauliflower for 1 minute, drain, and set them aside.
4. Place a large skillet over medium-high heat and melt the 2 tablespoons of butter.
5. Sauté the onion and garlic until tender, about 3 minutes. Whisk in the flour and cook, stirring constantly, for 1 minute.
6. Whisk in the milk and cook, stirring constantly, until the sauce has thickened, about 4 minutes.
7. Remove the skillet from the heat and whisk in the goat cheese and nutmeg.
8. Add the broccoli and cauliflower, then spoon the mixture into a 1½-quart casserole dish.
9. Sprinkle the almond mixture over the top and bake until the casserole is heated through, about 30 minutes.

Per Serving
Calories: 224 | fat: 7g | protein: 11g | carbs: 14g | fiber: 5g | sugar: 6g| sodium: 178mg

Sautéed Low Sodium Chicken Broccoli

Prep time: 10 minutes | Cook time: 10 minutes | Serves 4

1 tablespoon extra-virgin olive oil
½ sweet onion, thinly sliced
2 teaspoons grated fresh ginger
1 teaspoon minced fresh garlic

2 heads broccoli, cut into small florets
¼ cup low-sodium chicken broth
Sea salt to taste
Freshly ground black pepper to taste

1. Place a large skillet over medium-high heat and add the oil.
2. Sauté the onion, ginger, and garlic until softened, about 3 minutes.
3. Add the broccoli florets and chicken broth, and sauté until the broccoli is tender, about 5 minutes.
4. Season with salt and pepper.
5. Serve immediately.

Per Serving
Calories: 102 | fat: 4g | protein: 5g | carbs: 14g | fiber: 5g | sugar: 4g| sodium: 109mg

Garlic spiced Mussels with Onions

Prep time: 10 minutes | Cook time: 10 minutes | Serves 4

2 pounds (907 g) mussels, cleaned
2 plum tomatoes, peeled, seeded and diced
1 cup onion, diced
2 tablespoons fresh parsley, diced

¼ cup dry white wine
3 cloves garlic, diced fine
3 tablespoons olive oil
2 tablespoons fresh breadcrumbs
¼ teaspoon crushed red pepper flakes

1. Heat oil in a large sauce pot over medium heat.
2. Add the onions and cook until soft, about 2 to 3 minutes. Add garlic and cook 1 minute more.
3. Stir in wine, tomatoes, and pepper flakes. Bring to a boil, stirring occasionally.
4. Add the mussels and cook 3 to 4 minutes, or until all the mussels have opened. Discard any mussels that do not open.
5. Once mussels open, transfer them to a serving bowl.
6. Add bread crumbs to the sauce and continue to cook, stirring frequently, until mixture thickens. Stir in parsley and pour evenly over mussels. Serve.

Per Serving
Calories: 341 | fat: 16.0g | protein: 29.2g | carbs: 18.1g | fiber: 2.0g | sugar: 4.0g | sodium: 682mg

Zucchini Pasta with Pine Nuts

Prep time: 20 minutes | Cook time: 15 minutes | Serves 4

2 cups packed fresh basil leaves
½ cup pine nuts
2 teaspoons minced garlic
Zest and juice of 1 lime
Pinch sea salt
Pinch freshly ground

black pepper
¼ cup extra-virgin olive oil
4 green or yellow zucchini, rinsed, dried, and julienned or spiralized
1 tomato, diced

1. Place the basil, pine nuts, garlic, lime zest, lime juice, salt, and pepper in a food processor or a blender and pulse until very finely chopped.
2. While the machine is running, add the olive oil in a thin stream until a thick paste forms.
3. In a large bowl, combine the zucchini noodles and tomato.
4. Add the pesto by the tablespoonful until you have the desired flavour. Serve the zucchini pasta immediately.
5. Store any leftover pesto in a sealed container in the refrigerator for up to 2 weeks.

Per Serving
Calories: 261 | fat: 23g | protein: 5g | carbs: 10g | fiber: 3g | sugar: 5g| sodium: 80mg

Hot & Spicy Squash with Spinach

Prep time: 20 minutes | Cook time: 60 minutes | Serves 4

1 spaghetti squash, halved and seeded
3 teaspoons extra-virgin olive oil, divided
¼ sweet onion, chopped
1 teaspoon minced garlic
2 cups fresh spinach

¼ cup chopped sun-dried tomatoes
¼ cup roasted, shelled sunflower seeds
Juice of ½ lemons
Sea salt to taste
Freshly ground black pepper to taste

1. Preheat the oven to 350°F (177°C). Line a baking sheet with parchment paper.
2. Place the squash on the baking sheet and brush the cut edges with 2 teaspoons of olive oil.
3. Bake the squash until it is tender and separates into strands with a fork, about 1 hour.
4. Let the squash cool for 5 minutes then use a fork to scrape out the strands from both halves of the squash. Cover the squash strands and set them aside.
5. Place a large skillet over medium-high heat and add the remaining 1 teaspoon of olive oil. Sauté the onion and garlic until softened and translucent, about 3 minutes.
6. Stir in the spinach and sun-dried tomatoes, and sauté until the spinach is wilted, about 4 minutes.
7. Remove the skillet from the heat and stir in the squash strands, sunflower seeds, and lemon juice.
8. Season with salt and pepper and serve warm.

Per Serving
Calories: 103 | fat: 6g | protein: 3g | carbs: 13g | fiber: 1g | sugar: 2g| sodium: 163mg

Chapter 8: Pork, Beef, and Lamb

Cheesy Pepper Mushroom Lamb Burger

Prep time: 15 minutes | Cook time: 15 minutes | Serves 4

8 ounces (227 g) grass-fed ground lamb
8 ounces (227 g) brown mushrooms, finely chopped
¼ teaspoon salt
¼ teaspoons freshly ground black pepper
¼ cup crumbled goat cheese
1 tablespoon minced fresh basil

1. In a large mixing bowl, combine the lamb, mushrooms, salt, and pepper, and mix well.
2. In a small bowl, mix the goat cheese and basil.
3. Form the lamb mixture into 4 patties, reserving about ½ cup of the mixture in the bowl. In each patty, make an indentation in the center and fill with 1 tablespoon of the goat cheese mixture.
4. Use the reserved meat mixture to close the burgers. Press the meat firmly to hold together.
5. Heat the barbecue or a large skillet over medium-high heat. Add the burgers and cook for 5 to 7 minutes on each side, until cooked through. Serve.

Per Serving
Calories: 172 | fat: 13.1g | protein: 11.1g | carbs: 2.9g | fiber: 0g | sugar: 1.0g | sodium: 155mg

Pork Apple Cabbage Skillet

Prep time: 10 minutes | Cook time: 20 minutes | Serves 4

1 pound (454 g) ground pork
1 red onion, thinly sliced
1 apple, peeled, cored, and thinly sliced
2 cups shredded cabbage
1 teaspoon dried
thyme
2 garlic cloves, minced
¼ cup apple cider vinegar
1 tablespoon Dijon mustard
½ teaspoon sea salt
⅛ teaspoon freshly ground black pepper

1. In a large skillet over medium-high heat, cook the ground pork, crumbling it with a spoon, until browned, about 5 minutes. Use a slotted spoon to transfer the pork to a plate.
2. Add the onion, apples, cabbage, and thyme to the fat in the pan. Cook, stirring occasionally, until the vegetables are soft, about 5 minutes.
3. Add the garlic and cook, stirring constantly, for 5 minutes.
4. Return the pork to the pan.
5. In a small bowl, whisk together the vinegar, mustard, salt, and pepper. Add to the pan. Bring to a simmer. Cook, stirring, until the sauce thickens, about 2 minutes.

Per Serving
Calories: 364 | fat: 24g | protein: 20g | carbs: 19g | fiber: 4g | sugar: 30g | sodium: 260mg

Low Sugar Beef Veggie Soup

Prep time: 10 minutes | Cook time: 15 minutes | Serves 4

1 pound (454 g) ground beef
1 onion, chopped
2 celery stalks, chopped
1 carrot, chopped
1 teaspoon dried
rosemary
6 cups low-sodium beef or chicken broth
½ teaspoon sea salt
⅛ teaspoon freshly ground black pepper
2 cups peas

1. In a large pot over medium-high heat, cook the ground beef, crumbling with the side of a spoon, until browned, about 5 minutes.
2. Add the onion, celery, carrot, and rosemary. Cook, stirring occasionally, until the vegetables start to soften, about 5 minutes.
3. Add the broth, salt, pepper, and peas. Bring to a simmer. Reduce the heat and simmer, stirring, until warmed through, about 5 minutes more.

Per Serving
Calories: 355 | fat: 17g | protein: 34g | carbs: 18g | fiber: 5g | sugar: 10.1g | sodium: 362mg

Diabetic Friendly Beef Broccoli Skillet

Prep time: 10 minutes | Cook time: 15 minutes | Serves 4

2 tablespoons extra-virgin olive oil
1 pound sirloin steak, cut into ¼-inch-thick strips
2 cups broccoli florets
1 garlic clove, minced
1 teaspoon peeled and grated fresh ginger
2 tablespoons reduced-sodium soy sauce
¼ cup beef broth
½ teaspoon Chinese hot mustard
Pinch red pepper flakes

1. In a large skillet over medium-high heat, heat the olive oil until it shimmers.
2. Add the beef. Cook, stirring, until it browns, 3 to 5 minutes. With a slotted spoon, remove the beef from the oil and set it aside on a plate.
3. Add the broccoli to the oil. Cook, stirring, until it is crisp-tender, about 4 minutes.
4. Add the garlic and ginger and cook, stirring constantly, for 30 seconds.
5. Return the beef to the pan, along with any juices that have collected.
6. In a small bowl, whisk together the soy sauce, broth, mustard, and red pepper flakes.
7. Add the soy sauce mixture to the skillet and cook, stirring, until everything warms through, about 3 minutes.

Per Serving
Calories: 227 | fat: 11g | protein: 27g | carbs: 5g | fiber: 1g | sugar: 8.8g | sodium: 375mg

Cauliflower Sirloin Steak Bowl

Prep time: 10 minutes | Cook time: 15 minutes | Serves 4

4 tablespoons extra-virgin olive oil, divided
1 head cauliflower, riced
1 pound (454 g) sirloin steak, cut into ¼-inch-thick strips
1 red bell pepper, seeded and sliced
1 onion, thinly sliced
2 garlic cloves, minced
Juice of 2 limes
1 teaspoon chili powder

1. In a large skillet over medium-high heat, heat 2 tablespoons of olive oil until it shimmers.
2. Add the cauliflower. Cook, stirring occasionally, until it softens, about 3 minutes. Set aside.
3. Wipe out the skillet with a paper towel. Add the remaining 2 tablespoons of oil to the skillet, and heat it on medium-high until it shimmers.
4. Add the steak and cook, stirring occasionally, until it browns, about 3 minutes. Use a slotted spoon to remove the steak from the oil in the pan and set aside.
5. Add the bell pepper and onion to the pan. Cook, stirring occasionally, until they start to brown, about 5 minutes.
6. Add the garlic and cook, stirring constantly, for 30 seconds.
7. Return the beef along with any juices that have collected and the cauliflower to the pan. Add the lime juice and chili powder.
8. Cook, stirring, until everything is warmed through, 2 to 3 minutes.

Per Serving
Calories: 310 | fat: 18g | protein: 27g | carbs: 13g | fiber: 3g | sugar: 9.5g | sodium: 93mg

Peppery Pork Roast and Carrots

Prep time: 5 minutes | Cook time: 40 minutes | Serves 4

1 pound (454 g) pork loin
1 tablespoon extra-virgin olive oil, divided
¼ teaspoons freshly ground black pepper
½ teaspoon dried rosemary
4 (6-inch) carrots, chopped into ½-inch rounds

1. Preheat the oven to 350ºF (180ºC).
2. Rub the pork loin with ½ tablespoon of oil. Season with the pepper and rosemary.
3. In a medium bowl, toss the carrots in the remaining ½ tablespoon of oil.
4. Place the pork and the carrots on a baking sheet in a single layer. Cook for 40 minutes.
5. Remove the baking sheet from the oven and let the pork rest for at least 10 minutes before slicing. Divide the pork and carrots into four equal portions.

Per Serving
Calories: 344 | fat: 10.1g | protein: 26.1g | carbs: 25.9g | fiber: 3.9g | sugar: 6.0g | sodium: 110mg

Spiced Ground Lamb with Cucumber Salad

Prep time: 10 minutes | Cook time: 15 minutes | Serves 4

¼ cup red wine vinegar
Pinch red pepper flakes
1 teaspoon sea salt, divided
2 cucumbers, peeled and chopped
½ red onion, finely chopped

1 pound (454 g) ground lamb
2 teaspoons ground coriander
1 teaspoon ground cumin
3 garlic cloves, minced
1 tablespoon fresh mint, chopped

1. Preheat the oven to 375°F (191°C). Line a rimmed baking sheet with parchment paper.
2. In a medium bowl, whisk together the vinegar, red pepper flakes, and ½ teaspoon of salt. Add the cucumbers and onion and toss to combine. Set aside.
3. In a large bowl, mix the lamb, coriander, cumin, garlic, mint, and remaining ½ teaspoon of salt. Form the mixture into 1-inch meatballs and place them on the prepared baking sheet.
4. Bake until the lamb reaches 140°F (60°C) internally, about 15 minutes.
5. Serve with the salad on the side.

Per Serving
Calories: 345 | fat: 27g | protein: 20g | carbs: 7g | fiber: 1g | sugar: 14.9g | sodium: 362mg

Delicious Apple Onion Pork Chops

Prep time: 15 minutes | Cook time: 30 minutes | Serves 4

¼ cup apple cider vinegar
2 tablespoons granulated sweetener
4 (4-ounce / 113-g) pork chops, about 1 inch thick
Sea salt and freshly ground black pepper, to taste

1 tablespoon extra-virgin olive oil
½ red cabbage, finely shredded
1 sweet onion, thinly sliced
1 apple, peeled, cored, and sliced
1 teaspoon chopped fresh thyme

1. In a small bowl, whisk together the vinegar and sweetener. Set it aside.
2. Season the pork with salt and pepper.
3. Place a large skillet over medium-high heat and add the olive oil.
4. Cook the pork chops until no longer pink, turning once, about 8 minutes per side.
5. Transfer the chops to a plate and set aside.
6. Add the cabbage and onion to the skillet and sauté until the vegetables have softened, about 5 minutes.
7. Add the vinegar mixture and the apple slices to the skillet and bring the mixture to a boil.
8. Reduce the heat to low and simmer, covered, for 5 additional minutes.
9. Return the pork chops to the skillet, along with any accumulated juices and thyme, cover, and cook for 5 more minutes.

Per Serving
Calories: 224 | fat: 8.1g | protein: 26.1g | carbs: 12.1g | fiber: 3.1g | sugar: 8.0g | sodium: 293mg

Orange Lamb Chops

Prep time: 10 minutes | Cook time: 20 minutes | Serves 4

4 (4-ounce / 113-g) lamb chops
1½ teaspoons chopped fresh rosemary
¼ teaspoon salt
¼ teaspoons freshly ground black pepper

1 cup frozen cherries, thawed
2 tablespoons orange juice
1 teaspoon extra-virgin olive oil

1. Season the lamb chops with the rosemary, salt, and pepper.
2. In a small saucepan over medium-low heat, combine the cherries and orange juice, and simmer, stirring regularly, until the sauce thickens, 8 to 10 minutes.
3. Heat a large skillet over medium-high heat. When the pan is hot, add the olive oil to lightly coat the bottom.
4. Cook the lamb chops for 3 to 4 minutes on each side until well-browned yet medium rare.
5. Serve, topped with the cherry glaze.

Per Serving
Calories: 355 | fat: 27.1g | protein: 19.8g | carbs: 5.9g | fiber: 1.0g | sugar: 4.0g | sodium: 200mg

Baked and Herbed Spicy Meatballs

Prep time: 10 minutes | Cook time: 15 minutes | Serves 4

½ pound (227 g) lean ground pork
½ pound (227 g) lean ground beef
1 sweet onion, finely chopped
¼ cup bread crumbs
2 tablespoons chopped

fresh basil
2 teaspoons minced garlic
1 egg
Pinch sea salt
Pinch freshly ground black pepper

1. Preheat the oven to 350ºF (180ºC).
2. Line a baking tray with parchment paper and set it aside.
3. In a large bowl, mix together the pork, beef, onion, bread crumbs, basil, garlic, egg, salt, and pepper until very well mixed.
4. Roll the meat mixture into 2-inch meatballs.
5. Transfer the meatballs to the baking sheet and bake until they are browned and cooked through, about 15 minutes.
6. Serve the meatballs with your favorite marinara sauce and some steamed green beans.

Per Serving
Calories: 333 | fat: 19.1g | protein: 24.1g | carbs: 12.9g | fiber: 0.9g | sugar: 2.9g | sodium: 189mg

Pepper Beef Roast with Shallot Sauce

Prep time: 10 minutes | Cook time: 1 hour 40 minutes | Serves 4

1½ pounds (680 g) top rump beef roast
Sea salt and freshly ground black pepper, to taste
3 teaspoons extra-virgin olive oil, divided
3 shallots, minced
2 teaspoons minced

garlic
1 tablespoon green peppercorns
2 tablespoons dry sherry
2 tablespoons all-purpose flour
1 cup sodium-free beef broth

1. Heat the oven to 300ºF (150ºC).
2. Season the roast with salt and pepper.
3. Place a large skillet over medium-high heat and add 2 teaspoons of olive oil.
4. Brown the beef on all sides, about 10 minutes in total, and transfer the roast to a baking dish.

5. Roast until desired doneness, about 1½ hours for medium. When the roast has been in the oven for 1 hour, start the sauce.
6. In a medium saucepan over medium-high heat, sauté the shallots in the remaining 1 teaspoon of olive oil until translucent, about 4 minutes.
7. Stir in the garlic and peppercorns, and cook for another minute. Whisk in the sherry to deglaze the pan.
8. Whisk in the flour to form a thick paste, cooking for 1 minute and stirring constantly.
9. Pour in the beef broth and whisk until the sauce is thick and glossy, about 4 minutes. Season the sauce with salt and pepper.
10. Serve the beef with a generous spoonful of sauce.

Per Serving
Calories: 331 | fat: 18.1g | protein: 36.1g | carbs: 3.9g | fiber: 0g | sugar: 1.0g | sodium: 208mg

Cheesy Crusted Pork Recipe

Prep time: 10 minutes | Cook time: 25 minutes | Serves 4

Nonstick cooking spray
4 bone-in, thin-cut pork chops
2 tablespoons butter
½ cup grated Parmesan cheese

3 garlic cloves, minced
¼ teaspoon salt
¼ teaspoon dried thyme
Freshly ground black pepper, to taste

1. Preheat the oven to 400ºF (205ºC). Line a baking sheet with parchment paper and spray with nonstick cooking spray.
2. Arrange the pork chops on the prepared baking sheet so they do not overlap.
3. In a small bowl, combine the butter, cheese, garlic, salt, thyme, and pepper. Press 2 tablespoons of the cheese mixture onto the top of each pork chop.
4. Bake for 18 to 22 minutes until the pork is cooked through and its juices run clear. Set the broiler to high, and then broil for 1 to 2 minutes to brown the tops.

Per Serving
Calories: 333 | fat: 16.1g | protein: 44.1g | carbs: 1.1g | fiber: 0g | sugar: 0g | sodium: 441mg

Classic Beef with Sour Cream and Parsley

Prep time: 10 minutes | Cook time: 30 minutes | Serves 4

1 teaspoon extra-virgin olive oil
1 pound (454 g) top sirloin, cut into thin strips
1 cup sliced button mushrooms
½ sweet onion, finely chopped
1 teaspoon minced garlic
1 tablespoon whole-wheat flour
½ cup low-sodium beef broth
¼ cup dry sherry
½ cup fat-free sour cream
1 tablespoon chopped fresh parsley
Sea salt and freshly ground black pepper, to taste

1. Place a large skillet over medium-high heat and add the oil.
2. Sauté the beef until browned, about 10 minutes, then remove the beef with a slotted spoon to a plate and set it aside.
3. Add the mushrooms, onion, and garlic to the skillet and sauté until lightly browned, about 5 minutes.
4. Whisk in the flour and then whisk in the beef broth and sherry.
5. Return the sirloin to the skillet and bring the mixture to a boil.
6. Reduce the heat to low and simmer until the beef is tender, about 10 minutes.
7. Stir in the sour cream and parsley. Season with salt and pepper.

Per Serving
Calories: 258 | fat: 14.1g | protein: 26.1g | carbs: 6.1g | fiber: 1.1g | sugar: 1.0g | sodium: 142mg

Whole-wheat Sandwiches with Pulled Pork

Prep time: 5 minutes | Cook time: 15 minutes | Serves 4

Avocado oil cooking spray
8 ounces (227 g) store-bought pulled pork
½ cup chopped green bell pepper
2 slices provolone cheese
4 whole-wheat sandwiches thins
2½ tablespoons apricot jelly

1. Heat the pulled pork according to the package instructions.
2. Heat a medium skillet over medium-low heat. When hot, coat the cooking surface with cooking spray.
3. Put the bell pepper in the skillet and cook for 5 minutes. Transfer to a small bowl and set aside.
4. Meanwhile, tear each slice of cheese into 2 strips, and halves the sandwich thins so you have a top and bottom.
5. Reduce the heat to low, and place the sandwich thins in the skillet cut-side down to toast, about 2 minutes.
6. Remove the sandwich thins from the skillet. Spread one-quarter of the jelly on the bottom half of each sandwich thin, and then place one-quarter of the cheese, pulled pork, and pepper on top.
7. Cover with the top half of the sandwich thin.

Per Serving
Calories: 250 | fat: 8.1g | protein: 16.1g | carbs: 34.1g | fiber: 6.1g | sugar: 8.0g | sodium: 510mg

Maple Dijon Pork Chops

Prep time: 5 minutes | Cook time: 25 minutes | Serves 4

¼ cup Dijon mustard
1 tablespoon pure maple syrup
2 tablespoons rice vinegar
4 bone-in, thin-cut pork chops

1. Preheat the oven to 400ºF (205ºC).
2. In a small saucepan, combine the mustard, maple syrup, and rice vinegar. Stir to mix and bring to a simmer over medium heat. Cook for about 2 minutes until just slightly thickened.
3. In a baking dish, place the pork chops and spoon the sauce over them, flipping to coat.
4. Bake, uncovered, for 18 to 22 minutes until the juices run clear.

Per Serving
Calories: 258 | fat: 7.1g | protein: 39.1g | carbs: 6.9g | fiber: 0g | sugar: 4.0g | sodium: 465mg

Amazing Beef Cauliflower Tacos

Prep time: 5 minutes | Cook time: 20 minutes | Serves 4

Avocado oil cooking spray
½ cup chopped white onion
1 cup chopped Portobello mushrooms
1 pound (454 g) 93% lean ground beef
½ teaspoon garlic powder
Pinch salt
1 (10-ounce / 283-g) bag frozen cauliflower rice
12 iceberg lettuce leaves
¾ cup shredded Cheddar cheese

1. Heat a large skillet over medium heat. When hot, coat the cooking surface with cooking spray and add the onion and mushrooms. Cook for 5 minutes, stirring occasionally.
2. Add the beef, garlic powder, and salt, stirring and breaking apart the meat as needed. Cook for 5 minutes.
3. Stir in the frozen cauliflower rice and increase the heat to medium-high. Cook for 5 minute more, or until the water evaporates.
4. For each portion, use three lettuce leaves. Spoon one-quarter of the filling onto the lettuce leaves, and top with one-quarter of the cheese.
5. Then, working from the side closest to you, roll up the lettuce to close the wrap. Repeat with the remaining lettuce leaves and filling.

Per Serving
Calories: 290 | fat: 15.1g | protein: 31.1g | carbs: 7.1g | fiber: 3.1g | sugar: 4.0g | sodium: 265mg

Bacon Zucchini with Parmesan cheese

Prep time: 10 minutes | Cook time: 25 minutes | Serves 4

6 slices bacon, cut into pieces
1 red onion, finely chopped
3 zucchini, cut into noodles
1 cup peas
½ teaspoon sea salt
3 garlic cloves, minced
3 large eggs, beaten
1 tablespoon heavy cream
Pinch red pepper flakes
½ cup grated Parmesan cheese (optional, for garnish)

1. In a large skillet over medium-high heat, cook the bacon until browned, about 5 minutes. With a slotted spoon, transfer the bacon to a plate.
2. Add the onion to the bacon fat in the pan and cook, stirring, until soft, 3 to 5 minutes.
3. Add the zucchini, peas, and salt. Cook, stirring, until the zucchini softens, about 3 minutes. Add the garlic and cook, stirring constantly, for 5 minutes.
4. In a small bowl, whisk together the eggs, cream, and red pepper flakes. Add to the vegetables.
5. Remove the pan from the stove top and stir for 3 minutes, allowing the heat of the pan to cook the eggs without setting them.
6. Return the bacon to the pan with Parmesan cheese and stir to mix.
7. Serve topped with Parmesan cheese, if desired.

Per Serving
Calories: 327 | fat: 24.1g | protein: 14.1g | carbs: 14.9g | fiber: 3.9g | sugar: 11.0g | sodium: 556mg

Simple Spanish Beef Lettuce Wraps

Prep time: 15 minutes | Cook time: 0 minutes | Serves 6

6 whole wheat flour tortillas (10-inch)
6 large romaine lettuce leaves
12 ounces (340 g) cooked deli roast beef, thinly sliced
1 cup diced red bell peppers
1 cup diced tomatoes
1 tablespoon red wine vinegar
1 teaspoon cumin
¼ tteaspoon freshly ground black pepper
1 tablespoon olive oil

1. Unfold the tortillas on a clean work surface, and then top each tortilla with a lettuce leaf. Divide the roast beef over the leaf.
2. Combine the remaining ingredients in a bowl. Stir to mix well. Pour the mixture over the beef.
3. Fold the tortillas over the fillings, and then roll them up. Serve immediately.

Per Serving
Calories: 295 | fat: 6.0g | protein: 19.0g | carbs: 43.0g | fiber: 6.0g | sugar: 3.0g | sodium: 600mg

Baked Honey Pork Loin with Veggies

Prep time: 5 minutes | Cook time: 40 minutes | Serves 4

1 pound (454 g) pork loin
½ teaspoons honey
½ teaspoon dried rosemary
¼ teaspoons freshly ground black pepper
1 tablespoon extra-virgin olive oil, divided
4 (6-inch) carrots, chopped into ½-inch rounds
2 small gold potatoes, chopped into 2-inch cubes

1. Preheat the oven to 350ºF (180ºC).
2. On a clean work surface, rub the pork with honey, rosemary, black pepper, and ½ tablespoon of olive oil. Brush the carrots and gold potatoes with remaining olive oil.
3. Place the pork, carrots, and potatoes in s single layer on a baking sheet.
4. Roast in the preheated oven for 40 minutes or until the pork is lightly browned and the vegetables are soft.
5. Remove them from the oven. Allow to cool for 10 minutes before serving.

Per Serving
Calories: 346 | fat: 9.9g | protein: 26.1g | carbs: 25.9g | fiber: 4.1g | sugar: 5.9g | sodium: 107mg

Garlic Honey Citrus Roasted Pork Tenderloin

Prep time: 10 minutes | Cook time: 30 minutes | Serves 4

¼ cup freshly squeezed orange juice
2 teaspoons orange zest
1 teaspoon low-sodium soy sauce
¼ teaspoon honey
1 teaspoon grated fresh ginger
2 teaspoons minced garlic
1½ pounds (680 g) pork tenderloin roast, fat trimmed
1 tablespoon extra-virgin olive oil

1. Combine the orange juice and zest, soy sauce, honey, ginger, and garlic in a large bowl. Stir to mix well. Dunk the pork in the bowl and press to coat well.
2. Wrap the bowl in plastic and refrigerate to marinate for at least 2 hours.

3. Preheat the oven to 400ºF (205ºC).
4. Remove the bowl from the refrigerator and discard the marinade.
5. Heat the olive oil in an oven-safe skillet over medium-high heat until shimmering.
6. Add the pork and sear for 5 minutes. Flip the pork halfway through the cooking time.
7. Arrange the skillet in the preheated oven and roast the pork for 25 minutes or until well browned. Flip the pork halfway through the cooking time.
8. Transfer the pork on a plate. Allow to cool before serving.

Per Serving
Calories: 228 | fat: 9.0g | protein: 34.0g | carbs: 4.0g | fiber: 0g | sugar: 3.0g | sodium: 486mg

The Best Homemade Beef Sloppy Joes

Prep time: 10 minutes | Cook time: 15 minutes | Serves 4

1 tablespoon extra-virgin olive oil
1 pound (454 g) 93% lean ground beef
1 medium red bell pepper, chopped
½ medium yellow onion, chopped
2 tablespoons low-sodium Worcestershire sauce
1 (15-ounce / 425-g) can low-sodium tomato sauce
2 tablespoons low-sodium, sugar-free ketchup
4 whole-wheat sandwiches thins, cut in half
1 cup cabbage, shredded

1. Heat the olive oil in a nonstick skillet over medium heat until shimmering.
2. Add the beef, bell pepper, and onion to the skillet and sauté for 8 minutes or until the beef is browned and the onion is translucent.
3. Pour the Worcestershire sauce, tomato sauce, and ketchup in the skillet. Turn up the heat to medium-high and simmer for 5 minutes.
4. Assemble the sandwich thin halves with beef mixture and cabbage to make the sloppy Joes, then serve warm.

Per Serving
Calories: 329 | fat: 8.9g | protein: 31.2g | carbs: 35.9g | fiber: 7.9g | sugar: 10.9g | sodium: 271mg

Chunky Chili Pork

Prep time: 4 hours 20 minutes | Cook time: 20 minutes | Serves 4

4 (5-ounce / 142-g) pork chops, about 1 inch thick
1 tablespoon chipotle chili powder
Juice and zest of 1 lime
2 teaspoons minced garlic
1 teaspoon ground cinnamon
1 tablespoon extra-virgin olive oil
Pinch sea salt
Lime wedges, for garnish

1. Combine all the ingredients, except for the lemon wedges, in a large bowl. Toss to combine well.
2. Wrap the bowl in plastic and refrigerate to marinate for at least 4 hours.
3. Preheat the oven to 400ºF (205ºC). Set a rack on a baking sheet.
4. Remove the bowl from the refrigerator and let sit for 15 minutes. Discard the marinade and place the pork on the rack.
5. Roast in the preheated oven for 20 minutes or until well browned. Flip the pork halfway through the cooking time.
6. Serve immediately with lime wedges.

Per Serving
Calories: 204 | fat: 9.0g | protein: 30.0g | carbs: 1.0g | fiber: 0g | sugar: 1.0g | sodium: 317mg

20 Minute Worcestershire sauce Pork

Prep time: 10 minutes | Cook time: 20 minutes | Serves 4

2 teaspoons Worcestershire sauce
1 tablespoon freshly squeezed lemon juice
¼ cup low-sodium chicken broth
2 teaspoons Dijon mustard
4 (5-ounce / 142-g) boneless pork top loin
chops, about 1 inch thick
Sea salt and freshly ground black pepper, to taste
1 teaspoon extra-virgin olive oil
2 teaspoons chopped fresh chives
1 teaspoon lemon zest

1. Combine the Worcestershire sauce, lemon juice, broth, and Dijon mustard in a bowl. Stir to mix well.
2. On a clean work surface, rub the pork chops with salt and ground black pepper.
3. Heat the olive oil in a nonstick skillet over medium-high heat until shimmering.
4. Add the pork chops and sear for 16 minutes or until well browned. Flip the pork halfway through the cooking time. Transfer to a plate and set aside.
5. Pour the sauce mixture in the skillet and cook for 2 minutes or until warmed through and lightly thickened. Mix in the chives and lemon zest.
6. Baste the pork with the sauce mixture and serve immediately.

Per Serving
Calories: 200 | fat: 8.0g | protein: 30.0g | carbs: 1.0g | fiber: 0g | sugar: 1.0g | sodium: 394mg

Coriander spiced Ground Lamb with Salad

Prep time: 10 minutes | Cook time: 15 minutes | Serves 4

Pinch red pepper flakes
1 teaspoon sea salt, divided
2 cucumbers, peeled and chopped
½ red onion, finely chopped
1 pound (454 g)
ground lamb
2 teaspoons ground coriander
1 teaspoon ground cumin
3 garlic cloves, minced
1 tablespoon fresh mint, chopped

1. Preheat the oven to 375ºF (190ºC). Line a rimmed baking sheet with parchment paper.
2. In a medium bowl, whisk together the vinegar, red pepper flakes, and ½ teaspoon of salt. Add the cucumbers and onion and toss to combine. Set aside.
3. In a large bowl, mix the lamb, coriander, cumin, garlic, mint, and remaining ½ teaspoon of salt. Form the mixture into 1-inch meatballs and place them on the prepared baking sheet.
4. Bake until the lamb reaches 140ºF (60ºC) internally, about 15 minutes.
5. Serve with the salad on the side.

Per Serving
Calories: 346 | fat: 27.1g | protein: 20.1g | carbs: 6.9g | fiber: 1.1g | sugar: 5.0g | sodium: 363mg

15 Minute Spicy Green Onion Beef Bowls

Prep time: 15 minutes | Cook time: 15 minutes | Serves 4

1 pound (454 g) lean ground beef
1 bunch green onions, sliced
¼ cup fresh ginger, grated
1 cup rice cauliflower
¼ cup toasted sesame
oil
5 cloves garlic, diced fine
2 tablespoons light soy sauce
2 teaspoons sesame seeds

1. Heat oil in a large, cast iron skillet over high heat. Add all but 2 tablespoons, of the onions and cook until soft and starting to brown, about 5 minutes.
2. Add beef, and cook, breaking up with a spatula, until no longer pink. About 8 minutes.
3. Add remaining and simmer for 2 to 3 minutes, stirring frequently. Serve over hot cauliflower rice garnished with sesame seeds and reserved green onions.

Per Serving
Calories: 385 | fat: 21.0g | protein: 40.1g | carbs: 24.1g | fiber: 2.0g | sugar: 11.0g | sodium: 209mg

Steak Fajita Bowls with Chili-Lime

Prep time: 10 minutes | Cook time: 15 minutes | Serves 4

4 tablespoons extra-virgin olive oil, divided
1 head cauliflower, riced
1 pound (454 g) sirloin steak, cut into ¼-inch-thick strips
1 red bell pepper, seeded and sliced
1 onion, thinly sliced
2 garlic cloves, minced
Juice of 2 limes
1 teaspoon chili powder

1. In a large skillet over medium-high heat, heat 2 tablespoons of olive oil until it shimmers.
2. Add the cauliflower. Cook, stirring occasionally, until it softens, about 3 minutes. Set aside.
3. Wipe out the skillet with a paper towel. Add the remaining 2 tablespoons of oil to the skillet, and heat it on medium-high until it shimmers.

4. Add the steak and cook, stirring occasionally, until it browns, about 3 minutes. Use a slotted spoon to remove the steak from the oil in the pan and set aside.
5. Add the bell pepper and onion to the pan. Cook, stirring occasionally, until they start to brown, about 5 minutes.
6. Add the garlic and cook, stirring constantly, for 30 seconds.
7. Return the beef along with any juices that have collected and the cauliflower to the pan.
8. Add the lime juice and chili powder. Cook, stirring, until everything is warmed through, 2 to 3 minutes.

Per Serving
Calories: 311 | fat: 18.1g | protein: 27.1g | carbs: 13.1g | fiber: 2.9g | sugar: 10.0g | sodium: 94mg

Hot n Spicy Lamb Racks with Garlic and Herbs

Prep time: 15 minutes | Cook time: 20 minutes | Serves 4

1 tablespoon olive oil, plus more for brushing the grill grates
1 tablespoon garlic, minced
½ teaspoon salt
Freshly ground black pepper, to taste
2 (1-inch) sprig fresh
rosemary
2 (1½-pounds / 680-g) French lamb racks, trimmed of fat, cut into four pieces with two bones, and leave one bone with an equal amount of meat

1. Combine all the ingredients in a large bowl. Toss to coat the lamb racks well.
2. Wrap the bowl in plastic and refrigerate to marinate for at least 2 hours.
3. Preheat the grill over medium heat. Brush the grill grates with olive oil.
4. Remove the bowl from the refrigerator, and arrange the lamb racks on the grill grates, bone side down.
5. Grill for 3 minutes until lightly browned, then flip the lamb racks, and cover and grill for 15 minutes or until it reaches your desired doneness.
6. Remove the lamb racks from the grill grates and serve hot.

Per Serving
Calories: 192 | fat: 9.9g | protein: 22.2g | carbs: 1.0g | fiber: 0g | sugar: 0g | sodium: 347mg

Local Beef Bowl with Tomato sauce

Prep time: 10 minutes | Cook time: 3 to 4 hours | Serves 10

1½ pounds (680 g) lean ground beef
1 onion, diced fine
1 red bell pepper, diced
1 small tomato, diced
¼ cup cilantro, diced fine
1 cup tomato sauce
3 cloves garlic, diced
fine
¼ cup green olives, pitted
2 bay leaves
1½ teaspoons cumin
¼ teaspoon garlic powder
Salt and ground black pepper, to taste

1. In a large skillet, over medium heat, brown ground beef. Season with salt and pepper. Drain fat. Add onion, bell pepper, and garlic and cook for 3 to 4 minutes.
2. Transfer to crock pot and add remaining. Cover and cook on high 3 hours.
3. Discard bay leaves. Taste and adjust seasonings as desired. Serve.

Per Serving
Calories: 256 | fat: 9.0g | protein: 35.1g | carbs: 6.1g | fiber: 1.0g | sugar: 3.0g | sodium: 227mg

Next-level Steak & Tomato Sandwich

Prep time: 10 minutes | Cook time: 10 minutes | Serves 4

2 tablespoons balsamic vinegar
2 teaspoons freshly squeezed lemon juice
1 teaspoon fresh parsley, chopped
2 teaspoons fresh oregano, chopped
2 teaspoons garlic, minced
2 tablespoons olive oil
1 pound (454 g) flank steak, trimmed of fat
4 whole-wheat pitas
1 tomato, chopped
2 cups lettuce, shredded
1 red onion, thinly sliced

1. Combine the balsamic vinegar, lemon juice, parsley, oregano, garlic, and olive oil in a bowl.
2. Dunk the steak in the bowl to coat well, then wrap the bowl in plastic and refrigerate for at least 1 hour.
3. Preheat the oven to 450ºF (235ºC).
4. Remove the bowl from the refrigerator. Discard the marinade and arrange the steak on a baking sheet lined with aluminum foil.
5. Broil in the preheated oven for 10 minutes for medium. Flip the steak halfway through the cooking time.
6. Remove the steak from the oven and allow cooling for 10 minutes. Slice the steak into strips.
7. Assemble the pitas with steak, tomato, lettuce, and onion to make the sandwich, and serve warm.

Per Serving
Calories: 345 | fat: 15.8g | protein: 28.1g | carbs: 21.9g | fiber: 3.1g | sugar: 18.8g | sodium: 295mg

Garlicky Tomato Beef with Chive Dumplings

Prep time: 15 minutes | Cook time: 1 hour | Serves 6

2 pounds (907 g) chuck steak, trim fat and cut into bite-sized pieces
3 onions, quartered
1 green pepper, chopped
1 red pepper, chopped
1 orange pepper, chopped
3 cups water
1 can tomatoes, chopped
1 cup low sodium beef broth
3 cloves garlic, diced fine
2 tablespoons tomato paste
1 tablespoon olive oil
1 tablespoon paprika
2 teaspoons hot smoked paprika
2 bay leaves
Salt and ground black pepper, to taste

1. Heat oil in a large soup pot over medium-high.
2. Add steak and cook until browned, stirring frequently. Add onions and cook 5 minutes, or until soft.
3. Add garlic and cook another minute, stirring frequently.
4. Add remaining. Stir well and bring to a boil. Reduce heat to medium-low and simmer 45 to 50 minutes, stirring occasionally.
5. Goulash is done when steak is tender. Stir and serve with Chive dumplings.

Per Serving
Calories: 412 | fat: 15.0g | protein: 53.1g | carbs: 14.1g | fiber: 3.0g | sugar: 8.0g | sodium: 159mg

Loaded Easy Cheesy Cauliflower Scallion Pot

Prep time: 15 minutes | Cook time: 20 minutes | Serves 6

6 slices bacon, cooked and crumbled, divided
3 scallions, sliced thin, divided
5 cup cauliflower
2 cup cheddar cheese, grated and divided

1 cup fat free sour cream
½ teaspoon salt
¼ teaspoon fresh cracked pepper
Nonstick cooking spray

1. Heat oven to 350ºF (180ºC). Spray casserole dish with cooking spray.
2. Steam cauliflower until just tender.
3. In a large bowl, combine cauliflower, sour cream, half the bacon, half the scallions and half the cheese. Stir in salt and pepper. Place in prepared baking dish and sprinkle remaining cheese over top.
4. Bake 18 to 20 minutes until heated through. Sprinkle remaining scallions and bacon over top and serve.

Per Serving
Calories: 333 | fat: 20.0g | protein: 21.1g | carbs: 15.1g | fiber: 4.0g | sugar: 6.0g | sodium: 681mg

Cheesy Ground Beef and Vegetable Fold

Prep time: 15 minutes | Cook time: 10 minutes | Serves 4

¾ pound (340 g) lean ground beef
2 tomatoes, seeded and diced
1 onion, diced
1 zucchini, grated
1 carrot, grated
¾ cup mushrooms, diced
½ cup Mozzarella cheese, grated

¼ cup cilantro, diced
4 (8-inch) whole wheat tortillas, warmed
2 cloves garlic, diced
2 teaspoons chili powder
¼ teaspoon salt
¼ teaspoon hot pepper sauce
Nonstick cooking spray

1. Heat oven to 400ºF (205ºC). Spray a large baking sheet with cooking spray.
2. Cook beef and onions in a large nonstick skillet over medium heat, until beef is no longer pink, drain fat. Transfer to a bowl and keep warm.
3. Add the mushrooms, zucchini, carrot, garlic, chili powder, salt and pepper sauce to the skillet and cook until vegetables are tender.
4. Stir in the tomatoes, cilantro and beef.
5. Lay the tortillas on the prepared pan. Cover half of each with beef mixture, and top with cheese.
6. Fold other half over filling. Bake 5 minutes. Flip over and bake 5 to 6 minute more or until cheese has melted. Cut into wedges and serve.

Per Serving
Calories: 320 | fat: 7.0g | protein: 33.1g | carbs: 31.1g | fiber: 5.0g | sugar: 5.0g | sodium: 575mg

Garlicky Pork Tacos with Cabbage and Onions

Prep time: 20 minutes | Cook time: 6 hours | Serves 16

2 pounds (907 g) pork shoulder, trim off excess fat
2 onions, diced fine
2 cups cabbages, shredded
16 (6-inch) low carb whole wheat tortillas

4 chipotle peppers in adobo sauce, puréed
1 cup light barbecue sauce
2 cloves garlic, diced fine
1½ teaspoons paprika

1. In a medium bowl, whisk together garlic, barbecue sauce and chipotles, cover and chill.
2. Place pork in the crock pot. Cover and cook on low 8 to 10 hours, or on high 4 to 6 hours.
3. Transfer pork to a cutting board. Use two forks and shred the pork, discarding the fat. Place pork back in the crock pot. Sprinkle with paprika then pour the barbecue sauce over mixture.
4. Stir to combine, cover and cook 1 hour. Skim off excess fat.
5. To assemble the tacos: place about ¼ cup of pork on warmed tortilla. Top with cabbage and onions and serve. Refrigerate any leftover pork up to 3 days.

Per Serving
Calories: 266 | fat: 14.0g | protein: 17.1g | carbs: 14.1g | fiber: 9.0g | sugar: 3.0g | sodium: 434mg

Ground Turkey with Cauliflower Rice

Prep time: 10 minutes | Cook time: 20 minutes | Serves 2

2 tablespoons extra-virgin olive oil
½ pound (227 g) ground turkey
1 onion, chopped
1 green bell pepper, seeded and chopped
½ teaspoon sea salt
1 small head cauliflower, grated
½ cup corn kernels
½ cup prepared salsa
½ cup shredded pepper Jack cheese

1. In a large non-stick skillet over medium-high heat, heat the olive oil until it shimmers.
2. Add the turkey. Cook, crumbling with a spoon, until browned, about 5 minutes.
3. Add the onion, bell pepper, and salt. Cook, stirring occasionally, until the vegetables soften, 4 to 5 minutes.
4. Add the cauliflower, corn, and salsa. Cook, stirring, until the cauliflower rice softens, about 3 minutes more.
5. Sprinkle with the cheese. Reduce heat to low, cover, and allow the cheese to melt, 2 or 3 minutes.

Per Serving
Calories: 448 | fat: 30g | protein: 30g | carbs: 18 g | fiber: 4g | sugar: 19.46g | sodium: 649mg

Low Sugar Ground Turkey Meat Balls

Prep time: 10 minutes | Cook time: 20 minutes | Serves 4

¼ cup tomato paste
1 tablespoon Worcestershire sauce
½ cup milk
½ cup whole-wheat bread crumbs
1 pound (454 g)
ground turkey
1 onion, grated
1 tablespoon Dijon mustard
1 teaspoon dried thyme
½ teaspoon sea salt

1. Preheat the oven to 375°F (190°C). Line a rimmed baking sheet with parchment paper.
2. In a small saucepan on medium-low heat, whisk together the tomato paste, and Worcestershire sauce. Bring to a simmer and then remove from the heat.
3. In a large bowl, combine the milk and bread crumbs. Let rest for 5 minutes.
4. Add the ground turkey, onion, mustard, thyme, and salt. Using your hands, mix well without over mixing.
5. Form into 1-inch meatballs and place on the prepared baking sheet. Brush the tops with the tomato paste mixture.
6. Bake until the meatballs reach 165°F (74°C) internally, about 15 minutes.

Per Serving
Calories: 285 | fat: 11g | protein: 24g | carbs: 22g | fiber: 2g | sugar: 19.7g | sodium: 465mg

Sirloin Steak & Broccoli Buddha Bowls

Prep time: 10 minutes | Cook time: 15 minutes | Serves 4

2 tablespoons extra-virgin olive oil
1 pound (454 g) sirloin steak, cut into ¼-inch-thick strips
2 cups broccoli florets
1 garlic clove, minced
1 teaspoon peeled and grated fresh ginger
2 tablespoons reduced-sodium soy sauce
¼ cup beef broth
½ teaspoon Chinese hot mustard
Pinch red pepper flakes

1. In a large skillet over medium-high heat, heat the olive oil until it shimmers.
2. Add the beef. Cook, stirring, until it browns, 3 to 5 minutes. With a slotted spoon, remove the beef from the oil and set it aside on a plate.
3. Add the broccoli to the oil. Cook, stirring, until it is crisp-tender, about 4 minutes.
4. Add the garlic and ginger and cook, stirring constantly, for 30 seconds.
5. Return the beef to the pan, along with any juices that have collected.
6. In a small bowl, whisk together the soy sauce, broth, mustard, and red pepper flakes.
7. Add the soy sauce mixture to the skillet and cook, stirring, until everything warms through, about 3 minutes.

Per Serving
Calories: 230 | fat: 11.1g | protein: 27.1g | carbs: 4.9g | fiber: 1.0g | sugar: 3.0g | sodium: 376mg

Ultimate Beef and Vegetables Pot

Prep time: 15 minutes | Cook time: 4 hours | Serves 4

1 tablespoon olive oil
2 medium celery stalks, halved lengthwise and cut into 3-inch pieces
4 medium carrots, scrubbed, halved lengthwise, and cut into 3-inch pieces
1 medium onion cut in eighths
1¼ pounds (567 g)
lean chuck roast, boneless, trimmed of fat
2 teaspoons Worcestershire sauce
1 tablespoon balsamic vinegar
2 tablespoons water
1 tablespoon onion soup mix
½ teaspoon ground black pepper

1. Grease a slow cooker with olive oil.
2. Put the celery, carrots, and onion in the slow cooker, then add the beef.
3. Top them with Worcestershire sauce, balsamic vinegar, and water, and then sprinkle with onion soup mix and black pepper.
4. Cover and cook on high for 4 hours.
5. Allow to cool for 20 minutes, and then serve them on a large plate.

Per Serving
Calories: 250 | fat: 6.0g | protein: 33.0g | carbs: 15.0g | fiber: 3.0g | sugar: 6.0g | sodium: 510mg

Aromatic Lamb Parsley Cutlets

Prep time: 4 hours 20 minutes | Cook time: 8 minutes | Serves 4

¼ cup freshly squeezed lime juice
2 tablespoons lime zest
2 tablespoons chopped fresh parsley
Sea salt and freshly
ground black pepper, to taste
1 tablespoon extra-virgin olive oil
12 lamb cutlets (about 1½ pounds / 680 g in total)

1. Combine the lime juice and zest, parsley, salt, black pepper, and olive oil in a large bowl. Stir to mix well.
2. Dunk the lamb cutlets in the bowl of the lime mixture, and then toss to coat well. Wrap the bowl in plastic and refrigerate to marinate for at least 4 hours.
3. Preheat the oven to 450ºF (235ºC) or broil. Line a baking sheet with aluminum foil.
4. Remove the bowl from the refrigerator and let sit for 10 minutes, and then discard the marinade. Arrange the lamb cutlets on the baking sheet.
5. Broil the lamb in the preheated oven for 8 minutes or until it reaches your desired doneness. Flip the cutlets with tongs to make sure they are cooked evenly.
6. Serve immediately.

Per Serving
Calories: 297 | fat: 18.8g | protein: 31.0g | carbs: 1.0g | fiber: 0g | sugar: 0g | sodium: 100mg

Best Ever Cheese Roasted Beef

Prep time: 15 minutes | Cook time: 35 minutes | Serves 4

4 slices low-salt deli roast beef, cut into ½-inch strips
4 slices Mozzarella cheese, cut in half
2 large green bell peppers, slice in half, remove seeds, and blanch in boiling water 1 minute
1½ cup sliced mushrooms
1 cup thinly sliced onion
1 tablespoon margarine
1 tablespoon vegetable oil
2 teaspoons garlic, diced fine
¼ teaspoon salt
¼ teaspoon black pepper

1. Heat oven to 400ºF (205ºC). Place peppers, skin side down, in baking dish.
2. Heat oil and margarine in a large skillet over medium heat. Once hot, add onions, mushrooms, garlic, salt, and pepper, and cook, stirring occasionally, 10 to 12 minutes or mushrooms are tender.
3. Remove from heat and stir in roast beef.
4. Place a piece of cheese inside each pepper and fill with meat mixture. Cover with foil and bake 20 minutes.
5. Remove the foil and top each pepper with remaining cheese. Bake another 5 minutes, or until cheese is melted.

Per Serving
Calories: 192 | fat: 12.0g | protein: 12.1g | carbs: 10.1g | fiber: 2.0g | sugar: 5.0g | sodium: 234mg

Coffee Flavoured Flank Steak

Prep time: 10 minutes | Cook time: 10 minutes | Serves 4

¼ cup whole coffee beans
2 teaspoons fresh rosemary, chopped
2 teaspoons fresh thyme, chopped
2 teaspoons garlic, minced
1 teaspoon freshly ground black pepper
2 tablespoons apple cider vinegar
2 tablespoons olive oil
1 pound (454 g) flank steak, trimmed of fat

1. Put the coffee beans, rosemary, thyme, garlic, and black pepper in a food processor. Pulse until well ground and combined.
2. Pour the mixture in a large bowl, and then pour the vinegar and olive oil in the bowl. Stir to mix well.
3. Dunk the steak in the mixture, then wrap the bowl in plastic and refrigerate to marinate for 2 hours.
4. Preheat the broiler to medium.
5. Remove the bowl from the refrigerator, and discard the marinade.
6. Place the marinated steak on a baking sheet lined with aluminum foil.
7. Broil in the preheated broiler for 10 minutes or until the steak reaches your desired doneness. Flip the steak halfway through the cooking time.
8. Remove the steak from the broiler. Allow cooling for a few minutes and slice to serve.

Per Serving
Calories: 316 | fat: 19.8g | protein: 31.1g | carbs: 0g | fiber: 0g | sugar: 0g | sodium: 78mg

Buttery Tenderloin Steaks with Gravy

Prep time: 10 minutes | Cook time: 15 minutes | Serves 4

4 beef tenderloin steaks
2 tablespoons blue cheese, crumbled
4½ teaspoon fresh parsley, diced
4½ teaspoon chives, diced
1½ teaspoons butter
½ cup low sodium beef broth
4½ teaspoon bread crumbs
1 tablespoon flour
¼ teaspoon pepper
Nonstick cooking spray

1. Heat oven to 350ºF (180ºC). Spray a large baking sheet with cooking spray.
2. In a small bowl, combine blue cheese, bread crumbs, parsley, chives, and pepper. Press onto one side of the steaks.
3. Spray a large skillet with cooking spray and place over medium-high heat.
4. Add steaks and sear 2 minutes per side. Transfer to prepared baking sheet and bake for 6 to 8 minutes, or steaks reach desired doneness.
5. Melt butter in a small saucepan over medium heat. Whisk in flour until smooth. Slowly whisk in broth. Bring to a boil, cook, stirring, 2 minutes or until thickened.
6. Plate the steaks and top with gravy. Serve.

Per Serving
Calories: 265 | fat: 10.0g | protein: 36.1g | carbs: 4.1g | fiber: 0g | sugar: 0g | sodium: 879mg

Cheesy Lettuce wraps with Mushroom and Beef

Prep time: 5 minutes | Cook time: 20 minutes | Serves 4

1 tablespoon avocado oil
1 cup Portobello mushrooms, chopped
½ cup white onion, chopped
1 pound (454 g) 93% lean ground beef
½ teaspoon garlic
powder
Salt, to taste
1 (10-ounce / 284-g) bag frozen cauliflower rice
¾ cup Cheddar cheese, shredded
12 iceberg lettuce leaves

1. Heath the avocado oil in a nonstick skillet over medium heat.
2. Add the mushrooms and onion to the skillet and sauté for 5 minutes until the mushrooms are soft and the onion starts to become translucent.
3. Add the beef, garlic powder, and salt to the skillet and sauté for another 5 minutes to brown the beef.
4. Increase the heat to medium-high, and then add the cauliflower rice and sauté for an additional 5 minutes.
5. Divide the mixture and cheese on all lettuce leaves with a spoon, then roll up the lettuce to seal the wrap and serve warm.

Per Serving
Calories: 289 | fat: 14.8g | protein: 31.2g | carbs: 6.9g | fiber: 3.1g | sugar: 3.8g | sodium: 262mg

Smoked Sausage Zucchini Vegetables

Prep time: 10 minutes | Cook time: 15 minutes | Serves 6

1 package smoked sausage, cut in ¼-inch slices
1 cup half-and-half
½ cup zucchini cut in matchsticks
½ cup carrots cut in matchsticks
½ cup red bell pepper cut in matchsticks
½ cup peas, frozen
¼ cup margarine

¼ cup onion, diced
2 tablespoons fresh parsley, diced
1 cup whole-wheat pasta, cooked and drained
⅓ cup reduced fat Parmesan cheese
1 clove garlic, diced fine
Salt and ground black pepper, to taste

1. Melt margarine in a large skillet over medium heat. Add onion and garlic and cook, stirring occasionally, 3 to 4 minutes or until onion is soft.
2. Increase heat to medium-high. Add sausage, zucchini, carrots, and red pepper. Cook, stirring frequently, 5 to 6 minutes, or until carrots are tender crisp.
3. Stir in peas and half-and-half, cook for 1 to 2 minutes until heated through. Stir in cheese, parsley, salt, and pepper. Add pasta and toss to mix. Serve.

Per Serving
Calories: 285 | fat: 15.0g | protein: 21.1g | carbs: 18.1g | fiber: 4.0g | sugar: 8.0g | sodium: 807mg

Supper Beef and Cauliflower Rice

Prep time: 10 minutes | Cook time: 25 minutes | Serves 4

¾ pound (340 g) lean ground beef
2 cup cauliflower rice, cooked
1 red bell pepper, sliced thin
½ yellow onion, diced
1 stalk celery, sliced thin

1 jalapeño pepper, seeds removed and diced fine
¼ cup fresh parsley, diced
½ cup low sodium beef broth
4 teaspoons Cajun seasoning

1. Place beef and 1½ teaspoons Cajun seasoning in a large skillet over medium-high heat. Cook, breaking apart with wooden spoon, until no longer pink, about 10 minutes.
2. Add vegetables, except cauliflower, and remaining Cajun seasoning. Cook, stirring occasionally, 6 to 8 minutes, or until vegetables are tender.
3. Add broth and stir, scraping brown bits from the bottom of the pan. Cook 2 to 3 minutes until mixture has thickened. Stir in cauliflower and cook just until heated through. Remove from heat, stir in parsley and serve.

Per Serving
Calories: 200 | fat: 6.0g | protein: 28.1g | carbs: 8.1g | fiber: 2.0g | sugar: 4.0g | sodium: 291mg

Moroccan Beef Carrot Stew

Prep time: 20 minutes | Cook time: 1 hour 40 minutes | Serves 8

2 tablespoons olive oil
1½ pounds (680 g) lean beef stew meat
2 carrots cut ½ inch thick slices
2 celery stalks, diced
1 onion, diced
2½ cup low-sodium beef broth
½ cup prunes, diced
1 cup hot water

2 (6-ounce / 170-g) sweet potatoes, peeled and diced into 1-inch chunks
1½ teaspoon ground cinnamon
1 teaspoon salt
1 teaspoon black pepper
¼ teaspoon parsley, chopped

1. Heat the olive oil in a stockpot over high heat.
2. Arrange the beef in a single layer in the pot and cook for 12 minutes or until browned on all sides. You may need to work in batches to avoid overcrowding. Transfer the beef to a plate and set aside.
3. Add carrots, celery, and onions to the pot and sauté for 5 minutes or until the onions are translucent.
4. Pour the beef broth over, and then put the beef back to the pot. Simmer for 1 hour.
5. Meanwhile, soak the prunes in hot water for 20 minutes, and then pat dry with paper towels. Reserve ½ cup of the prune water.
6. Add the prunes, prune water, sweet potatoes, cinnamon, salt, and black pepper to the pot. Cover and simmer for 20 minutes until potatoes are soft.
7. Spoon the stew in a large bowl, then serve with chopped parsley on top.

Per Serving
Calories: 196 | fat: 4.9g | protein: 19.1g | carbs: 17.8g | fiber: 3.1g | sugar: 7.9g | sodium: 205mg

Chapter 9: Soups and Stews

Authentic Gazpacho

Prep time: 15 minutes | Cook time: 0 minutes | Serves 4

3 pounds (1.4 kg) ripe tomatoes, chopped
1 cup low-sodium tomato juice
½ red onion, chopped
1 cucumber, peeled, seeded, and chopped
1 red bell pepper, seeded and chopped
2 celery stalks, chopped
2 tablespoons chopped

fresh parsley
2 garlic cloves, chopped
2 tablespoons extra-virgin olive oil
2 tablespoons red wine vinegar
1 teaspoon honey
½ teaspoon salt
¼ teaspoons freshly ground black pepper

1. In a blender jar, combine the tomatoes, tomato juice, onion, cucumber, bell pepper, celery, parsley, garlic, olive oil, vinegar, honey, salt, and pepper. Pulse until blended but still slightly chunky.
2. Adjust the seasonings as needed and serve.
3. To store, transfer to a nonreactive, airtight container and refrigerate for up to 3 days.

Per Serving
Calories: 172 | fat: 8.1g | protein: 5.1g | carbs: 23.9g | fiber: 6.1g | sugar: 16.0g | sodium: 333mg

Delicious Low Sodium Beef Chili Stew

Prep time: 15 minutes | Cook time: 1 hour 30 minutes | Serves 6

1½ pound (680 g) beef round steak, cut into ½-inch pieces
1¾ cup tomatoes, diced
1 cup carrots, sliced
1 cup onion, diced
¼ cup sweet red pepper, diced
1 jalapeno, seeded and diced
2 tablespoons cilantro,

diced
1¾ cup low sodium beef broth
1 clove garlic, diced
2 tablespoons flour
2 tablespoons water
1 tablespoon vegetable oil
1½ teaspoons chili powder
½ teaspoon salt

1. Heat the oil in a large pot over medium-high heat. Add the steak and cook until brown on all sides.

2. Add the broth, carrots, onion, red pepper, jalapeno, garlic, and seasonings and bring to a low boil. Reduce heat to low, cover and simmer 45 minutes, stirring occasionally.
3. Add the tomatoes and continue cooking 15 minutes.
4. Stir the flour and water together in a measuring up until smooth.
5. Add to stew with the cilantro and continue cooking another 20 to 30 minutes or until stew has thickened. Serve.

Per Serving
Calories: 313 | fat: 13.0g | protein: 39.2g | carbs: 9.1g | fiber: 2.2g | sugar: 4.1g | sodium: 306mg

Quick and Easy Chicken Ham Bone Soup

Prep time: 15 minutes | Cook time: 20 minutes | Serves 6

3 cups low-sodium chicken broth, divided
1 medium onion, chopped
3 garlic cloves, minced
1 bunch collard greens or mustard greens including stems,

roughly chopped
1 fresh ham bone
5 carrots, peeled and cut into 1-inch rounds
2 fresh thyme sprigs
3 bay leaves
Freshly ground black pepper, to taste

1. Select the Sauté setting on an electric pressure cooker, and combine ½ cup of chicken broth, the onion, and garlic and cook for 3 to 5 minutes, or until the onion and garlic are translucent.
2. Add the collard greens, ham bone, carrots, and remaining 2½ cups of broth, the thyme, and bay leaves.
3. Close and lock the lid and set the pressure valve to sealing.
4. Change to the Manual/Pressure Cook setting, and cook for 15 minutes.
5. Once cooking is complete, quick-release the pressure. Carefully remove the lid. Discard the bay leaves.
6. Serve with Skillet Bivalves.

Per Serving
Calories: 100 | fat: 4.1g | protein: 6.1g | carbs: 9.9g | fiber: 3.1g | sugar: 4.0g | sodium: 200mg

Traditional Mixed Chicken Pork Soup

Prep time: 5 minutes | Cook time: 25 minutes | Serves 6

1 yellow onion, diced fine
1½ cup pork, cook and shred
1 fresh lime cut in wedges
½ bunch cilantro, chopped
1 (15-ounce / 425-g) can hominy, drain
1 (4-ounce / 113-g) can green chilies, diced
3 ounces (85 g) tomato paste

3 cup low sodium chicken broth
2 cup water
2 tablespoons vegetable oil
2 tablespoons flour
2 tablespoons chili powder
¾ teaspoon salt
½ teaspoon cumin
½ teaspoon garlic powder
¼ teaspoon cayenne pepper

1. Heat oil in a large pot over medium heat. Add onion and cook 3 to 5 minutes, or until it softens.
2. Add the flour and chili powder and cook 2 minutes more, stirring continuously.
3. Add water, tomato paste, and seasonings. Whisk mixture until tomato paste dissolves. Bring to a simmer and let thicken, about 2 to 3 minutes.
4. Stir in broth, pork, chilies, and hominy and cook until heated through, about 10 minutes.
5. Ladle into bowls and garnish with a lime wedge and chopped cilantro.

Per Serving
Calories: 235 | fat: 8.0g | protein: 11.2g | carbs: 33.1g | fiber: 9.2g | sugar: 12.1g | sodium: 913mg

Creamy Smooth Asparagus Veggie Soup

Prep time: 10 minutes | Cook time: 20 minutes | Serves 4

2 pounds (907 g) fresh asparagus remove the bottom and cut into small pieces
1 yellow onion, diced
1 small lemon, zest and juice
1 teaspoon fresh

thyme, diced fine
4 cup low sodium vegetable broth
3 tablespoons olive oil
3 cloves garlic, diced fine
Salt and ground black pepper, to taste

1. Heat oil in a large saucepan over medium-high heat. Add asparagus and onion and cook, stirring occasionally, until nicely browned, about 5 minutes. Add garlic and cook 1 minute more.
2. Stir in remaining and bring to a boil. Reduce heat, and simmer 12 to 15 minutes or until asparagus is soft.
3. Use an immersion blender and process until smooth. Salt and ground black pepper, to taste and serve.

Per Serving
Calories: 170 | fat: 11.0g | protein: 6.2g | carbs: 17.1g | fiber: 6.2g | sugar: 7.1g | sodium: 185mg

Quick Onion Tomato Veggie Soup

Prep time: 10 minutes | Cook time: 15 minutes | Serves 4

1 tablespoon extra-virgin olive oil
1 medium onion, chopped
2 carrots, finely chopped
3 garlic cloves, minced
4 cups low-sodium vegetable broth

1 (28-ounce / 794-g) can crushed tomatoes
½ teaspoon dried oregano
¼ teaspoon dried basil
4 cups chopped baby kale leaves
¼ teaspoon salt

1. In a large pot, heat the oil over medium heat.
2. Add the onion and carrots to the pan. Sauté for 3 to 5 minutes until they begin to soften. Add the garlic and sauté for 30 seconds more, until fragrant.
3. Add the vegetable broth, tomatoes, oregano, and basil to the pot and bring to a boil. Reduce the heat to low and simmer for 5 minutes.
4. Using an immersion blender, purée the soup.
5. Add the kale and simmer for 3 more minutes. Season with the salt. Serve immediately.

Per Serving
Calories: 172 | fat: 5.1g | protein: 6.1g | carbs: 30.9g | fiber: 9.1g | sugar: 13.0g | sodium: 583mg

Low Carb Leek Veggie Soup

Prep time: 10 minutes | Cook time: 20 minutes | Serves 2

Avocado oil cooking spray
2½ cups chopped leeks (2 to 3 leeks)
2½ cups cauliflower florets
1 garlic clove, peeled
⅓ cup low-sodium vegetable broth
½ cup half-and-half
¼ teaspoon salt
¼ teaspoons freshly ground black pepper

1. Heat a large stockpot over medium-low heat. When hot, coat the cooking surface with cooking spray. Put the leeks and cauliflower into the pot.
2. Increase the heat to medium and cover the pan. Cook for 10 minutes, stirring halfway through.
3. Add the garlic and cook for 5 minutes.
4. Add the broth and deglaze the pan, stirring to scrape up the browned bits from the bottom.
5. Transfer the broth and vegetables to a food processor or blender and add the half-and-half, salt, and pepper. Blend well.

Per Serving
Calories: 174 | fat: 7.1g | protein: 6.1g | carbs: 23.9g | fiber: 5.1g | sugar: 8.0g | sodium: 490mg

Cheesy Beef Tomato Soup

Prep time: 5 minutes | Cook time: 25 minutes | Serves 4

Avocado oil cooking spray
½ cup diced white onion
½ cup diced celery
½ cup sliced Portobello mushrooms
1 pound (454 g) 93% lean ground beef
1 (15-ounce / 425-g) can no-salt-added diced tomatoes
2 cups low-sodium beef broth
⅓ cup half-and-half
¾ cup shredded sharp Cheddar cheese

1. Heat a large stockpot over medium-low heat. When hot, coat the cooking surface with cooking spray. Put the onion, celery, and mushrooms into the pot. Cook for 7 minutes, stirring occasionally.
2. Add the ground beef and cook for 5 minutes, stirring and breaking apart as needed.
3. Add the diced tomatoes with their juices and the broth. Increase the heat to medium-high and simmer for 10 minutes.
4. Remove the pot from the heat and stir in the half-and-half.
5. Serve topped with the cheese.

Per Serving
Calories: 332 | fat: 18.1g | protein: 33.1g | carbs: 8.9g | fiber: 2.1g | sugar: 5.0g | sodium: 320mg

Sweet Potato Beef Soup for Four

Prep time: 20 minutes | Cook time: 30 minutes | Serves 4

2 teaspoons olive oil
1 tablespoon garlic, minced
1 sweet onion, chopped
2 carrots, peeled, diced
1 sweet potato, peeled, diced
4 celery stalks, with greens, chopped
2 cups cooked beef, diced
1 cup cooked pearl barley
8 cups low-sodium beef broth
2 teaspoons hot sauce
2 bay leaves
1 cup kale, shredded
2 teaspoons fresh thyme, chopped
Salt and freshly ground black pepper, to taste

1. Heat the olive oil in a stockpot over medium-high heat.
2. Add the garlic and onion to the pot and sauté for 3 minutes or until the onion is translucent and the garlic is fragrant.
3. Add the carrot, sweet potato, and celery to the pot and sauté for 5 minutes more.
4. Add the beef, barley, beef broth, hot sauce, and bay leaves to the pot.
5. Bring to a boil, and then reduce the heat to low and simmer for 15 minutes until the beef is browned and the vegetables are tender.
6. Discard the bay leaves, and then add the kale and thyme to the pot. Sprinkle with salt and black pepper, and simmer for an additional 5 minutes.
7. Pour the soup in a large bowl, then serve warm.

Per Serving
Calories: 697 | fat: 23.9g | protein: 54.6g | carbs: 76.6g | fiber: 5.7g | sugar: 11.9g | sodium: 282mg

Classic Spicy Macaroni Bowl

Prep time: 10 minutes | Cook time: 20 minutes | Serves 4

2 tablespoons extra-virgin olive oil
1 onion, chopped
1 red bell pepper, seeded and chopped
2 garlic cloves, minced
2 cups green beans (fresh or frozen; halved if fresh)
6 cups low-sodium

vegetable broth
1 (14-ounce / 397-g) can crushed tomatoes
1 tablespoon Italian seasoning
½ cup dried whole-wheat elbow macaroni
½ teaspoon sea salt
Pinch red pepper flakes (or to taste)

1. In a large pot over medium-high heat, heat the olive oil until it shimmers. Add the onion and bell pepper and cook, stirring occasionally, until they soften, about 3 minutes.
2. Add the garlic and cook, stirring constantly, for 30 seconds.
3. Add the green beans, vegetable broth, tomatoes, and Italian seasoning and bring to a boil.
4. Add the elbow macaroni, salt, and red pepper flakes. Cook, stirring occasionally, until the macaroni is soft, about 8 minutes.

Per Serving
Calories: 200 | fat: 7.1g | protein: 5.1g | carbs: 28.9g | fiber: 7.1g | sugar: 12.8g | sodium: 478mg

Simple Veggie Bacon Soup

Prep time: 10 minutes | Cook time: 15 minutes | Serves 4

2 tablespoons extra-virgin olive oil
3 slices pepper bacon, chopped
1 onion, chopped
1 red bell pepper, seeded and chopped
1 fennel bulb, chopped

3 tablespoons flour
5 cups low-sodium or unsalted chicken broth
6 ounces (170 g) chopped canned clams, undrained
½ teaspoon sea salt
½ cup milk

1. In a large pot over medium-high heat, heat the olive oil until it shimmers. Add the bacon and cook, stirring, until browned, about 4 minutes.
2. Remove the bacon from the fat with a slotted spoon, and set it aside on a plate.

3. Add the onion, bell pepper, and fennel to the fat in the pot. Cook, stirring occasionally, until the vegetables are soft, about 5 minutes.
4. Add the flour and cook, stirring constantly, for 1 minute.
5. Add the broth, clams, and salt. Bring to a simmer. Cook, stirring, until the soup thickens, about 5 minutes more.
6. Stir in the milk and return the bacon to the pot. Cook, stirring, 1 minute more.

Per Serving
Calories: 336 | fat: 20.1g | protein: 20.1g | carbs: 20.9g | fiber: 3.1g | sugar: 11.4g | sodium: 495mg

Everyday Lentil Carrot Vegetable Soup

Prep time: 10 minutes | Cook time: 55 minutes | Serves 8

1 teaspoon olive oil
1 tablespoon garlic, minced
1 sweet onion, chopped
3 carrots, peeled and diced
4 celery stalks, with the greens, chopped
2 bay leaves
3 cups red lentils,

picked over, washed, and drained
4 cups low-sodium vegetable soup
3 cups water
2 teaspoons fresh thyme, chopped
Salt and freshly ground black pepper, to taste

1. Heat the olive oil in a stockpot over medium-high heat.
2. Add the garlic and onion to the pot and sauté for 3 minutes until the onion is translucent.
3. Add the carrots and celery to the pot and sauté for 5 minutes.
4. Add the bay leaves, lentils, vegetables soup, and water to the pot. Bring to a boil.
5. Turn down the heat to low and simmer for 45 minutes until lentils are tender and soup starts to have a thick consistency.
6. Pour the soup in a large bowl. Discard the bay leaves, and top with thyme, salt, and black pepper before serving.

Per Serving
Calories: 285 | fat: 1.9g | protein: 20.1g | carbs: 46.8g | fiber: 24.2g | sugar: 3.8g | sodium: 417mg

Mom's Special Vegetable Beef Soup

Prep time: 10 minutes | Cook time: 15 minutes | Serves 4

1 pound (454 g) ground beef
1 onion, chopped
2 celery stalks, chopped
1 carrot, chopped
1 teaspoon dried rosemary
6 cups low-sodium beef or chicken broth
½ teaspoon sea salt
⅛ Teaspoon freshly ground black pepper
2 cups peas

1. In a large pot over medium-high heat, cook the ground beef, crumbling with the side of a spoon, until browned, about 5 minutes.
2. Add the onion, celery, carrot, and rosemary. Cook, stirring occasionally, until the vegetables start to soften, about 5 minutes.
3. Add the broth, salt, pepper, and peas. Bring to a simmer. Reduce the heat and simmer, stirring, until warmed through, about 5 minutes more.

Per Serving
Calories: 356 | fat: 17.1g | protein: 34.1g | carbs: 17.9g | fiber: 5.1g | sugar: 12.6g | sodium: 363mg

Homemade Cinnamon Lamb Sweet Potato Stew

Prep time: 20 minutes | Cook time: 2 hours 15 minutes | Serves 4

2 tablespoons olive oil
1½ pounds (680 g) lamb shoulder, cut into 1-inch chunks
1 teaspoon ground cinnamon
1 teaspoon ground cumin
1 tablespoon fresh ginger, grated
2 teaspoons garlic, minced
¼ teaspoon ground cloves
½ sweet onion, chopped
2 cups low-sodium beef broth
2 sweet potatoes, peeled, diced
2 teaspoons chopped fresh parsley, for garnish
Salt and freshly ground black pepper, to taste

1. Preheat the oven to 300ºF (150ºC). Heat the olive oil in an oven-safe skillet over medium-high heat.
2. Brown the lamb shoulder in the skillet for 6 minutes. Shake the skillet periodically.
3. Add the cinnamon, cumin, ginger, garlic, cloves, and onion to the skillet and sauté for 5 minutes or until aromatic.
4. Add the beef broth and sweet potatoes to the skillet. Bring to a boil. Stir constantly.
5. Put the skillet lid on and cook in the preheated oven for 2 hours until the lamb is fork-tender.
6. Divide the stew among four bowls, then top with parsley, salt, and pepper. Give it a stir before serving.

Per Serving
Calories: 488 | fat: 24.1g | protein: 40.6g | carbs: 30.5g | fiber: 3.2g | sugar: 7.5g | sodium: 182mg

Quick and Easy Green Pea Carrot Soup

Prep time: 8 minutes | Cook time: 15 minutes | Serves 4

1½ cups dried green split peas, rinsed and drained
4 cups vegetable broth or water
2 celery stalks, chopped
1 medium onion, chopped
2 carrots, chopped
3 garlic cloves, minced
1 teaspoon herbes de Provence
1 teaspoon liquid smoke
Kosher salt and freshly ground black pepper, to taste
Shredded carrot, for garnish (optional)

1. In the electric pressure cooker, combine the peas, broth, celery, onion, carrots, garlic, herbs de Provence, and liquid smoke.
2. Close and lock the lid of the pressure cooker. Set the valve to sealing.
3. Cook on high pressure for 15 minutes.
4. When the cooking is complete, hit Cancel and allow the pressure to release naturally for 10 minutes, then quick release any remaining pressure.
5. Once the pin drops, unlock and remove the lid.
6. Stir the soup and season with salt and pepper.
7. Spoon into serving bowls and sprinkle shredded carrots on top (if using).

Per Serving
Calories: 285 | fat: 1.1g | protein: 19.1g | carbs: 51.9g | fiber: 21.1g | sugar: 9.0g | sodium: 61mg

Summer Squash Bonnet Chili Soup

Prep time: 15 minutes | Cook time: 45 minutes | Serves 8

2 pounds (907 g) calabaza squash, peeled and chopped
1 large tomato, chopped
1 medium onion, chopped
1 medium green bell pepper, chopped
1 scotch bonnet chili, deseeded and minced
8 scallions, chopped
3 sprigs fresh thyme
1 tablespoon minced ginger root
8 cups low-sodium vegetable broth
Juice of 1 lime
¼ cup chopped cilantro
Salt, to taste
¼ cup toasted pepitas

1. Put the calabaza squash, tomato, onion, bell pepper, scotch bonnet, scallions, thyme, and ginger roots in a saucepan, then pour in the vegetable broth.
2. Bring to a boil over medium-high heat. Reduce the heat to low, then simmer for 45 minutes or until the vegetables are soft. Stir constantly.
3. Add the lime juice, cilantro, and salt. Pour the soup in a large bowl, then discard the thyme sprigs and garnish with pepitas before serving.

Per Serving
Calories: 50 | fat: 0g | protein: 2.0g | carbs: 12.0g | fiber: 4.0g | sugar: 5.0g | sodium: 20mg

Buttercup Squash Soup with Ground Nutmeg

Prep time: 15 minutes | Cook time: 33 minutes | Serves 6

2 tablespoons extra-virgin olive oil
1 medium onion, chopped
1½ pounds (680 g) buttercup squash, peeled, deseeded, and cut into 1-inch chunks
4 cups vegetable broth
½ teaspoon kosher salt
¼ teaspoon ground white pepper
Ground nutmeg, to taste

1. Heat the olive oil in a pot over medium-high heat until shimmering.
2. Add the onion and sauté for 3 minutes or until translucent.

3. Add the buttercup squash, vegetable broth, salt, and pepper. Stir to mix well. Bring to a boil.
4. Reduce the heat to low and simmer for 30 minutes or until the buttercup squash is soft.
5. Pour the soup in a food processor, then pulse to purée until creamy and smooth.
6. Pour the soup in a large serving bowl, then sprinkle with ground nutmeg and serve.

Per Serving (1¹⁄₃ Cups)
Calories: 110 | fat: 5.0g | protein: 1.0g | carbs: 18.0g | fiber: 4.0g | sugar: 4.0g | sodium: 166mg

Left Over Turkey Avocado Carrot Soup

Prep time: 25 minutes | Cook time: 3 hours 7 minutes | Serves 8

2 tablespoons avocado oil
1 pound (454 g) ground turkey
28 ounces (1.3 kg) tomatoes, diced
2 tablespoons sugar-free tomato paste
4 cups low-sodium chicken broth
1 (15-ounce / 425-g) package frozen
peppers and onions (about 2½ cups)
1 (15-ounce / 425-g) package frozen chopped carrots (about 2½ cups)
⅓ cup dry barley
2 bay leaves
1 teaspoon kosher salt
¼ teaspoons freshly ground black pepper

1. Heat the avocado oil in a pot over medium-high heat.
2. Add the turkey and sauté for 7 minutes or until lightly browned.
3. Add the tomatoes, tomato paste, and chicken broth. Stir to mix well.
4. Add the peppers and onions, carrots, barley, bay leaves, salt, and pepper. Stir to mix well.
5. Bring to a boil. Reduce the heat to low, then cover the pot and simmer for 3 hours.
6. Once the simmering is finished, allow to cool for 20 minutes, then discard the bay leaves and pour the soup in a large bowl to serve.

Per Serving (1¼ Cups)
Calories: 253 | fat: 12.0g | protein: 19.0g | carbs: 21.0g | fiber: 7.0g | sugar: 7.0g | sodium: 560mg

Homemade Chicken Mustard Greens Soup

Prep time: 15 minutes | Cook time: 5 hours | Serves 4

½ pound (227 g) ground pork
4 cup mustard greens, torn
4 scallions, sliced thin
2 teaspoons fresh ginger, peeled and grated fine
4 cup low sodium chicken broth
2 tablespoons soy sauce
1 tablespoon vegetable

oil
2 cloves garlic, diced fine
1 teaspoon peppercorns, crushed
1 teaspoon fish sauce
¾ teaspoon red pepper flakes,
½ teaspoon cumin seeds, chopped coarse
Sea salt and black pepper, to taste

1. In a large bowl, combine pork, garlic, ginger, and spices. Season with salt and pepper. Use your hands to combine all thoroughly.
2. Heat oil in a large skillet over medium heat. Form pork into 1-inch balls and cook in oil till brown on all sides. Use a slotted spoon to transfer the meatballs to a crock pot.
3. Add remaining and stir. Cover and cook on low for 4 to 5 hours or until meatballs are cooked through. Serve.

Per Serving

Calories: 157 | fat: 6.0g | protein: 19.0g | carbs: 7.1g | fiber: 2.0g | sugar: 2.1g | sodium: 571mg

Crockpot Cabbage Cauliflower Soup

Prep time: 15 minutes | Cook time: 6 hours | Serves 6

6 bacon strips, cut into 1-inch pieces
3 cup cauliflower, separated into florets
2 cup cabbage, sliced thin
2 celery stalks, peeled and diced

1 onion, diced
1 carrot, peeled and diced
5 cup low sodium chicken broth
2 cloves garlic, diced fine
¼ teaspoon thyme

1. Cook bacon in a large skillet over medium-high heat until almost crisp. Remove from skillet and place on paper towels to drain.
2. Add the celery, garlic, and onion to the skillet and cook, stirring frequently, about 5 minutes. Use a slotted spoon to transfer to the crock pot.
3. Add the bacon, broth, cabbage, carrot, and thyme to the crock pot. Cover and cook on low for 4 to 5 hours or until the carrots are tender.
4. Add the cauliflower and cook until tender, about 1 to 2 hours. Serve.

Per Serving

Calories: 150 | fat: 8.0g | protein: 10.0g | carbs: 8.1g | fiber: 3.0g | sugar: 3.1g | sodium: 216mg

My Favorite Roma Tomato Chicken Stew

Prep time: 15 minutes | Cook time: 1 hour 40 minutes | Serves 6

3½ pounds (1.6 kg) chicken, whole pieces with bones in
6 Roma tomatoes
2 scallions, diced white and green parts
1 onion, sliced thin
1 cup carrots, sliced
2 cups water
⅛ Cup vegetable oil

3 tablespoons parsley
2 cloves garlic, diced fine
1 tablespoon paprika
1½ teaspoons thyme
¼ teaspoon curry powder
1 bay leaf
Salt and ground black pepper, to taste

1. Season chicken with salt and pepper on both sides. Place the tomatoes, onion, and scallions in a food processor and pulse until puréed.
2. In a large soup pot, heat the oil over medium heat. Add chicken and brown on both sides.
3. Pour the tomato mixture over the chicken and add the remaining. Bring to a low boil.
4. Reduce heat to low, cover, and simmer 60 to 90 minutes until the chicken is cooked through and the carrots are tender. Discard bay leaf before serving. Serve as is or over cauliflower rice.

Per Serving

Calories: 481 | fat: 13.0g | protein: 78.0g | carbs: 9.1g | fiber: 2.0g | sugar: 5.1g | sodium: 235mg

Spicy Thai Curried Shrimp Bowl

Prep time: 10 minutes | Cook time: 10 minutes | Serves 4

1 tablespoon coconut oil
1 tablespoon Thai red curry paste
½ onion, sliced
3 garlic cloves, minced
2 cups chopped carrots
½ cup whole unsalted peanuts

4 cups low-sodium vegetable broth
½ cup unsweetened plain almond milk
½ pound (227 g) shrimp, peeled and deveined
Minced fresh cilantro, for garnish

1. In a large pan, heat the oil over medium-high heat until shimmering.
2. Add the curry paste and cook, stirring constantly, for 1 minute. Add the onion, garlic, carrots, and peanuts to the pan, and continue to cook for 2 to 3 minutes until the onion begins to soften.
3. Add the broth and bring to a boil. Reduce the heat to low and simmer for 5 to 6 minutes until the carrots are tender.
4. Using an immersion blender or in a blender, purée the soup until smooth and return it to the pot. With the heat still on low, add the almond milk and stir to combine. Add the shrimp to the pot and cook for 2 to 3 minutes until cooked through.
5. Garnish with cilantro and serve.

Per Serving
Calories: 240 | fat: 14.1g | protein: 14.1g | carbs: 16.9g | fiber: 5.1g | sugar: 6.0g | sodium: 620mg

Simple Low-sodium Beef broth Taco Soup

Prep time: 5 minutes | Cook time: 20 minutes | Serves 4

Avocado oil cooking spray
1 medium red bell pepper, chopped
½ cup chopped yellow onion
1 pound (454 g) 93% lean ground beef
1 teaspoon ground cumin
½ teaspoon salt

½ teaspoon chili powder
½ teaspoon garlic powder
2 cups low-sodium beef broth
1 (15-ounce / 425 g) can no-salt-added diced tomatoes
1½ cups frozen corn
⅓ cup half-and-half

1. Heat a large stockpot over medium-low heat. When hot, coat the cooking surface with cooking spray. Put the pepper and onion in the pan and cook for 5 minutes.
2. Add the ground beef, cumin, salt, chili powder, and garlic powder. Cook for 5 to 7 minutes, stirring and breaking apart the beef as needed.
3. Add the broth, diced tomatoes with their juices, and corn. Increase the heat to medium-high and simmer for 10 minutes.
4. Remove from the heat and stir in the half-and-half.

Per Serving
Calories: 321 | fat: 12.1g | protein: 30.1g | carbs: 22.9g | fiber: 4.1g | sugar: 7.0g | sodium: 457mg

Low Carb Chicken Bowl with Bacon

Prep time: 5 minutes | Cook time: 30 minutes | Serves 6

1½ pounds (680 g) chicken breast, boneless, skinless and cut in 1-inch pieces
½ pound (227 g) bacon, chopped
3 cup half-and-half
4 chipotle peppers in adobo sauce, diced fine

2 tablespoons cilantro, diced
6 cup low sodium chicken broth
1 teaspoon salt
½ teaspoon onion powder
½ teaspoon garlic powder
½ teaspoon pepper

1. Place a large saucepan over medium-high heat. Add bacon and cook until crisp. Transfer to a paper towel lined plate.
2. Add the chicken and cook until browned on all sides.
3. Add the broth and seasonings and simmer for 10 to 15 minutes, or until the chicken is cooked through.
4. Stir in the half-and-half and chipotles and simmer 5 minutes more. Serve topped with the bacon and cilantro.

Per Serving
Calories: 500 | fat: 32.0g | protein: 46.0g | carbs: 7.1g | fiber: 1.1g | sugar: 0g | sodium: 827mg

Curried Coconut Carrot Soup with Cilantro

Prep time: 10 minutes | Cook time: 5 minutes | Serves 6

1 tablespoon extra-virgin olive oil
1 small onion, coarsely chopped
2 celery stalks, coarsely chopped
1½ teaspoons curry powder
1 teaspoon ground cumin
1 teaspoon minced fresh ginger
6 medium carrots, roughly chopped
4 cups low-sodium vegetable broth
¼ teaspoon salt
1 cup canned coconut milk
¼ teaspoons freshly ground black pepper
1 tablespoon chopped fresh cilantro

1. Heat an Instant Pot to high and add the olive oil.
2. Sauté the onion and celery for 2 to 3 minutes. Add the curry powder, cumin, and ginger to the pot and cook until fragrant, about 30 seconds.
3. Add the carrots, vegetable broth, and salt to the pot. Close and seal, and set for 5 minutes on high. Allow the pressure to release naturally.
4. In a blender jar, carefully purée the soup in batches and transfer back to the pot.
5. Stir in the coconut milk and pepper, and heat through. Top with the cilantro and serve.

Per Serving
Calories: 146 | fat: 11.1g | protein: 2.1g | carbs: 12.9g | fiber: 3.1g | sugar: 4.0g | sodium: 240mg

Creamy Tender Beef Barley Soup

Prep time: 10 minutes | Cook time: 1 hour 20 minutes | Serves 6

1 pound (454 g) beef stew meat, cubed
¼ teaspoon salt
¼ teaspoons freshly ground black pepper
1 tablespoon extra-virgin olive oil
8 ounces (227 g) sliced mushrooms
1 onion, chopped
2 carrots, chopped
3 celery stalks, chopped
6 garlic cloves, minced
½ teaspoon dried thyme
4 cups low-sodium beef broth
1 cup water
½ cup pearl barley

1. Season the meat with the salt and pepper.
2. In an Instant Pot, heat the oil over high heat. Add the meat and brown on all sides. Remove the meat from the pot and set aside.
3. Add the mushrooms to the pot and cook for 1 to 2 minutes, until they begin to soften. Remove the mushrooms and set aside with the meat.
4. Add the onion, carrots, and celery to the pot. Sauté for 3 to 4 minutes until the vegetables begin to soften.
5. Add the garlic and continue to cook until fragrant, about 30 seconds longer.
6. Return the meat and mushrooms to the pot, and then add the thyme, beef broth, and water. Set the pressure to high and cook for 15 minutes. Let the pressure release naturally.
7. Open the Instant Pot and add the barley. Use the slow cooker function on the Instant Pot, affix the lid (vent open), and continue to cook for 1 hour until the barley is cooked through and tender. Serve.

Per Serving
Calories: 250 | fat: 9.1g | protein: 21.1g | carbs: 18.9g | fiber: 4.1g | sugar: 3.0g | sodium: 515mg

Rich Beef Sirloin Burgundy Stew

Prep time: 15 minutes | Cook time: 8 hours | Serves 4

1 pound (454 g) sirloin steak, cut into bite size pieces
2 carrots, peeled and cut into 1-inch pieces
1 cup mushrooms, sliced
¾ cup pearl onions, thawed if frozen
½ cup low sodium beef broth
3 cloves garlic, diced
2 tablespoons olive oil
1 bay leaf
1 teaspoon marjoram
½ teaspoon salt
½ teaspoon thyme
¼ teaspoon pepper

1. Heat the oil in a large skillet over medium-high heat. Add steak and brown on all sides. Transfer to a crock pot.
2. Add remaining and stir to combine. Cover and cook on low 7 to 8 hours or until steak is tender and vegetables are cooked through. Discard the bay leaf before serving.

Per Serving
Calories: 352 | fat: 14.0g | protein: 36.0g | carbs: 8.1g | fiber: 1.0g | sugar: 3.1g | sodium: 470mg

Chapter 10: Poultry

Citrusy Chicken Skillet

Prep time: 10 minutes | Cook time: 15 minutes | Serves 4

3 tablespoons extra-virgin olive oil
4 chicken breast halves or thighs, pounded slightly to even thickness
½ teaspoon sea salt
⅛ teaspoon freshly ground black pepper
¼ cup freshly squeezed lemon juice
2 tablespoons capers, rinsed
2 tablespoons salted butter, very cold, cut into pieces

1. In a large skillet over medium-high heat, heat the olive oil until it shimmers.
2. Season the chicken with the salt and pepper. Add it to the hot oil and cook until opaque with an internal temperature of 165°F (74°C), about 5 minutes per side.
3. Transfer the chicken to a plate and tent loosely with foil to keep warm. Keep the pan on the heat. Add the lemon juice to the pan, using the side of a spoon to scrape any browned bits from the bottom of the pan.
4. Add the capers. Simmer until the liquid is reduced by half, about 3 minutes. Reduce the heat to low.
5. Whisk in the butter, one piece at a time, until incorporated.
6. Return the chicken to the pan, turning once to coat with the sauce. Serve with additional sauce spooned over the top.

Per Serving
Calories: 281 | fat: 17g | protein: 26g | carbs: 2g | fiber: 1g | sugar: 1.62g | sodium: 386mg

Chinese Satay Chicken Stir Fry Skillet

Prep time: 10 minutes | Cook time: 15 minutes | Serves 4

3 tablespoons extra-virgin olive oil
1 pound (454 g) chicken breasts or thighs, cut into ¾-inch pieces
½ teaspoon sea salt
2 cups broccoli florets
1 red bell pepper,
seeded and chopped
6 scallions, green and white parts, sliced on the bias (cut diagonally into thin slices)
1 head cauliflower, riced
Peanut Sauce

1. In a large skillet over medium-high heat, heat the olive oil until it shimmers.
2. Season the chicken with the salt. Add the chicken to the oil and cook, stirring occasionally, until opaque, about 5 minutes.
3. Remove the chicken from the oil with a slotted spoon and set it aside on a plate. Return the pan to the heat.
4. Add the broccoli, bell pepper, and scallions. Cook, stirring, until the vegetables are crisp-tender, 3 to 5 minutes. Add the cauliflower and cook for 3 minutes more.
5. Return the chicken to the skillet. Stir in the Peanut Sauce.
6. Bring to a simmer and reduce heat to medium-low. Simmer to heat through, about 2 minutes more.

Per Serving
Calories: 381 | fat: 20g | protein: 33g | carbs: 19g | fiber: 5g | sugar: 7.75g | sodium: 396mg

Crispy Oven Baked Chicken Bites

Prep time: 10 minutes | Cook time: 15 minutes | Serves 4

1 cup whole-wheat bread crumbs
1 tablespoon dried thyme
1 teaspoon garlic powder
1 teaspoon paprika
½ teaspoon sea salt
3 large eggs, beaten
1 tablespoon Dijon mustard
1 pound (454 g) chicken, cut into ½-inch-thick pieces and pounded to even thickness

1. Preheat the oven to 375°F (190°C). Line a rimmed baking sheet with parchment paper.
2. In a medium bowl, whisk together the bread crumbs, thyme, garlic powder, paprika, and salt.
3. In another bowl, whisk together the eggs and mustard.
4. Dip each piece of chicken in the egg mixture and then in the bread crumb mixture. Place on the prepared baking sheet.
5. Bake until the chicken reaches an internal temperature of 165°F (74°C) and the bread crumbs are golden, about 15 minutes.

Per Serving
Calories: 277 | fat: 6.1g | protein: 34.1g | carbs: 16.9g | fiber: 3.1g | sugar: 8.8g | sodium: 488mg

Delicious Chicken Edamame Stir Fry

Prep time: 10 minutes | Cook time: 10 minutes | Serves 4

3 tablespoons extra-virgin olive oil
1 pound chicken breasts or thighs, cut into ¾-inch pieces
2 cups edamame or pea pods
3 garlic cloves, chopped
1 tablespoon peeled and grated fresh

ginger
2 tablespoons reduced-sodium soy sauce
Juice of 2 limes
1 teaspoon sesame oil
2 teaspoons toasted sesame seeds
1 tablespoon chopped fresh cilantro

1. In a large skillet over medium-high heat, heat the olive oil until it shimmers.
2. Add the chicken to the oil and cook, stirring occasionally, until opaque, about 5 minutes.
3. Add the edamame and cook, stirring occasionally, until crisp-tender, 3 to 5 minutes.
4. Add the garlic and ginger and cook, stirring constantly, for 30 seconds.
5. In a small bowl, whisk together the soy sauce, lime juice, and sesame oil. Add the sauce mixture to the pan. Bring to a simmer, stirring, and cook for 2 minutes.
6. Remove from heat and garnish with the sesame seeds and cilantro.

Per Serving
Calories: 331 | fat: 17g | protein: 31g | carbs: 11g | fiber: 5g | sugar: 8.13g | sodium: 342mg

Original Orange Chicken with Scallions

Prep time: 10 minutes | Cook time: 10 minutes | Serves 4

3 tablespoons extra-virgin olive oil
1 pound chicken breasts or thighs, cut into ¾-inch pieces
1 teaspoon peeled and grated fresh ginger
2 garlic cloves, minced
Juice and zest of 1

orange
1 teaspoon corn-starch
½ teaspoon sriracha (or to taste)
Sesame seeds (optional, for garnish)
Thinly sliced scallion (optional, for garnish)

1. In a large skillet over medium-high heat, heat the olive oil until it shimmers.
2. Add the chicken to the oil and cook, stirring occasionally, until opaque, about 5 minutes.
3. Add the ginger and garlic and cook, stirring constantly, for 30 seconds.
4. In a small bowl, whisk together the orange juice and zest, corn-starch, and sriracha. Add the sauce mixture to the chicken and cook, stirring, until the sauce thickens, about 2 minutes.
5. Serve garnished with sesame seeds and sliced scallions, if desired.

Per Serving
Calories: 245 | fat: 12g | protein: 26g | carbs: 9g | fiber: 1g | sugar: 6.63g | sodium: 75mg

Low Carb Peppery Chicken Breasts

Prep time: 15 minutes | Cook time: 30 minutes | Serves 4

1 cup chopped roasted red pepper
2 ounces (57 g) goat cheese
4 Kalamata olives, pitted, finely chopped
1 tablespoon chopped

fresh basil
4 (5-ounce / 142-g) boneless, skinless chicken breasts
1 tablespoon extra-virgin olive oil

1. Preheat the oven to 400ºF (205ºC).
2. In a small bowl, stir together the red pepper, goat cheese, olives, and basil until well mixed.
3. Place the filling in the refrigerator for about 15 minutes to firm it up.
4. Cut a slit horizontally in each chicken breast to create a pocket in the middle.
5. Evenly divide the filling between the chicken breast pockets and secure them closed with wooden toothpicks.
6. Place a large skillet over medium-high heat and add the olive oil.
7. Brown the chicken breasts on both sides, about 10 minutes in total.
8. Transfer to the oven. Bake the chicken breasts until the chicken is cooked through, about 20 minutes.
9. Let the chicken breasts rest for 10 minutes, remove the toothpicks, and serve.

Per Serving
Calories: 246 | fat: 9.1g | protein: 35.1g | carbs: 3.0g | fiber: 1.1g | sugar: 2.0g | sodium: 280mg

Best-Ever Whole Wheat Turkey Burger

Prep time: 10 minutes | Cook time: 20 minutes | Serves 4

1½ pounds (680 g) lean ground turkey
½ cup bread crumbs
½ sweet onion, chopped
1 carrot, peeled, grated
1 teaspoon minced

garlic
1 teaspoon chopped fresh thyme
Sea salt and freshly ground black pepper, to taste
Nonstick cooking spray

1. In a large bowl, mix together the turkey, bread crumbs, onion, carrot, garlic, and thyme until very well mixed.
2. Season the mixture lightly with salt and pepper.
3. Shape the turkey mixture into 4 equal patties.
4. Place a large skillet over medium-high heat and coat it lightly with cooking spray.
5. Cook the turkey patties until golden and completely cooked through, about 10 minutes per side.
6. Serve the burgers plain or with your favorite toppings on a whole-wheat bun.

Per Serving
Calories: 320 | fat: 15.1g | protein: 32.1g | carbs: 11.9g | fiber: 1.1g | sugar: 2.0g | sodium: 271mg

Actually Delicious Turkey Peppers

Prep time: 15 minutes | Cook time: 50 minutes | Serves 4

1 teaspoon extra-virgin olive oil, plus more for greasing the baking dish
1 pound (454 g) ground turkey breast
½ sweet onion, chopped
1 teaspoon minced garlic

1 tomato, diced
½ teaspoon chopped fresh basil
Sea salt and freshly ground black pepper, to taste
4 red bell peppers, tops cut off, seeded
2 ounces (57 g) low-sodium feta cheese

1. Preheat the oven to 350ºF (180ºC).
2. Lightly grease a baking dish with olive oil and set it aside.
3. Place a large skillet over medium heat and add 1 teaspoon of olive oil.

4. Add the turkey to the skillet and cook until it is no longer pink, stirring occasionally to break up the meat and brown it evenly, about 6 minutes.
5. Add the onion and garlic and sauté until softened and translucent, about 3 minutes.
6. Stir in the tomato and basil. Season with salt and pepper.
7. Place the peppers cut-side up in the baking dish. Divide the filling into four equal portions and spoon it into the peppers.
8. Sprinkle the feta cheese on top of the filling.
9. Add ¼ cup of water to the dish and cover with aluminum foil.
10. Bake the peppers until they are soft and heated through, about 40 minutes.

Per Serving
Calories: 282 | fat: 14.1g | protein: 24.1g | carbs: 14.0g | fiber: 4.1g | sugar: 9.0g | sodium: 270mg

Secret Ingredient Turkey Cauliflower Rice

Prep time: 10 minutes | Cook time: 20 minutes | Serves 4

3 tablespoons extra-virgin olive oil
1 pound (454 g) ground turkey
1 onion, chopped
1 green bell pepper, seeded and chopped

½ teaspoon sea salt
1 small head cauliflower, grated
1 cup corn kernels
½ cup prepared salsa
1 cup shredded pepper Jack cheese

1. In a large nonstick skillet over medium-high heat, heat the olive oil until it shimmers.
2. Add the turkey. Cook, crumbling with a spoon, until browned, about 5 minutes.
3. Add the onion, bell pepper, and salt. Cook, stirring occasionally, until the vegetables soften, 4 to 5 minutes.
4. Add the cauliflower, corn, and salsa. Cook, stirring, until the cauliflower rice softens, about 3 minutes more.
5. Sprinkle with the cheese. Reduce heat to low, cover, and allow the cheese to melt, 2 or 3 minutes.

Per Serving
Calories: 449 | fat: 30.1g | protein: 30.1g | carbs: 17.9g | fiber: 4.1g | sugar: 8.7g | sodium: 650mg

Oregano Chicken Arugula Salad Sandwich

Prep time: 10 minutes | Cook time: 0 minutes | Serves 3

3 slices 100% whole-wheat bread, toasted
3 tablespoons red pepper hummus
3 cups arugula
¾ cup cucumber slices

1 cup rotisserie chicken, shredded
¼ cup sliced red onion
Oregano, for garnish (optional)

1. Place the toasted bread slices on a clean work surface, and spoon 1 tablespoon of red pepper hummus on each slice of bread.
2. Top each bread slice evenly with arugula, cucumber slices, chicken, and red onion.
3. Serve garnished with the oregano, if desired.

Per Serving
Calories: 227 | fat: 6.1g | protein: 23.1g | carbs: 24.8g | fiber: 4.1g | sugar: 4.1g | sodium: 330mg

Healthy Chicken Salad with Whole Wheat Sandwiches

Prep time: 10 minutes | Cook time: 10 minutes | Serves 4

2 (4-ounce / 113-g) boneless, skinless chicken breasts
⅛ teaspoon freshly ground black pepper
1½ tablespoons plain low-fat Greek yogurt
¼ cup halved purple

seedless grapes
¼ cup chopped pecans
2 tablespoons chopped celery
4 whole-wheat sandwiches thins
Avocado oil cooking spray

1. Heat a small skillet over medium-low heat. When hot, coat the cooking surface with cooking spray.
2. Season the chicken with the pepper. Place the chicken in the skillet and cook for 6 minutes. Flip and cook for 3 to 5 minute more, or until cooked through.
3. Remove the chicken from the skillet and let cool for 5 minutes.
4. Chop or shred the chicken.
5. Combine the chicken, yogurt, grapes, pecans, and celery.
6. Cut the sandwich thins in half, so there is a top and bottom.
7. Divide the chicken salad into four equal portions, spoon one portion on each of the bottom halves of the sandwich thins, and cover with the top halves.

Per Serving
Calories: 251 | fat: 8.1g | protein: 23.1g | carbs: 23.9g | fiber: 6.1g | sugar: 4.0g | sodium: 210mg

Easy Turkey Broth with Cabbage & Sweet Potato

Prep time: 15 minutes | Cook time: 30 minutes | Serves 4

1 tablespoon olive oil
2 celery stalks, chopped
2 teaspoons fresh garlic, minced
1 sweet onion, chopped
1 sweet potato, peeled, diced
4 cups green cabbage, finely shredded

8 cups low-sodium chicken broth
2 bay leaves
1 cup cooked turkey, chopped
2 teaspoons fresh thyme, chopped
Salt and freshly ground black pepper, to taste

1. Heat the olive oil in a large saucepan over medium-high heat until shimmering.
2. Add the celery, garlic, and onion to the saucepan and sauté for 3 minutes until the onion is translucent.
3. Add the sweet potato and cabbage to the saucepan and sauté for 3 minutes to soft the vegetables a little. Pour the chicken broth in the saucepan and add the bay leaves. Bring to a boil.
4. Turn down the heat to low, then simmer for 20 minutes or until the vegetables are tender. Add the turkey and thyme to the pan and simmer for 4 minutes until the turkey is heated through.
5. Pour the turkey broth in a large bowl, and discard the bay leaves. Sprinkle with salt and black pepper to taste before serving warm.

Per Serving
Calories: 328 | fat: 10.8g | protein: 24.1g | carbs: 29.8g | fiber: 4.3g | sugar: 12.7g | sodium: 710mg

Homemade Chicken Lettuce Sandwiches

Prep time: 5 minutes | Cook time: 0 minutes | Serves 4

Dressing:

4 tablespoons plain low-fat Greek yogurt
4 teaspoons Dijon mustard
4 teaspoons freshly squeezed lemon juice

4 teaspoons shredded Parmesan cheese
¼ teaspoon freshly ground black pepper
⅛ teaspoon garlic powder

Sandwiches:

2 cups shredded rotisserie chicken
1½ cup chopped romaine lettuce
12 cherry tomatoes,

halved
4 whole-wheat sandwiches thins
¼ cup thinly sliced red onion (optional)

Make the Dressing
1. In a small bowl, whisk together the yogurt, mustard, lemon juice, Parmesan cheese, black pepper, and garlic powder.

Make the Sandwiches
2. In a large bowl, combine the chicken, lettuce, and tomatoes. Add the dressing and stir until evenly coated. Divide the filling into four equal portions.
3. Slice the sandwich thins so there is a top and bottom half for each. Put one portion of filling on each of the bottom halves and cover with the top halves.

Per Serving
Calories: 243 | fat: 5.1g | protein: 28.1g | carbs: 24.9g | fiber: 8.1g | sugar: 4.0g | sodium: 360mg

Healthy Balsamic Chicken Kale Salad

Prep time: 5 minutes | Cook time: 15 minutes | Serves 4

4 (4-ounce / 113-g) boneless, skinless chicken breasts
¼ teaspoon salt
1 tablespoon freshly ground black pepper
2 tablespoons unsalted butter
1 tablespoon extra-

virgin olive oil
8 cups stemmed and roughly chopped kale, loosely packed (about 2 bunches)
½ cup balsamic vinegar
20 cherry tomatoes, halved

1. Season both sides of the chicken breasts with the salt and pepper.
2. Heat a large skillet over medium heat. When hot, heat the butter and oil. Add the chicken and cook for 8 to 10 minutes, flipping halfway through. When cooked all the way through, remove the chicken from the skillet and set aside.
3. Increase the heat to medium-high. Put the kale in the skillet and cook for 3 minutes, stirring every minute.
4. Add the vinegar and the tomatoes and cook for another 3 to 5 minutes.
5. Divide the kale and tomato mixture into four equal portions, and top each portion with 1 chicken breast.

Per Serving
Calories: 294 | fat: 11.1g | protein: 31.1g | carbs: 17.9g | fiber: 3.1g | sugar: 4.0g | sodium: 330mg

Cayenne Garlic Roasted Chicken Legs

Prep time: 10 minutes | Cook time: 35 minutes | Serves 6

1 teaspoon ground paprika
1 teaspoon garlic powder
½ teaspoon ground coriander
½ teaspoon ground

cumin
½ teaspoon salt
¼ teaspoon ground cayenne pepper
6 chicken legs
1 teaspoon extra-virgin olive oil

1. Preheat the oven to 400ºF (205ºC).
2. Combine the coriander, cumin, paprika, garlic powder, salt, and cayenne pepper in a bowl. Dunk the chicken legs in the mixture to coat well.
3. Heat the olive oil in an oven-safe skillet over medium heat.
4. Add the chicken legs and sear for 9 minutes or until browned and crisp. Flip the legs halfway through the cooking time.
5. Place the skillet in the oven and roast for 14 minutes or until the internal temperature of the chicken legs reaches at least 165ºF (74ºC).
6. Remove the chicken legs from the oven and serve warm.

Per Serving
Calories: 278 | fat: 15.8g | protein: 30.1g | carbs: 0.8g | fiber: 0g | sugar: 0g | sodium: 254mg

Baked Turkey Tomato Meatballs

Prep time: 10 minutes | Cook time: 20 minutes | Serves 4

¼ cup tomato paste
1 tablespoon honey
1 tablespoon Worcestershire sauce
½ cup milk
½ cup whole-wheat bread crumbs
1 pound (454 g)

ground turkey
1 onion, grated
1 tablespoon Dijon mustard
1 teaspoon dried thyme
½ teaspoon sea salt

1. Preheat the oven to 375°F (190°C). Line a rimmed baking sheet with parchment paper.
2. In a small saucepan on medium-low heat, whisk together the tomato paste, honey, and Worcestershire sauce. Bring to a simmer and then remove from the heat.
3. In a large bowl, combine the milk and bread crumbs. Let rest for 5 minutes.
4. Add the ground turkey, onion, mustard, thyme, and salt. Using your hands, mix well without over mixing.
5. Form into 1-inch meatballs and place on the prepared baking sheet. Brush the tops with the tomato paste mixture.
6. Bake until the meatballs reach 165°F (74°C) internally, about 15 minutes.

Per Serving
Calories: 286 | fat: 11.1g | protein: 24.1g | carbs: 21.9g | fiber: 2.1g | sugar: 13.6g | sodium: 464mg

Easy Lemony Chicken

Prep time: 10 minutes | Cook time: 15 minutes | Serves 4

3 tablespoons extra-virgin olive oil
4 chicken breast halves or thighs, pounded slightly to even thickness
½ teaspoon sea salt
⅛ teaspoon freshly

ground black pepper
¼ cup freshly squeezed lemon juice
2 tablespoons capers, rinsed
2 tablespoons salted butter, cold, cut into pieces

1. In a large skillet over medium-high heat, heat the olive oil until it shimmers.
2. Season the chicken with the salt and pepper. Add it to the hot oil and cook until opaque with an internal temperature of 165°F (74°C), about 5 minutes per side.
3. Transfer the chicken to a plate and tent loosely with foil to keep warm. Keep the pan on the heat.
4. Add the lemon juice to the pan, using the side of a spoon to scrape any browned bits from the bottom of the pan.
5. Add the capers. Simmer until the liquid is reduced by half, about 3 minutes. Reduce the heat to low.
6. Whisk in the butter, one piece at a time, until incorporated.
7. Return the chicken to the pan, turning once to coat with the sauce. Serve with additional sauce spooned over the top.

Per Serving
Calories: 282 | fat: 17.1g | protein: 26.1g | carbs: 1.9g | fiber: 1.0g | sugar: 0.9g | sodium: 388mg

Budgeted Honey Turkey Balls

Prep time: 20 minutes | Cook time: 20 minutes | Serves 6

1 pound (454 g) lean ground turkey
1 egg, beaten
2 tablespoons tamari
2 teaspoons mirin
¼ cup scallions, both white and green parts,

finely chopped
1 teaspoon fresh ginger, grated
2 garlic cloves, minced
1 tablespoon honey
1 teaspoon toasted sesame oil

1. Preheat the oven to 400°F (205°C).
2. Combine the ground turkey, beaten egg, tamari, mirin, scallions, ginger, garlic, honey, and sesame oil in a bowl. Stir to mix well.
3. Use a tablespoon to shape the turkey mixture into balls, and then arrange the balls on a baking sheet lined with parchment paper.
4. Bake the balls in the preheated oven for 20 minutes until the balls are well browned. Flip the balls with a spatula halfway through the cooking time.
5. Remove the balls from the oven and serve hot.

Per Serving
Calories: 156 | fat: 7.8g | protein: 16.1g | carbs: 4.8g | fiber: 0g | sugar: 3.9g | sodium: 267mg

Garlic Soy Chicken with Pea Pods Stir-Fry

Prep time: 10 minutes | Cook time: 10 minutes | Serves 4

3 tablespoons extra-virgin olive oil
1 pound (454 g) chicken breasts or thighs, cut into ¾-inch pieces
2 cups edamame or pea pods
3 garlic cloves, chopped
1 tablespoon peeled

and grated fresh ginger
2 tablespoons reduced-sodium soy sauce
Juice of 2 limes
1 teaspoon sesame oil
2 teaspoons toasted sesame seeds
1 tablespoon chopped fresh cilantro

1. In a large skillet over medium-high heat, heat the olive oil until it shimmers.
2. Add the chicken to the oil and cook, stirring occasionally, until opaque, about 5 minutes.
3. Add the edamame and cook, stirring occasionally, until crisp-tender, 3 to 5 minutes.
4. Add the garlic and ginger and cook, stirring constantly, for 30 seconds.
5. In a small bowl, whisk together the soy sauce, lime juice, and sesame oil.
6. Add the sauce mixture to the pan. Bring to a simmer, stirring, and cook for 2 minutes.
7. Remove from heat and garnish with the sesame seeds and cilantro.

Per Serving
Calories: 332 | fat: 17.1g | protein: 31.1g | carbs: 10.9g | fiber: 5.1g | sugar: 5.0g | sodium: 341mg

One Pan Chicken Thighs with Peaches & Greens

Prep time: 10 minutes | Cook time: 30 minutes | Serves 4

4 boneless, skinless chicken thighs
Juice of 1 lime
½ cup white vinegar
2 garlic cloves, smashed
1 cup frozen peaches
½ cup water
Pinch ground cinnamon

Pinch ground cloves
Pinch ground nutmeg
⅛ teaspoon vanilla extract
½ cup low-sodium chicken broth
1 bunch dandelion greens cut into ribbons
1 medium onion, thinly sliced

1. Set oven to broil. In a bowl, combine the chicken, lime juice, vinegar, and garlic, coating the chicken thoroughly.
2. Meanwhile, to make the peach glaze, in a small pot, combine the peaches, water, cinnamon, cloves, nutmeg, and vanilla. Cook over medium heat, stirring often, for 10 minutes, or until the peaches have softened.
3. In a large cast iron skillet, bring the broth to a simmer over medium heat. Add the greens, and sauté for 5 minutes, or until the greens are wilted.
4. Add the onion and cook, stirring occasionally, for 3 minutes, or until slightly reduced. Add the chicken and cover with the peach glaze.
5. Transfer the pan to the oven, and broil for 10 to 12 minutes, or until the chicken is golden brown.

Per Serving
Calories: 201 | fat: 4.9g | protein: 24.1g | carbs: 13.9g | fiber: 4.1g | sugar: 6.0g | sodium: 156mg

Olive Chicken with Lime Aioli

Prep time: 15 minutes | Cook time: 45 minutes | Serves 6

4 pounds (1.8 kg) chicken, spatchcocked
3 tablespoons

blackened seasoning
2 tablespoons olive oil

Lime Aioli:

Juice and zest of 1 lime
¼ teaspoon kosher

salt
¼ teaspoon ground black pepper

1. Preheat the grill to medium high heat.
2. On a clean work surface, rub the chicken with blackened seasoning and olive oil.
3. Place the chicken on the preheated grill, skin side up, and grill for 45 minutes or until the internal temperature of the chicken reaches at least 165ºF (74ºC).
4. Meanwhile, combine the ingredients for the aioli in a small bowl and stir to mix well.
5. Once the chicken is fully grilled, transfer it to a large plate and baste with the lime aioli. Allow to cool and serve.

Per Serving
Calories: 436 | fat: 16.3g | protein: 61.8g | carbs: 6.8g | fiber: 0.7g | sugar: 1.5g | sodium: 653mg

Quinoa with Creamy Chicken & Broccoli

Prep time: 5 minutes | Cook time: 15 minutes | Serves 4

½ cup uncooked quinoa
4 (4-ounce / 113-g) boneless, skinless chicken breasts
1 teaspoon garlic powder, divided
¼ teaspoon salt

¼ teaspoons freshly ground black pepper
1 tablespoon avocado oil
3 cups fresh or frozen broccoli, cut into florets
1 cup half-and-half

1. Put the quinoa in a pot of salted water. Bring to a boil. Reduce the heat to low and simmer for 15 minutes or until the quinoa is soft and has a white "tail". Cover and turn off the heat. Let sit for 5 minutes.
2. On a clean work surface, rub the chicken breasts with ½ teaspoon of garlic powder, salt, and pepper.
3. Heat the avocado oil in a nonstick skillet over medium-low heat.
4. Add the chicken and broccoli in the skillet and cook for 9 minutes or until the chicken is browned and the broccoli is tender.
5. Flip the chicken and shake the skillet halfway through the cooking time.
6. Pour the half-and-half in the skillet, and sprinkle with remaining garlic powder. Turn up the heat to high and simmer for 2 minutes until creamy.
7. Divide the rice, chicken breasts, broccoli florets, and the sauce remains in the skillet in four bowls and serve warm.

Per Serving
Calories: 305 | fat: 9.8g | protein: 33.1g | carbs: 21.8g | fiber: 3.1g | sugar: 3.9g | sodium: 270mg

Cauliflower Rice Chicken with Teriyaki Sauce

Prep time: 5 minutes | Cook time: 20 minutes | Serves 4

1 tablespoon sesame oil
4 (4-ounce / 113-g) boneless, skinless chicken breasts cut into bite-size cubes

1 (12-ounce / 340-g) bag frozen cauliflower rice
1 (12-ounce / 340-g) bag frozen broccoli

Teriyaki Sauce:

¼ teaspoon garlic powder
½ cup water
1 tablespoon corn-starch

1 tablespoon rice vinegar
2 tablespoons honey
2 tablespoons tamari
Pinch ground ginger

1. Put all the ingredients for the teriyaki sauce in a saucepan, then whisk to combine well.
2. Bring to a boil over medium heat, then let boil for 1 minute until thickened. Transfer the sauce in a bowl and set aside until ready to use.
3. Heat the sesame oil in a nonstick skillet over medium-low heat.
4. Add the chicken to the skillet and cook for 6 minutes until browned on all sides. Remove the chicken from the skillet and set aside.
5. Put the cauliflower rice and broccoli in a microwave-safe bowl, then add 1 tablespoon of water and sprinkle with salt. Microwave for 2 minutes or until they are soft.
6. Divide the chicken, cauliflower rice, and broccoli among four bowls, and then serve with teriyaki sauce on top.

Per Serving
Calories: 250 | fat: 6.7g | protein: 29.1g | carbs: 19.9g | fiber: 5.2g | sugar: 11.8g | sodium: 416mg

Chicken Cucumber Lettuce Wraps

Prep time: 10 minutes | Cook time: 0 minutes | Serves 4

8 romaine lettuce leaves
1½ cups shredded rotisserie chicken
1 avocado, sliced
2 hard-boiled eggs,

sliced
1 medium tomato, sliced
4 teaspoons honey mustard

1. Divide the rotisserie chicken, sliced avocado, sliced tomato, and eggs among the lettuce leaves.
2. Drizzle with honey mustard, and then roll the lettuce up before serving.

Per Serving
Calories: 229 | fat: 10.8g | protein: 24.2g | carbs: 7.8g | fiber: 4.2g | sugar: 2.8g | sodium: 158mg

Honey Citrus Chicken Skillet

Prep time: 10 minutes | Cook time: 10 minutes | Serves 4

3 tablespoons extra-virgin olive oil
1 pound (454 g) chicken breasts or thighs, cut into ¾-inch pieces
1 teaspoon peeled and grated fresh ginger
2 garlic cloves, minced
1 tablespoon honey
Juice and zest of 1 orange
1 teaspoon cornstarch
½ teaspoon sriracha (or to taste)
Sesame seeds (optional, for garnish)
Thinly sliced scallion (optional, for garnish)

1. In a large skillet over medium-high heat, heat the olive oil until it shimmers. Add the chicken to the oil and cook, stirring occasionally, until opaque, about 5 minutes.
2. Add the ginger and garlic and cook, stirring constantly, for 30 seconds.
3. In a small bowl, whisk together the honey, orange juice and zest, cornstarch, and sriracha.
4. Add the sauce mixture to the chicken and cook, stirring, until the sauce thickens, about 2 minutes.
5. Serve garnished with sesame seeds and sliced scallions, if desired.

Per Serving
Calories: 246 | fat: 12.1g | protein: 26.1g | carbs: 8.9g | fiber: 1.1g | sugar: 6.7g | sodium: 76mg

Scallions Chicken and Peanut Butter Sauce

Prep time: 15 minutes | Cook time: 0 minutes | Serves 4

Filling:
1½ cups cooked chicken breast, shredded
1 cup shredded green cabbage
1 cup bean sprouts
½ cup carrots, shredded
¼ cup chopped fresh cilantro
¼ cup chopped scallions, both white and green parts

Sauce:
2 tablespoons water
2 tablespoons natural peanut butter
1 garlic clove, minced
1 tablespoon rice wine vinegar
¼ teaspoon salt
4 (8-inch) low-carb whole-wheat tortillas

1. Put the chicken breast, cabbage, bean sprouts, carrots, cilantro, and scallion in a large bowl. Gently toss to combine well and set aside.
2. Mix the water, peanut butter, garlic, rice vinegar, and salt together in a separate bowl. Stir well with a fork until blended.
3. Arrange each tortilla on a clean work surface. Evenly divide the chicken and vegetable mixture among the tortillas, then spread 1 tablespoon of the sauce over the filling.
4. Fold each tortilla in half to enclose filling and roll up. Serve immediately.

Per Serving
Calories: 212 | fat: 8.2g | protein: 21.2g | carbs: 17.1g | fiber: 10.2g | sugar: 3.1g | sodium: 358mg

Zucchini Noodles with Spaghetti Turkey Recipe

Prep time: 5 minutes | Cook time: 20 minutes | Serves 2

1 (10-ounce / 284-g) package zucchini noodles, rinsed and patted dry
2 tablespoons olive oil, divided
1 pound (454 g) 93%
lean ground turkey
½ teaspoon dried oregano
1 cup low-sodium spaghetti sauce
½ cup Cheddar cheese, shredded

1. Preheat the broiler to high.
2. Warm 1 tablespoon olive oil over in an oven-safe skillet over medium heat.
3. Add the zucchini noodles to the skillet and cook for 3 minutes until soft. Stir the zucchini noodles frequently.
4. Drizzle the remaining olive oil over, and then add the ground turkey and oregano to the skillet. Cook for 8 minutes until the turkey is well browned.
5. Pour the spaghetti sauce over the turkey and stir to coat well.
6. Spread the Cheddar on top, and then broil in the preheated broiler for 5 minutes until the cheese is melted and frothy.
7. Remove them from the broiler and serve warm.

Per Serving
Calories: 337 | fat: 20.8g | protein: 28.2g | carbs: 20.7g | fiber: 3.2g | sugar: 3.8g | sodium: 214mg

Crispy Coconut Chicken

Prep time: 10 minutes | Cook time: 20 minutes | Serves 6

4 chicken breasts each cut lengthwise into 3 strips
½ teaspoon salt
¼ teaspoons freshly ground black pepper
2 eggs

2 tablespoons unsweetened plain almond milk
½ cup coconut flour
1 cup unsweetened coconut flakes

1. Preheat the oven to 400ºF (205ºC).
2. On a clean work surface, rub the chicken with salt and black pepper.
3. Whisk together the eggs and almond milk in a bowl. Put the coconut flour in another bowl. Put the coconut flakes in a third bowl.
4. Dunk the chicken in the bowl of flour to coat, and then dredge in the egg mixture, and then dip in coconut flakes. Shake the excess off.
5. Arrange the well coated chicken in a baking pan lined with parchment paper. Bake in the preheated oven for 16 minutes.
6. Flip the chicken halfway through the cooking time or until well browned.
7. Remove the chicken from the oven and serve in a plate.

Per Serving
Calories: 218 | fat: 12.8g | protein: 20.1g | carbs: 8.8g | fiber: 6.1g | sugar: 1.8g | sodium: 345mg

Mexican inspired Turkey Patties with Veggies

Prep time: 15 minutes | Cook time: 6 minutes | Serves 7

1 pound (454 g) lean ground turkey
1 tablespoon chili powder
½ teaspoon garlic powder
¼ teaspoon ground black pepper

7 mini whole-wheat hamburger buns
7 tomato slices
3½ slices reduced-fat pepper Jack cheese, cut in half
½ mashed avocado

1. Preheat the grill to high heat.
2. Combine the ground turkey, chili powder, garlic powder, and black pepper in a large bowl. Stir to mix well.

3. Divide and shape the mixture into 7 patties, then arrange the patties on the preheated grill grates.
4. Grill for 6 minutes or until well browned. Flip the patties halfway through.
5. Assemble the patties with buns, tomato slices, cheese slices, and mashed avocado to make the sliders, and then serve immediately.

Per Serving
Calories: 225 | fat: 9.0g | protein: 17.0g | carbs: 21.0g | fiber: 4.0g | sugar: 6.0g | sodium: 230mg

8 Ingredient Chicken Veggie Roast

Prep time: 10 minutes | Cook time: 40 minutes | Serves 6

¼ cup olive oil, divided
½ head cabbage, cut into 2-inch chunks
1 sweet potato, peeled and cut into 1-inch chunks
1 onion, peeled and cut into eighths
4 garlic cloves, peeled

and lightly crushed
2 teaspoons fresh thyme, minced
Salt and freshly ground black pepper, to taste
2½ pounds (1.1 kg) bone-in chicken thighs and drumsticks

1. Preheat the oven to 450ºF (235ºC). Coat a baking pan with 1 tablespoon of olive oil.
2. Place the cabbage, sweet potato, onion, and garlic in the baking pan. Sprinkle with thyme, salt, and black pepper, and drizzle 1 tablespoon of olive oil on top. Set aside.
3. On a clean work surface, rub the chicken with salt and black pepper.
4. Heat 2 tablespoons olive oil in a large skillet over medium-high heat.
5. Add the chicken to the skillet and cook for 10 minutes or until lightly browned on both sides. Flip the chicken halfway through the cooking time.
6. Put the chicken over the vegetables in the baking pan, then roast in the preheated oven for 30 minutes until an instant-read thermometer inserted in the thickest part of the chicken registers at least 165ºF (74ºC).
7. Remove them from the oven and serve hot on a large platter.

Per Serving
Calories: 542 | fat: 33.8g | protein: 43.1g | carbs: 13.8g | fiber: 4.1g | sugar: 4.9g | sodium: 210mg

Traditional Peru Chicken Broth Sherry Dish

Prep time: 10 minutes | Cook time: 25 minutes | Serves 4

1 onion, diced
1 red pepper, diced
2 cup chicken breast, cooked and cubed
1 cup cauliflower, grated
1 cup peas, thaw
2 tablespoons cilantro, diced
½ teaspoon lemon zest

14½ ounces (411 g) low sodium chicken broth
¼ cup black olives, sliced
¼ cup sherry
1 clove garlic, diced
2 teaspoons olive oil
¼ teaspoon salt
¼ teaspoon cayenne pepper

1. Heat oil in a large skillet over medium-high heat. Add pepper, onion and garlic and cook 1 minute.
2. Add the cauliflower and cook, stirring frequently, until light brown, 4 to 5 minutes.
3. Stir in broth, sherry, zest and seasonings. Bring to a boil. Reduce heat, cover and simmer 15 minutes.
4. Stir in the chicken, peas and olives. Cover and simmer another 3 to 6 minutes or until heated through. Serve garnished with cilantro.

Per Serving
Calories: 162 | fat: 5.0g | protein: 14.2g | carbs: 13.1g | fiber: 4.2g | sugar: 5.1g | sodium: 307mg

Coconut Curry Chicken Recipe

Prep time: 15 minutes | Cook time: 35 minutes | Serves 4

2 teaspoons olive oil
3 (5-ounce / 142-g) boneless, skinless chicken breasts cut into 1-inch chunks
1 tablespoon garlic, minced
2 tablespoons curry powder
1 tablespoon fresh

ginger, grated
1 cup coconut milk
2 cups low-sodium chicken broth
1 sweet potato, diced
1 carrot, peeled and diced
2 tablespoons fresh cilantro, chopped

1. Heat the olive oil in a saucepan over medium-high heat until shimmering.

2. Add the chicken to the saucepan and sauté for 10 minutes until browned on all sides.
3. Add the garlic, curry powder, and ginger to the saucepan and sauté for 3 minutes until fragrant.
4. Pour the coconut milk and chicken broth in the saucepan, then add the sweet potato and carrot to the saucepan. Stir to mix well. Bring to a boil.
5. Turn down the heat to low, and then simmer for 20 minutes until tender. Stir periodically.
6. Pour them in a large bowl and spread the cilantro on top before serving.

Per Serving
Calories: 328 | fat: 16.9g | protein: 29.1g | carbs: 14.8g | fiber: 1.1g | sugar: 3.9g | sodium: 274mg

Five Spiced Roasted Duck Legs & Cabbage Slaw

Prep time: 10 minutes | Cook time: 1 hour 30 minutes | Serves 4

4 duck legs
3 plum tomatoes, diced
1 red chili, deseeded and sliced
½ small Savoy cabbage, quartered
2 teaspoons fresh

ginger, grated
3 cloves garlic, sliced
2 tablespoons soy sauce
2 tablespoons honey
1 teaspoon five-spice powder

1. Heat oven to 350ºF (180ºC).
2. Place the duck in a large skillet over low heat and cook until brown on all sides and most of the fat is rendered, about 10 minutes. Transfer duck to a deep baking dish. Drain off all but 2 tablespoons of the fat.
3. Add ginger, garlic, and chili to the skillet and cook 2 minutes until soft. Add soy sauce, tomatoes and 2 tablespoons water and bring to a boil.
4. Rub the duck with the five spice seasoning. Pour the sauce over the duck and drizzle with the honey. Cover with foil and bake 1 hour. Add the cabbage for the last 10 minutes.

Per Serving
Calories: 212 | fat: 5.0g | protein: 25.2g | carbs: 19.1g | fiber: 3.2g | sugar: 14.1g | sodium: 365mg

Citrus Honey Chicken with Cilantro

Prep time: 15 minutes | Cook time: 30 minutes | Serves 4

1 tablespoon grated fresh ginger
Sea salt, to taste
4 chicken thighs, bone-in, skinless
1 tablespoon extra-virgin olive oil
Juice and zest of ½ orange

Juice and zest of ½ lemons
1 tablespoon low-sodium soy sauce
Pinch red pepper flakes, to taste
2 tablespoons honey
1 tablespoon chopped fresh cilantro

1. In a large bowl, combine the ginger and salt. Dunk the chicken thighs and toss to coat well.
2. Heat the olive oil in a nonstick skillet over medium-high heat until shimmering.
3. Add the chicken thighs and cook for 10 minutes or until well browned. Flip halfway through the cooking time.
4. Meanwhile, combine the orange juice and zest, lemon juice and zest, soy sauce, red pepper flakes, and honey. Stir to mix well.
5. Pour the mixture in the skillet. Reduce the heat to low, then cover and braise for 20 minutes. Add tablespoons of water if too dry.
6. Serve the chicken thighs garnished with cilantro.

Per Serving
Calories: 114 | fat: 5.0g | protein: 9.0g | carbs: 9.0g | fiber: 0g | sugar: 9.0g | sodium: 287mg

Delicious Herb Chicken in 30 minutes

Prep time: 15 minutes | Cook time: 30 minutes | Serves 4

4 (4-ounce / 113-g) boneless, skinless chicken breasts
Salt and freshly ground black pepper, to taste
1 tablespoon extra-virgin olive oil
½ sweet onion,

chopped
2 teaspoons chopped fresh thyme
1 cup low-sodium chicken broth
¼ cup heavy whipping cream
1 scallion, white and green parts, chopped

1. Preheat the oven to 375ºF (190ºC).
2. On a clean work surface, rub the chicken with salt and pepper.
3. Heat the olive oil in an oven-safe skillet over medium-high heat until shimmering.
4. Put the chicken in the skillet and cook for 10 minutes or until well browned. Flip halfway through. Transfer onto a platter and set aside.
5. Add the onion to the skillet and sauté for 3 minutes or until translucent.
6. Add the thyme and broth and simmer for 6 minutes or until the liquid reduces in half.
7. Mix in the cream, then put the chicken back to the skillet.
8. Arrange the skillet in the oven and bake for 10 minutes.
9. Remove the skillet from the oven and serve them with scallion.

Per Serving
Calories: 287 | fat: 14.0g | protein: 34.0g | carbs: 4.0g | fiber: 1.0g | sugar: 1.0g | sodium: 184mg

Chicken Veggie Pan with Cauliflower Rice

Prep time: 15 minutes | Cook time: 25 minutes | Serves 2

2 chicken breast halves, boneless and skinless
1 cup cauliflower rice, cooked
⅓ cup green bell pepper, julienned
¼ cup celery, diced
¼ cup onion, diced

14½ ounces (411 g) stewed tomatoes, diced
1 teaspoon sunflower oil
1 teaspoon chili powder
½ teaspoon thyme
⅛ Teaspoon pepper

1. Heat oil in a small skillet over medium heat.
2. Add chicken and cook 5 to 6 minutes per side or cooked through. Transfer to plate and keep warm.
3. Add the pepper, celery, onion, tomatoes, and seasonings.
4. Bring to a boil. Reduce heat, cover, and simmer 10 minutes or until vegetables start to soften.
5. Add chicken back to pan to heat through. Serve over cauliflower rice.

Per Serving
Calories: 361 | fat: 14.0g | protein: 45.2g | carbs: 14.1g | fiber: 4.0g | sugar: 8.0g | sodium: 335mg

Chicken & Roasted Vegetable Zucchini Wrap

Prep time: 10 minutes | Cook time: 20 minutes | Serves 4

1 red bell pepper, seeded and cut into 1-inch-wide strips
½ small eggplants cut into ¼-inch-thick slices
½ small red onion, sliced
1 medium zucchini, cut lengthwise into strips
1 tablespoon extra-

virgin olive oil
Salt and freshly ground black pepper, to taste
4 whole-wheat tortilla wraps
2 (8-ounce / 227-g) cooked chicken breasts, sliced

1. Preheat the oven to 400ºF (205ºC). Line a baking sheet with aluminium foil.
2. Combine the bell pepper, eggplant, red onion, zucchini, and olive oil in a large bowl. Toss to coat well.
3. Pour the vegetables into the baking sheet, then sprinkle with salt and pepper.
4. Roast in the preheated oven for 20 minutes or until tender and charred.
5. Unfold the tortillas on a clean work surface, and then divide the vegetables and chicken slices on the tortillas.
6. Wrap and serve immediately.

Per Serving
Calories: 483 | fat: 25.0g | protein: 20.0g | carbs: 45.0g | fiber: 3.0g | sugar: 4.0g | sodium: 730mg

The Best Veggie Turkey Ever

Prep time: 10 minutes | Cook time: 45 minutes | Serves 4

1 pound (454 g) lean ground turkey
2 carrots, peeled and diced
2 stalks of celery, diced
1 onion, diced
1 zucchini, diced
1 red pepper, diced
1 (14-ounce / 397-g) can tomato sauce
1 can black beans, drained and rinsed

1 can kidney beans, drained and rinsed
3 cups water
3 garlic cloves, diced fine
1 tablespoon chili powder
1 tablespoon olive oil
2 teaspoons salt
1 teaspoon pepper
1 teaspoon cumin
1 teaspoon coriander
1 bay leaf

1. Heat oil in a heavy bottom soup pot over medium-high heat. Add turkey and onion and cook until no longer pink, 5 to 10 minutes.
2. Add the vegetables and cook, stirring occasionally, 5 minutes. Add the garlic and spices and cook, stirring, 2 minutes.
3. Add the remaining and bring to a boil. Reduce heat to low and simmer for 30 minutes.

Per Serving
Calories: 220 | fat: 9.0g | protein: 25.2g | carbs: 14.1g | fiber: 4.0g | sugar: 6.0g | sodium: 1447mg

Chicken Sesame Noodles Bowl with Tahini sauce

Prep time: 10 minutes | Cook time: 15 minutes | Serves 6

8 ounces (227 g) soba noodles
2 boneless, skinless chicken breasts, halved lengthwise
¼ cup tahini
1 tablespoon tamari
1 (1-inch) piece fresh ginger, finely grated
2 tablespoons rice vinegar

1 teaspoon toasted sesame oil
¼c cup water
1 large cucumber, deseeded and diced
1 scallion's bunch, green parts only, cut into 1-inch segments
1 tablespoon sesame seeds

1. Preheat the broiler to high.
2. Add the soba noodles in a pot of salted boiling water and cook for 5 minutes or until al dente. Transfer to a plate and pat dry with paper towels.
3. Place the chicken in a single layer on a baking sheet. Broil in the preheated broiler for 6 to 7 minutes or until the chicken is fork-tender. Transfer the chicken to a bowl and shred with forks.
4. Combine the tahini, tamari, ginger, rice vinegar, sesame oil, and water in a small bowl. Stir to combine well.
5. Put the soba noodles, chicken, cucumber, and scallions in a large bowl.
6. Top them with the tahini sauce, then toss to combine well. Serve with sesame seeds on top.

Per Serving
Calories: 253 | fat: 7.8g | protein: 16.1g | carbs: 34.8g | fiber: 2.2g | sugar: 1.8g | sodium: 479mg

Spicy Garlic Corn Starch Chicken

Prep time: 15 minutes | Cook time: 3 to 4 hours | Serves 6

2 pounds (907 g) chicken thighs, boneless and skinless
2 tablespoons fresh ginger, grated
4 cloves garlic, diced fine
¼ cup lite soy sauce

2 tablespoons Korean chili paste
2 tablespoons toasted sesame oil
2 teaspoons cornstarch
Pinch of red pepper flakes

1. Add the soy sauce, chili paste, sesame oil, ginger, garlic and pepper flakes to the crock pot, stir to combine. Add the chicken and turn to coat in the sauce.
2. Cover and cook on low 3–4 hours or till chicken is cooked through.
3. When the chicken is cooked, transfer it to a plate.
4. Pour the sauce into a medium saucepan. Whisk the cornstarch and ¼ cup cold water until smooth. Add it to the sauce. Cook over medium heat, stirring constantly, about 5 minutes, or until sauce is thick and glossy.
5. Use 2 forks and shred the chicken. Add it to the sauce and stir to coat. Serve.

Per Serving
Calories: 400 | fat: 16.0g | protein: 44.2g | carbs: 18.1g | fiber: 0g | sugar: 13.0g | sodium: 583mg

Cheesy Chicken with Garlic & Italian Seasoning

Prep time: 10 minutes | Cook time: 45 minutes | Serves 6

3 chicken breasts, boneless, skinless and halved lengthwise
6 ounces (170 g) low fat cream cheese, soft
2 cup baby spinach
1 cup Mozzarella cheese, grated

2 tablespoons olive oil, divided
3 cloves garlic, diced fine
1 teaspoon Italian seasoning
Nonstick cooking spray

1. Heat oven to 350ºF (180ºC). Spray a glass baking dish with cooking spray.
2. Lay chicken breast cutlets in baking dish. Drizzle 1 tablespoon oil over chicken. Sprinkle evenly with garlic and Italian seasoning.

3. Spread cream cheese over the top of chicken.
4. Heat remaining tablespoon of oil in a small skillet over medium heat. Add spinach and cook until spinach wilts, about 3 minutes.
5. Place evenly over cream cheese layer. Sprinkle Mozzarella over top.
6. Bake for 35 to 40 minutes, or until chicken is cooked through. Serve.

Per Serving
Calories: 362 | fat: 25.0g | protein: 31.2g | carbs: 3.1g | fiber: 0g | sugar: 0g | sodium: 376mg

Creamy Chicken with Cauliflower

Prep time: 10 minutes | Cook time: 40 minutes | Serves 6

4 slices bacon, cooked and crumbled
3 cups cauliflower
3 cups chicken, cooked and chopped
3 cups broccoli florets
2 cups reduced fat cheddar cheese, grated
1 cup fat free sour

cream
4 tablespoons margarine, soft
1 teaspoon salt
½ teaspoon black pepper
½ teaspoon garlic powder
½ teaspoon paprika
Nonstick cooking spray

1. In a large saucepan add 4 to 5 cups of water and bring to a boil. Add the cauliflower and cook about 4 to 5 minutes, or until it is tender drain well. Repeat with broccoli.
2. Heat oven to 350ºF (180ºC). Spray a baking dish with cooking spray.
3. In a medium bowl, mash the cauliflower with the margarine, sour cream and seasonings. Add remaining, saving ½ the cheese, and mix well.
4. Spread mixture in prepared baking dish and sprinkle remaining cheese on top.
5. Bake 20 to 25 minutes, or until heated through and cheese has melted. Serve.

Per Serving
Calories: 345 | fat: 15.0g | protein: 28.2g | carbs: 10.1g | fiber: 2.2g | sugar: 4.1g | sodium: 990mg

Cheesy Chicken with Spinach and Tomatoes

Prep time: 10 minutes | Cook time: 15 minutes | Serves 4

1½ pounds (680 g) chicken breasts, boneless, skinless and sliced thin
1 cup spinach, chopped
1 cup half-and-half
½ cup reduced fat Parmesan cheese
½ cup low sodium chicken broth
½ cup sun dried tomatoes
2 tablespoons olive oil
1 teaspoon Italian seasoning
1 teaspoon garlic powder

1. Heat oil in a large skillet over medium-high heat. Add chicken and cook 3 to 5 minutes per side, or until browned and cooked through. Transfer to a plate.
2. Add half-and-half, broth, cheese and seasonings to the pan. Whisk constantly until sauce starts to thicken.
3. Add spinach and tomatoes and cook, stirring frequently, until spinach starts to wilt, about 2 to 3 minutes.
4. Add chicken back to the pan and cook just long enough to heat through.

Per Serving
Calories: 463 | fat: 23.0g | protein: 55.2g | carbs: 6.1g | fiber: 1.0g | sugar: 0g | sodium: 441mg

Chicken Patties with Roasted Tomato Salsa

Prep time: 10 minutes | Cook time: 10 minutes | Serves 8

2 cup chicken breast, cooked, divided
1 zucchini cut in ¾-inch pieces
¼ cup cilantro, diced
⅓ cup bread crumbs
2 teaspoons olive oil
½ teaspoon salt
¼ teaspoon pepper
Roasted Tomato Salsa:
6 plum tomatoes
1¼ cups cilantro
2 teaspoons olive oil
1 teaspoon adobo
sauce
½ teaspoon salt, divided
Nonstick cooking spray

1. Place 1½ cups chicken and zucchini into a food processor. Cover and process until coarsely chopped.
2. Add bread crumbs, pepper, cilantro, remaining chicken, and salt. Cover and pulse until chunky.
3. Heat oil in a large skillet over medium-high heat. Shape chicken mixture into 8 patties and cook 4 minutes per side, or until golden brown.
4. Meanwhile, combine the ingredients for the salsa in a small bowl.
5. Serve the patties topped with salsa.

Per Serving
Calories: 147 | fat: 7.0g | protein: 12.2g | carbs: 10.1g | fiber: 2.0g | sugar: 5.0g | sodium: 461mg

Creamy Chicken with Green Chillies & Cilantro

Prep time: 20 minutes | Cook time: 45 minutes | Serves 12

1 onion, diced
4 cup chicken breast, cooked and cubed
1 cup fat free sour cream
1 cup skim milk
4 ounces (113 g) low fat cream cheese
½ cup reduced fat cheddar cheese, grated
2 tablespoons cilantro, diced
12 (6-inch) flour tortillas, warm
1 can low fat condensed cream of chicken soup
¼ cup pecans, toasted
2 tablespoons green chilies, diced
1 tablespoon water
1 teaspoon cumin
¼ teaspoon pepper
⅛ teaspoon salt
Nonstick cooking spray

1. Heat oven to 350ºF (180ºC). Spray a baking dish with cooking spray.
2. Spray a nonstick skillet with cooking spray and place over medium heat. Add onion and cook until tender.
3. In a large bowl, beat cream cheese, water, cumin, salt, and pepper until smooth. Stir in the onion, chicken, and pecans.
4. Spoon ⅓ cup chicken mixture down the middle of each tortilla. Roll up and place, seam side down, in prepared baking dish.
5. In a medium bowl, combine soup, sour cream, milk, and chilies and pour over enchiladas.
6. Cover with foil and bake 40 minutes. Uncover and sprinkle cheese over top and bake another 5 minutes until cheese is melted.
7. Sprinkle with cilantro and serve.

Per Serving
Calories: 321 | fat: 13.0g | protein: 21.2g | carbs: 27.1g | fiber: 2.0g | sugar: 4.0g | sodium: 684mg

Creamy Curried Apple Chicken

Prep time: 15 minutes | Cook time: 30 minutes | Serves 4

1 pound (454 g) chicken breasts, boneless, skinless, cut in 1-inch cubes
2 tart apples peel and slice
1 sweet onion cut in half and slice
1 jalapeno, seeded and diced
2 tablespoons cilantro, diced
½ teaspoon ginger, grated
14½ ounces (411 g) tomatoes, diced and drained
½ cup water
3 cloves garlic, diced
2 tablespoons sunflower oil
1 teaspoon salt
1 teaspoon coriander
½ teaspoon turmeric
¼ teaspoon cayenne pepper

1. Heat oil in a large skillet over medium-high heat. Add chicken and onion, and cook until onion is tender. Add garlic and cook 1 more minute.
2. Add apples, water and seasonings and stir to combine. Bring to a boil.
3. Reduce heat and simmer 12 to 15 minutes, or until chicken is cooked through, stirring occasionally.
4. Stir in tomatoes, jalapeno, and cilantro and serve.

Per Serving
Calories: 372 | fat: 16.0g | protein: 34.2g | carbs: 23.1g | fiber: 5.0g | sugar: 15.0g | sodium: 705mg

Baked Pineapple Chicken

Prep time: 15 minutes | Cook time: 3 hours | Serves 8

8 chicken thighs bone-in and skin-on
1 red bell pepper, diced
1 red onion, diced
2 tablespoons fresh parsley, chopped
2 tablespoons margarine
8 ounces (227 g) can pineapple chunks
8 ounces (227 g) can crushed pineapple
1 cup pineapple juice
½ cup low sodium chicken broth
¼ cup water
3 tablespoons light soy sauce
2 tablespoons apple cider vinegar
2 tablespoons honey
2 tablespoons cornstarch
1 teaspoon garlic powder
1 teaspoon Sriracha
½ teaspoon ginger
½ teaspoon sesame seeds
Salt and ground black pepper, to taste to taste

1. Season chicken with salt and pepper.
2. Melt butter in a large skillet over medium heat.
3. Add chicken, skin side down, and sear both sides until golden brown. Add chicken to the crock pot.
4. In a large bowl, combine pineapple juice, broth, Splenda, soy sauce, honey, vinegar, Sriracha, garlic powder, and ginger. Pour over chicken.
5. Top with kinds of pineapple. Cover and cook on high 2 hours. Baste the chicken occasionally.
6. Mix the cornstarch and water together until smooth. Stir into chicken and add the pepper and onion, cook another 60 minutes, or until sauce has thickened. Serve garnished with parsley and sesame seeds.

Per Serving
Calories: 300 | fat: 13.0g | protein: 17.2g | carbs: 24.1g | fiber: 1.0g | sugar: 18.0g | sodium: 280mg

Italian Mushroom Chicken Dish

Prep time: 10 minutes | Cook time: 25 minutes | Serves 4

4 boneless chicken breasts
½ pound (227 g) mushrooms, sliced
1 tablespoon margarine
¼ cup flour
1 tablespoon oil
Pinch of white pepper
Pinch of oregano
Pinch of basil

1. On a shallow plate, combine flour and seasonings.
2. Dredge the chicken in the flour mixture to coat both sides.
3. In a large skillet, over medium heat, heat oil until hot. Add chicken and cook until brown on both sides, about 15 minutes. Transfer chicken to a plate.
4. Reduce heat to low and add mushrooms. Cook about 5 minutes. Scrape bottom of pan to loosen any flour. Stir in reserved flour mixture.
5. Simmer until mixture starts to thicken, stirring constantly. Add the chicken back to the pan and cook an additional 5 minutes. Serve.

Per Serving
Calories: 328 | fat: 14.0g | protein: 21.2g | carbs: 9.1g | fiber: 1.0g | sugar: 1.0g | sodium: 190mg

Chapter 11: Dinner Recipes: Salads

Rise and Shine Veggie Salad

Prep time: 10 minutes | Cook time: 0 minutes | Serves 4

1 cup cherry tomatoes, halved
1 large cucumber, chopped
1 small red onion, thinly sliced
1 avocado, diced
2 tablespoons chopped

fresh dill
2 tablespoons extra-virgin olive oil
Juice of 1 lemon
¼ teaspoon salt
¼ teaspoon freshly ground black pepper

1. In a large mixing bowl, combine the tomatoes, cucumber, onion, avocado, and dill.
2. In a small bowl, combine the oil, lemon juice, salt, and pepper, and mix well.
3. Drizzle the dressing over the vegetables and toss to combine. Serve.

Per Serving
Calories: 152 | fat: 12.1g | protein: 2.1g | carbs: 10.9g | fiber: 4.1g | sugar: 4.0g | sodium: 129mg

Homemade Red & Green Cabbage Slaw

Prep time: 15 minutes | Cook time: 0 minutes | Serves 6

2 cups finely chopped green cabbage
2 cups finely chopped red cabbage
2 cups grated carrots
3 scallions, both white and green parts, sliced

2 tablespoons extra-virgin olive oil
2 tablespoons rice vinegar
1 garlic clove, minced
¼ teaspoon salt

1. In a large bowl, toss together the green and red cabbage, carrots, and scallions.
2. In a small bowl, whisk together the oil, vinegar, honey, garlic, and salt.
3. Pour the dressing over the veggies and mix to thoroughly combine.
4. Serve immediately, or cover and chill for several hours before serving.

Per Serving
Calories: 81 | fat: 5.1g | protein: 1.1g | carbs: 69.9g | fiber: 3.1g | sugar: 6.0g | sodium: 124mg

High Protein Kidney Bean Cucumber Salad

Prep time: 10 minutes | Cook time: 0 minutes | Serves 4

3 cups diced cucumber
1 (15-ounce / 425-g) can low-sodium dark red kidney beans, drained and rinsed
2 avocados, diced
1½ cup diced tomatoes

1 cup cooked corn
¾ cup sliced red onion
1 tablespoon extra-virgin olive oil
1 tablespoon apple cider vinegar

1. In a large bowl, combine the cucumber, kidney beans, avocados, tomatoes, corn, onion, olive oil, and vinegar.

Per Serving
Calories: 320 | fat: 16.1g | protein: 10.1g | carbs: 35.9g | fiber: 14.1g | sugar: 7.0g | sodium: 117mg

Crunchy Kale and Chickpea Salad Recipe

Prep time: 10 minutes | Cook time: 0 minutes | Serves 6

1 (15-ounce / 425-g) can chickpeas packed in water, rinsed and drained
2 cups shredded kale
1 English cucumber, shredded
1 red bell pepper, seeded and cut into very thin strips
2 tablespoons balsamic

vinegar
1 tablespoon chopped fresh oregano
Sea salt and freshly ground black pepper, to taste
½ cup chopped fresh parsley
½ cup crumbled low-sodium feta cheese

1. In a large bowl, toss together the chickpeas, kale, cucumber, pepper, vinegar, and oregano.
2. Season with salt and pepper.
3. Sprinkle on the parsley and feta, and serve.

Per Serving
Calories: 193 | fat: 5.1g | protein: 10.1g | carbs: 30.1g | fiber: 8.1g | sugar: 6.0g | sodium: 169mg

Delicious Cayenne Pepper Tomato Mushroom Salad

Prep time: 10 minutes | Cook time: 0 minutes | Serves 4

4 sun-dried tomatoes cut in half
3 cup torn leaf lettuce
1½ cup broccoli florets
1 cup mushrooms, sliced
⅓ cup radishes, sliced
2 tablespoons water
1 tablespoon balsamic vinegar

1 teaspoon vegetable oil
¼ teaspoon chicken bouillon granules
¼ teaspoon parsley
¼ teaspoon dry mustard
⅛ teaspoon cayenne pepper

1. Place tomatoes in a small bowl and pour boiling water over, just enough to cover. Let stand 5 minutes, drain.
2. Chop tomatoes and place in a large bowl. Add lettuce, broccoli, mushrooms, and radishes.
3. In a jar with a tight fitting lid, add remaining and shake well. Pour over salad and toss to coat. Serve.

Per Serving
Calories: 55 | fat: 2.1g | protein: 3.0g | carbs: 9.1g | fiber: 2.0g | sugar: 1.9g | sodium: 19mg

Easy Corn Avocado Salad

Prep time: 10 minutes | Cook time: 0 minutes | Serves 8

2 avocados cut into ½-inch cubes
1 pint cherry tomatoes cut in half
2 cups fresh corn kernels, cooked
½ cup red onion, diced fine

¼ cup cilantro, chopped
1 tablespoon fresh lime juice
½ teaspoon lime zest
2 tablespoons olive oil
¼ teaspoon salt
¼ teaspoon pepper

1. In a large bowl, combine corn, avocado, tomatoes, and onion.
2. In a small bowl, whisk together remaining until combined. Pour over salad and toss to coat.
3. Cover and chill 2 hours. Serve.

Per Serving
Calories: 240 | fat: 18.1g | protein: 4.0g | carbs: 20.1g | fiber: 7.0g | sugar: 3.9g | sodium: 77mg

Sunday Creamy Veggie Salad

Prep time: 10 minutes | Cook time: 0 minutes | Serves 8

1 head broccoli, separated into florets
1 head cauliflower, separated into florets
1 red onion, sliced thin

2 cup cherry tomatoes, halved
½ cup fat free sour cream
1 tablespoon Splenda

1. In a large bowl combine vegetables.
2. In a small bowl, whisk together sour cream and Splenda. Pour over vegetables and toss to mix.
3. Cover and refrigerate at least 1 hour before serving.

Per Serving
Calories: 153 | fat: 10.1g | protein: 2.0g | carbs: 12.1g | fiber: 2.0g | sugar: 4.9g | sodium: 264mg

Bacon Cheese and Green Onion Salad

Prep time: 15 minutes | Cook time: 15 minutes | Serves 8

2 pounds (907 g) cauliflower, separated into small florets
6 to 8 slices bacon, chopped and fried crisp
6 boiled eggs, cooled, peeled, and chopped
1 cup sharp cheddar

cheese, grated
½ cup green onion, sliced
2 teaspoons yellow mustard
1½ teaspoons onion powder, divided
Salt and fresh-ground black pepper to taste

1. Place cauliflower in a vegetable steamer, or a pot with a steamer insert, and steam 5 to 6 minutes.
2. Drain the cauliflower and set aside.
3. In a small bowl, whisk together mustard, 1 teaspoon onion powder, salt, and pepper.
4. Pat cauliflower dry with paper towels and place in a large mixing bowl. Add eggs, salt, pepper, remaining ½ teaspoon onion powder, and then dressing. Mix gently to combine together.
5. Fold in the bacon, cheese, and green onion. Serve warm or cover and chill before serving.

Per Serving
Calories: 248 | fat: 17.1g | protein: 17.0g | carbs: 8.1g | fiber: 3.0g | sugar: 2.9g | sodium: 384mg

Chilled Crab Egg Slaw

Prep time: 10 minutes | Cook time: 0 minutes | Serves 4

½ pound (227 g) cabbage, shredded
½ pound (227 g) red cabbage, shredded
2 hard-boiled eggs, chopped
Juice of ½ lemon
2 (6-ounce / 170-g) cans crabmeat, drained
1 teaspoon celery seeds
Salt and ground black pepper, to taste

1. In a large bowl, combine both kinds of cabbage.
2. In a small bowl, combine lemon juice, and celery seeds. Add to cabbage and toss to coat.
3. Add crab and eggs and toss to mix, season with salt and pepper. Cover and refrigerate 1 hour before serving.

Per Serving
Calories: 381 | fat: 24.1g | protein: 18.0g | carbs: 25.1g | fiber: 8.0g | sugar: 12.9g | sodium: 266mg

Feel Cool Watermelon Mint Salad

Prep time: 10 minutes | Cook time: 0 minutes | Serves 6

4 cups watermelon cut in 1-inch cubes
3 cup arugula
1 lemon, zested
½ cup feta cheese, crumbled
¼ cup fresh mint,
chopped
1 tablespoon fresh lemon juice
3 tablespoons olive oil
Fresh ground black pepper, to taste
Salt, to taste

1. Combine oil, zest, juice and mint in a large bowl. Stir together.
2. Add watermelon and gently toss to coat. Add remaining and toss to combine. Taste and adjust seasoning as desired.
3. Cover and chill at least 1 hour before serving.

Per Serving
Calories: 150 | fat: 11.1g | protein: 4.0g | carbs: 10.1g | fiber: 1.0g | sugar: 6.9g | sodium: 145mg

Holiday Special Pomegranate Almonds Salad

Prep time: 10 minutes | Cook time: 0 minutes | Serves 6

3 slices bacon, cooked crisp and crumbled
3 cup Brussels sprouts, shredded
3 cup kale, shredded
1½ cup pomegranate
seeds
½ cup almonds, toasted and chopped
¼ cup reduced fat Parmesan cheese, grated
Citrus Vinaigrette:
1 orange, zested and juiced
1 lemon, zested and juiced
¼ cup extra virgin olive oil
1 teaspoon Dijon mustard
1 teaspoon honey
1 clove garlic, crushed
Salt and ground black pepper, to taste

1. Combine the ingredient for the citrus vinaigrette in a small bowl.
2. Toss the remaining ingredients with the vinaigrette in a large bowl.
3. Serve garnished with more cheese if desired.

Per Serving
Calories: 255 | fat: 18.1g | protein: 9.0g | carbs: 15.1g | fiber: 5.0g | sugar: 4.9g | sodium: 176mg

Blue Cheese Mixed Green Salad

Prep time: 15 minutes | Cook time: 0 minutes | Serves 8

10 ounces (283 g) mixed greens
3 pears, chopped
½ cup blue cheese, crumbled
2 cup pecan halves
1 cup dried cranberries
½ cup olive oil
6 tablespoons champagne vinegar
2 tablespoons Dijon mustard
¼ teaspoon salt

1. In a large bowl combine greens, pears, cranberries and pecans.
2. Whisk remaining, except blue cheese, together in a small bowl Pour over salad and toss to coat. Serve topped with blue cheese crumbles.

Per Serving
Calories: 326 | fat: 26.1g | protein: 5.0g | carbs: 20.1g | fiber: 6.0g | sugar: 9.9g | sodium: 294mg

Autumn Pear Walnut Salad

Prep time: 10 minutes | Cook time: 0 minutes | Serves 2

2 tablespoons apple cider vinegar
1 teaspoon peeled and grated fresh ginger
½ teaspoon Dijon mustard
2 tablespoons extra-

virgin olive oil
½ teaspoon sea salt
4 cups baby spinach
½ pear, cored, peeled, and chopped
¼ cup chopped walnuts

1. Combine the vinegar, ginger, mustard, olive oil, and salt in a small bowl. Stir to mix well.
2. Combine the remaining ingredients in a large serving bowl, and then toss to combine well.
3. Pour the vinegar dressing in the bowl of salad and toss before serving.

Per Serving
Calories: 229 | fat: 20.4g | protein: 3.5g | carbs: 10.7g | fiber: 3.4g | sugar: 4.9g | sodium: 644mg

Traditional Spinach Sofrito Steak Salad

Prep time: 10 minutes | Cook time: 15 minutes | Serves 4

4 ounces (113 g) recaíto cooking base
2 (4-ounce / 113-g) flank steaks
8 cups fresh spinach, loosely packed

½ cup sliced red onion
2 cups diced tomato
2 avocados, diced
2 cups diced cucumber
⅓ cup crumbled feta

1. Heat a large skillet over medium-low heat. When hot, pour in the recaíto cooking base, add the steaks, and cover. Cook for 8 to 12 minutes.
2. Meanwhile, divide the spinach into four portions. Top each portion with one-quarter of the onion, tomato, avocados, and cucumber.
3. Remove the steak from the skillet, and let it rest for about 2 minutes before slicing. Place one-quarter of the steak and feta on top of each portion.

Per Serving
Calories: 346 | fat: 18.1g | protein: 25.1g | carbs: 17.9g | fiber: 8.1g | sugar: 6.0g | sodium: 380mg

Maple dressed Black Rice Walnut Salad

Prep time: 15 minutes | Cook time: 25 minutes | Serves 8

Rice:
1 cup black rice (forbidden rice), rinsed and still wet
Dressing:
3 tablespoons extra-virgin olive oil
2 tablespoons freshly squeezed lemon juice
2 tablespoons white wine vinegar or rice

vinegar
1 tablespoon honey or pure maple syrup
1 tablespoon sesame oil

Salad:
1 (8-ounce / 227-g) bag frozen shelled edamame, thawed (about 1½ cups)
2 scallions, both white and green parts, thinly

sliced
¼ cup chopped walnuts
Kosher salt and freshly ground black pepper, to taste

Make the Rice
1. In the electric pressure cooker, combine the rice and 1 cup of water.
2. Close and lock the lid of the pressure cooker. Set the valve to sealing.
3. Cook on high pressure for 22 minutes.
4. When the cooking is complete, hit Cancel and allow the pressure to release naturally for 10 minutes, then quick release any remaining pressure.
5. Once the pin drops, unlock and remove the lid.
6. Fluff the rice with a fork and let it cool.

Make the Dressing
7. While the rice is cooking, make the dressing. In a small jar with a screw-top lid, combine the olive oil, lemon juice, vinegar, honey or maple syrup, and sesame oil. Shake until well combined.

Make the salad
8. Shake up the dressing. In a large bowl, toss the rice and dressing. Stir in the edamame, scallions, and walnuts.
9. Season with salt and pepper.

Per Serving
Calories: 171 | fat: 11.1g | protein: 5.1g | carbs: 14.9g | fiber: 2.1g | sugar: 3.0g | sodium: 11mg

Lettuce Walnut Salad with Honey

Prep time: 5 minutes | Cook time: 0 minutes | Serves 4

Salad:
8 cups mixed greens or preferred lettuce, loosely packed
4 cups arugula, loosely packed
2 peaches, sliced ½
cup thinly sliced red onion
½ cup chopped walnuts or pecans
½ cup crumbled feta

Dressing:
4 teaspoons extra-virgin olive oil
4 teaspoons honey

Make the Salad
1. Combine the mixed greens, arugula, peaches, red onion, walnuts, and feta in a large bowl. Divide the salad into four portions.
2. Drizzle the dressing over each individual serving of salad.

Make the Dressing
3. In a small bowl, whisk together the olive oil and honey.

Per Serving
Calories: 264 | fat: 18.1g | protein: 8.1g | carbs: 21.9g | fiber: 5.1g | sugar: 16.0g | sodium: 223mg

Honeyed Rainbow Fruit Baby Spinach Salad

Prep time: 15 minutes | Cook time: 0 minutes | Serves 5

1 (15-ounce / 425-g) can low-sodium black beans, drained and rinsed
1 avocado, diced
1 cup cherry
2 tomatoes, halved
1 cup chopped baby spinach
½ cup finely chopped red bell pepper
¼ cup finely chopped jicama
½ cup chopped
scallions, both white and green parts
¼ cup chopped fresh cilantro
2 tablespoons freshly squeezed lime juice
1 tablespoon extra-virgin olive oil
2 garlic cloves, minced
1 teaspoon honey
¼ teaspoon salt
¼ teaspoons freshly ground black pepper

1. In a large bowl, combine the black beans, avocado, tomatoes, spinach, bell pepper, jicama, scallions, and cilantro.

2. In a small bowl, mix the lime juice, oil, garlic, honey, salt, and pepper. Add to the salad and toss.
3. Chill for 1 hour before serving.

Per Serving
Calories: 168 | fat: 7.1g | protein: 6.1g | carbs: 21.8g | fiber: 9.1g | sugar: 3.0g | sodium: 236mg

Best Ever Green Salad with Honeyed Black Berry

Prep time: 15 minutes | Cook time: 20 minutes | Serves 4

Vinaigrette:
1 pint blackberries
2 tablespoons red wine vinegar
1 tablespoon honey
3 tablespoons extra-
virgin olive oil
¼ teaspoon salt
Freshly ground black pepper

Salad:
1 sweet potato, cubed
1 teaspoon extra-virgin olive oil
8 cups salad greens (baby spinach, spicy
greens, romaine)
½ red onion, sliced
¼ cup crumbled goat cheese

Make the Vinaigrette
1. In a blender jar, combine the blackberries, vinegar, honey, oil, salt, and pepper, and process until smooth. Set aside.

Make the Salad
2. Preheat the oven to 425ºF (220ºC). Line a baking sheet with parchment paper.
3. In a medium mixing bowl, toss the sweet potato with the olive oil.
4. Transfer to the prepared baking sheet and roast for 20 minutes, stirring once halfway through, until tender. Remove and cool for a few minutes.
5. In a large bowl, toss the greens with the red onion and cooled sweet potato, and drizzle with the vinaigrette.
6. Serve topped with 1 tablespoon of goat cheese per serving.

Per Serving
Calories: 197 | fat: 12.1g | protein: 3.1g | carbs: 20.9g | fiber: 6.1g | sugar: 10.0g | sodium: 185mg

Nutty Fruity Spinach Chicken Salad

Prep time: 5 minutes | Cook time: 0 minutes | Serves 4

Salad:

8 cups baby spinach
2 cups shredded rotisserie chicken
½ cup sliced strawberries or other

berries
½ cup sliced almonds
1 avocado, sliced
¼ cup crumbled feta (optional)

Dressing:

2 tablespoons extra-virgin olive oil
2 teaspoons honey

2 teaspoons balsamic vinegar

Make the Salad

1. In a large bowl, combine the spinach, chicken, strawberries, and almonds.
2. Pour the dressing over the salad and lightly toss.
3. Divide into four equal portions and top each with sliced avocado and 1 tablespoon of crumbled feta (if using).

Make the Dressing

4. In a small bowl, whisk together the olive oil, honey, and balsamic vinegar.

Per Serving

Calories: 340 | fat: 22.1g | protein: 25.1g | carbs: 12.9g | fiber: 6.1g | sugar: 6.0g | sodium: 133mg

Delicious Scallions and Three Bean Salad

Prep time: 10 minutes | Cook time: 0 minutes | Serves 8

1 (15-ounce / 425-g) can low-sodium chickpeas, drained and rinsed
1 (15-ounce / 425-g) can low-sodium kidney beans, drained and rinsed
1 (15-ounce / 425-g) can low-sodium white beans, drained and rinsed
1 red bell pepper, seeded and finely chopped

¼ cup chopped scallions, both white and green parts
¼ cup finely chopped fresh basil
3 garlic cloves, minced
2 tablespoons extra-virgin olive oil
1 tablespoon red wine vinegar
1 teaspoon Dijon mustard
¼ teaspoons freshly ground black pepper

1. In a large mixing bowl, combine the chickpeas, kidney beans, white beans, bell pepper, scallions, basil, and garlic. Toss gently to combine.
2. In a small bowl, combine the olive oil, vinegar, mustard, and pepper. Toss with the salad.
3. Cover and refrigerate for an hour before serving, to allow the flavors to mix.

Per Serving

Calories: 194 | fat: 5.1g | protein: 10.1g | carbs: 28.9g | fiber: 8.1g | sugar: 3.0g | sodium: 245mg

Easy Creamy Broccoli Yogurt Salad

Prep time: 10 minutes | Cook time: 0 minutes | Serves 4

2 cups broccoli, separated into florets
4 slices bacon, chopped and cooked crisp
½ cup cheddar cheese, cubed
¼ cup low-fat Greek yogurt
⅛ cup red onion, diced fine

⅛ Cup almonds, sliced
1 tablespoon lemon juice
1 tablespoon apple cider vinegar
1 tablespoon granulated sugar substitute
¼ teaspoon salt
¼ teaspoon pepper

1. In a large bowl, combine broccoli, onion, cheese, bacon, and almonds.
2. In a small bowl, whisk remaining together till combined.
3. Pour dressing over broccoli mixture and stir. Cover and chill at least 1 hour before serving.

Per Serving

Calories: 220 | fat: 14.1g | protein: 11.0g | carbs: 12.1g | fiber: 2.0g | sugar: 5.9g | sodium: 508mg

Kale, Cantaloupe, and Chicken Salad

Prep time: 10 minutes | Cook time: 0 minutes | Serves 3

Salad:

4 cups chopped kale, packed
1½ cups diced cantaloupe

1½ cups shredded rotisserie chicken
½ cup sliced almonds
¼ cup crumbled feta

Dressing:

½ teaspoons honey
2 tablespoons extra-virgin olive oil

2 teaspoons apple cider vinegar or freshly squeezed lemon juice

Make the Salad

1. Divide the kale into three portions. Layer ⅓ of the cantaloupe, chicken, almonds, and feta on each portion.
2. Drizzle some of the dressing over each portion of salad. Serve immediately.

Make the Dressing

3. In a small bowl, whisk together the honey, olive oil, and vinegar.

Per Serving

Calories: 395 | fat: 22.1g | protein: 27.1g | carbs: 23.9g | fiber: 4.1g | sugar: 12.0g | sodium: 235mg

Honeyed Mozzarella Prosciutto Salad

Prep time: 15 minutes | Cook time: 0 minutes | Serves 4

6 Mozzarella balls, quartered
1 medium cantaloupe, peeled and cut into small cubes
4 ounces (113 g) prosciutto, chopped

1 tablespoon fresh lime juice
1 tablespoon fresh mint, chopped
2 tablespoons extra virgin olive oil
½ teaspoon honey

1. In a large bowl, whisk together oil, lime juice, honey, and mint.
2. Season with salt and pepper to taste.
3. Add the cantaloupe and Mozzarella and toss to combine.
4. Arrange the mixture on a serving plate and add prosciutto. Serve.

Per Serving

Calories: 241 | fat: 16.1g | protein: 18.0g | carbs: 6.1g | fiber: 0g | sugar: 3.9g | sodium: 701mg

Zucchini Cherry Tomato Salad

Prep time: 10 minutes | Cook time: 0 minutes | Serves 4

1 cup cottage cheese
Juice of ½ lemons
2 tablespoons chopped fresh chives
2 tablespoons chopped fresh dill
2 scallions, white and

green parts, finely chopped
1 garlic clove, minced
½ teaspoon sea salt
2 zucchinis cut into sticks
8 cherry tomatoes

1. In a small bowl, mix the cottage cheese, lemon juice, chives, dill, scallions, garlic, and salt.
2. Serve with the zucchini sticks and cherry tomatoes for dipping.

Per Serving

Calories: 92 | fat: 4.1g | protein: 7.1g | carbs: 6.9g | fiber: 1.1g | sugar: 5.3g | sodium: 388mg

Asian Kale Salad with Paprika Peanuts

Prep time: 15 minutes | Cook time: 0 minutes | Serves 6

2 bunches baby kale, thinly sliced
½ head green savoy

cabbage, cored and thinly sliced

Dressing:

¼ cup apple cider vinegar
Juice of 1 lemon
1 teaspoon ground cumin
¼ teaspoon smoked

paprika
1 cup toasted peanuts
1 medium red bell pepper, thinly sliced
1 garlic clove, thinly sliced

1. Toss the kale with cabbage in a large bowl. Set aside.
2. Make the dressing: In a separate bowl, whisk together the vinegar, lemon juice, cumin, and paprika until completely mixed.
3. Pour the dressing into the bowl of greens and using your hands to massage the greens until thickly coated.
4. Add the peanuts, bell peppers, and garlic to the bowl. Gently toss to combine well.
5. Serve chilled or at room temperature.

Per Serving

Calories: 200 | fat: 12.3g | protein: 9.8g | carbs: 16.8g | fiber: 4.8g | sugar: 4.2g | sodium: 45mg

Best Ever Scallion Slaw

Prep time: 5 minutes | Cook time: 0 minutes | Serves 8

1 (1-pound / 454-g) bag coleslaw mix
5 scallions, sliced
1 cup sunflower seeds
1 cup almonds, sliced
3 ounces (85 g) ramen
noodles, broken into small pieces
¾ cup vegetable oil
½ cup Splenda
⅓ cup vinegar

1. In a large bowl, combine coleslaw, sunflower seeds, almonds, and scallions.
2. Whisk together the oil, vinegar and Splenda in a large measuring cup.
3. Pour over salad, and stir to combine.
4. Stir in ramen noodles, cover and chill 2 hours.

Per Serving
Calories: 355 | fat: 26.1g | protein: 5.0g | carbs: 24.1g | fiber: 3.1g | sugar: 9.9g | sodium: 22mg

Asparagus Egg Salad with Vinaigrette

Prep time: 5 minutes | Cook time: 5 minutes | Serves 1

1 hard-boiled egg, peeled and sliced
1⅔ cups asparagus, chopped
2 slices bacon, cooked crisp and crumbled
1 teaspoon extra virgin
olive oil
1 teaspoon red wine vinegar
½ teaspoon Dijon mustard
Pinch salt and pepper, to taste

1. Bring a pot of water to a boil. Add the asparagus and cook 2 to 3 minutes or until tender-crisp. Drain and add cold water to stop the cooking process.
2. In a small bowl, whisk together, mustard, oil, vinegar, and salt and pepper to taste.
3. Place the asparagus on a plate, top with egg and bacon. Drizzle with vinaigrette and serve.

Per Serving
Calories: 357 | fat: 25.1g | protein: 25.0g | carbs: 10.1g | fiber: 5.1g | sugar: 4.9g | sodium: 492mg

Italian Tomato Mozzarella Salad

Prep time: 10 minutes | Cook time: 0 minutes | Serves 4

3 medium tomatoes cut into 8 slices
2 (1-ounce / 28-g) slices Mozzarella cheese, cut into strips
¼ cup fresh basil,
sliced thin
2 teaspoons extra-virgin olive oil
⅛ teaspoon salt
Pinch black pepper

1. Place tomatoes and cheese on serving plates. Sprinkle with salt and pepper. Drizzle oil over and top with basil. Serve.

Per Serving
Calories: 78 | fat: 5.1g | protein: 5.0g | carbs: 4.1g | fiber: 1.0g | sugar: 1.9g | sodium: 84mg

Crunchy Dates with Maple Shallot Vinaigrette

Prep time: 5 minutes | Cook time: 10 minutes | Serves 4

2 green onions, diced
2 Medjool dates, pitted and diced fine
1 honey crisp apple, sliced thin
2 cup celery, sliced
½ cup celery leaves, diced
¼ cup walnuts, chopped

Maple Shallot Vinaigrette:
1 tablespoon shallot, diced fine
2 tablespoons apple cider vinegar
1 tablespoon spicy
brown mustard
1 tablespoon olive oil
2 teaspoon sugar-free maple syrup

1. Heat oven to 375ºF (190ºC). Place walnuts on a cookie sheet and bake 10 minutes, stirring every few minutes, to toast.
2. Meanwhile, combine the ingredients for the vinaigrette in a small bowl. Stir to mix well.
3. When the baking is complete, in a large bowl, combine the baked walnuts with the remaining ingredients and toss to mix.
4. Drizzle vinaigrette over and toss to coat. Serve immediately.

Per Serving
Calories: 172 | fat: 8.1g | protein: 3.0g | carbs: 25.1g | fiber: 4.0g | sugar: 14.9g | sodium: 95mg

Baked Chicken Avocado Salad

Prep time: 10 minutes | Cook time: 20 minutes | Serves 6

1 pound (454 g) chicken breast, boneless and skinless
2 avocados
1 to 2 jalapeno peppers, seeded and diced
⅓ cup onion, diced
3 tablespoons cilantro, diced
2 tablespoons fresh lime juice
2 cloves garlic, diced
1 tablespoon olive oil
Salt and ground black pepper, to taste

1. Heat oven to 400ºF (205ºC). Line a baking sheet with foil.
2. Season chicken with salt and pepper and place on prepared pan.
3. Bake 20 minutes, or until chicken is cooked through. Let cool completely.
4. Once chicken has cooled, shred or dice and add to a large bowl.
5. Add remaining and mix well, mashing the avocado as you mix it in. Taste and season with salt and pepper as desired. Serve immediately.

Per Serving
Calories: 325 | fat: 22.1g | protein: 23.0g | carbs: 12.1g | fiber: 7.0g | sugar: 0.9g | sodium: 79mg

Raw Veggie Salad

Prep time: 15 minutes | Cook time: 0 minutes | Serves 4

1 cucumber, chopped
1 pint cherry tomatoes cut in half
3 radishes, chopped
1 yellow bell pepper chopped
½ cup fresh parsley, chopped
3 tablespoons lemon juice
1 tablespoon olive oil
Salt, to taste

1. Place all in a large bowl and toss to combine. Serve immediately, or cover and chill until ready to serve.

Per Serving
Calories: 71 | fat: 4.1g | protein: 2.0g | carbs: 9.1g | fiber: 2.0g | sugar: 4.9g | sodium: 98mg

Simple Pickled Onion Salad

Prep time: 10 minutes | Cook time: 0 minutes | Serves 2

½ cucumber, peeled and sliced
¼ cup red onion, sliced thin
1 tablespoon olive oil
1 tablespoon white vinegar
1 teaspoon dill

1. Place all in a medium bowl and toss to combine. Serve.

Per Serving
Calories: 80 | fat: 7.1g | protein: 1.0g | carbs: 4.1g | fiber: 1.0g | sugar: 1.9g | sodium: 2mg

Cheesy Shrimp Cherry Tomato Salad

Prep time: 20 minutes | Cook time: 4 minutes | Serves 8

2 tablespoons extra virgin olive oil, divided
1 pound (454 g) large shrimps, peeled and deveined
2 avocados, peeled and cubed
2 ears fresh corn, kernels sliced off
2 cups cherry tomatoes, halved
3 ounces (85 g) reduced-fat feta
cheese, cubed
1 tablespoon balsamic vinegar
¼ teaspoon cumin
¼ teaspoon celery seeds
¼ cup slivered fresh basil
1 tablespoon fresh lemon juice
⅛ teaspoon salt
¼ teaspoons freshly ground black pepper

1. Heat 1 tablespoon of olive oil in a nonstick skillet over medium heat until shimmering.
2. Add the shrimps and grill for 4 minutes or until opaque. Flip the shrimps halfway through the cooking time.
3. Combine the remaining ingredients in a large salad bowl, then add the shrimps and toss to combine well.
4. Serve immediately.

Per Serving
Calories: 195 | fat: 10.0g | protein: 17.0g | carbs: 12.0g | fiber: 4.0g | sugar: 3.0g | sodium: 440mg

Chapter 12: Snacks and Appetizers

Cinnamon Apple Wheat Pitas

Prep time: 10 minutes | Cook time: 2 minutes | Serves 2

½ apple, cored and chopped
½ teaspoon cinnamon
¼ cup almond butter
1 whole-wheat pita, halved

1. Combine the apple, cinnamon, and almond butter in a bowl. Stir to mix well.
2. Heat the pita in a nonstick skillet over medium heat until lightly browned on both sides.
3. Remove the pita from the skillet. Allow to cool for a few minutes. Spoon the mixture in the halved pita pockets, then serve.

Per Serving
Calories: 315 | fat: 20.3g | protein: 8.2g | carbs: 31.3g | fiber: 7.2g | sugar: 20.6g | sodium: 175mg

Pepper Cauliflower with Hot Sauce

Prep time: 5 minutes | Cook time: 10 minutes | Serves 4

1 egg
½ head of cauliflower, separated into florets
1 cup panko bread crumbs
1 cup low-fat ranch dressing
½ cup hot sauce
½ teaspoon salt
½ teaspoon garlic powder
Black pepper, to taste
Nonstick cooking spray

1. Heat oven to 400ºF (205ºC). Spray a baking sheet with cooking spray.
2. Place the egg in a medium bowl and mix in the salt, pepper and garlic. Place the panko crumbs into a small bowl.
3. Dip the florets first in the egg then into the panko crumbs. Place in a single layer on prepared pan.
4. Bake for 8 to 10 minutes, stirring halfway through, until cauliflower is golden brown and crisp on the outside.
5. In a small bowl stir the dressing and hot sauce together. Use for dipping.

Per Serving
Calories: 133 | fat: 5.1g | protein: 6.1g | carbs: 15.1g | fiber: 1.1g | sugar: 4.0g | sodium: 1778mg

Nutty Butter Cake

Prep time: 5 minutes | Cook time: 0 minutes | Serves 6

½ cup reduced-fat cream cheese, soft
½ cup almonds,
ground fine
¼ cup almond butter
2 drops liquid stevia

1. In a large bowl, beat cream cheese, almond butter and stevia on high speed until mixture is smooth and creamy. Cover and chill 30 minutes.
2. Use your hands to shape the mixture into 12 balls.
3. Place the ground almonds in a shallow plate. Roll the balls in the nuts completely covering all sides. Store in an airtight container in the refrigerator.

Per Serving
Calories: 70 | fat: 4.9g | protein: 5.1g | carbs: 3.1g | fiber: 1g | sugar: 0g | sodium: 73mg

Creamy Spinach Crab with Melba Toast

Prep time: 10 minutes | Cook time: 2 hours | Serves 10

1 package frozen chopped spinach, thawed and squeezed nearly dry
8 ounces (227 g) reduced-fat cream cheese
6.5 ounces (184 g) can crabmeat, drained and shredded
6 ounces (170 g) jar marinated artichoke hearts, drained and diced fine
¼ teaspoon hot pepper sauce
Melba toast or whole grain crackers (optional)

1. Remove any shells or cartilage from crab.
2. Place all in a small crock pot. Cover and cook on high for 1½ to 2 hours, or until heated through and cream cheese is melted. Stir after 1 hour.
3. Serve with Melba toast or whole grain crackers. Serving size is ¼ cup.

Per Serving
Calories: 105 | fat: 8.1g | protein: 5.0g | carbs: 7.1g | fiber: 1.1g | sugar: 2.9g | sodium: 185mg

Sticky and Crispy Soy Chicken Wings

Prep time: 5 minutes | Cook time: 30 minutes | Serves 3

24 chicken wings
6 tablespoons soy sauce
6 tablespoons Chinese

5 spice
Salt and ground black pepper, to taste
Nonstick cooking spray

1. Heat oven to 350°F (180°C). Spray a baking sheet with cooking spray.
2. Combine the soy sauce, 5 spice, salt, and pepper in a large bowl. Add the wings and toss to coat.
3. Pour the wings onto the prepared pan. Bake for 15 minutes. Turn chicken over and cook another 15 minutes until chicken is cooked through.
4. Serve warm.

Per Serving
Calories: 180 | fat: 10.9g | protein: 12.1g | carbs: 8.1g | fiber: 0g | sugar: 1.0g | sodium: 1210mg

Vanilla flavoured Banana-Walnut Cookies

Prep time: 10 minutes | Cook time: 15 minutes | Makes 18 Cookies

1½ cup banana, mashed
2 cup oat
1 cup raisins

1 cup walnuts
1/3 cup sunflower oil
1 teaspoon vanilla
½ teaspoon salt

1. Heat oven to 350°F (180°C).
2. In a large bowl, combine oats, raisins, walnuts, and salt.
3. In a medium bowl, mix banana, oil, and vanilla. Stir into oat mixture until combined. Let rest 15 minutes.
4. Drop by rounded tablespoonful onto 2 ungreased cookie sheets. Bake 15 minutes, or until a light golden brown. Cool and store in an airtight container. Serving size is 2 cookies.

Per Serving (1 Cookie)
Calories: 150 | fat: 8.9g | protein: 3.1g | carbs: 16.1g | fiber: 1.9g | sugar: 6.0g | sodium: 65mg

Bacon Cucumber Lettuce Salad

Prep time: 15 minutes | Cook time: 0 minutes | Serves 4

3 slices bacon, cooked crisp and crumbled
1 large cucumber
½ cup lettuce, diced fine
½ cup baby spinach, diced fine
¼ cup tomato, diced

fine
½ tablespoon plus ½ teaspoon fat-free mayonnaise
¼ teaspoon black pepper
1/8 teaspoon salt

1. Peel the cucumber and slice in half lengthwise. Use a spoon to remove the seeds.
2. In a medium bowl, combine remaining and stir well.
3. Spoon the bacon mixture into the cucumber halves. Cut into 2-inch pieces and serve.

Per Serving
Calories: 100 | fat: 5.9g | protein: 6.1g | carbs: 4.1g | fiber: 1.1g | sugar: 2.0g | sodium: 179mg

Quick and Easy Butter Pecan Bowl

Prep time: 5 minutes | Cook time: 10 minutes | Serves 6

1½ teaspoons butter
1½ cup pecan halves
2½ tablespoons Splenda, divided
1 teaspoons cinnamon

¼ teaspoons ginger
1/8 teaspoons cardamom
1/8 teaspoons salt

1. In a small bowl, stir together 1½ teaspoons Splenda, cinnamon, ginger, cardamom and salt. Set aside.
2. Melt butter in a medium skillet over medium-low heat. Add pecans, and two tablespoons Splenda. Reduce heat to low and cook, stirring occasionally, until sweetener melts, about 5 to 8 minutes.
3. Add spice mixture to the skillet and stir to coat pecans. Spread mixture to parchment paper and let cool for 10 to 15 minutes. Store in an airtight container. Serving size is ¼ cup.

Per Serving
Calories: 173 | fat: 16.1g | protein: 2.1g | carbs: 8.1g | fiber: 2.1g | sugar: 6.0g | sodium: 52mg

Tahini Cauliflower Bowl with Favorite Veggies

Prep time: 5 minutes | Cook time: 15 minutes | Serves 6

3 cup cauliflower florets
3 tablespoons fresh lemon juice
5 cloves garlic, divided
5 tablespoons olive oil, divided
2 tablespoons water

1½ tablespoons Tahini paste
1¼ teaspoons salt, divided
Smoked paprika and extra olive oil for serving

1. In a microwave safe bowl, combine cauliflower, water, 2 tablespoons oil, ½ teaspoon salt, and 3 whole cloves garlic. Microwave on high 15 minutes, or until cauliflower is soft and darkened.
2. Transfer mixture to a food processor or blender and process until almost smooth.
3. Add tahini paste, lemon juice, remaining garlic cloves, remaining oil, and salt. Blend until almost smooth.
4. Place the hummus in a bowl and drizzle lightly with olive oil and a sprinkle or two of paprika. Serve with your favorite raw vegetables.

Per Serving
Calories: 108 | fat: 10.1g | protein: 2.1g | carbs: 5.1g | fiber: 2.1g | sugar: 1.0g | sodium: 506mg

Quick and Easy Parmesan Bites

Prep time: 5 minutes | Cook time: 5 minutes | Serves 2

1 cup grated Parmesan cheese

1. Preheat the oven to 400ºF (205ºC). Line a rimmed baking sheet with parchment paper.
2. Spread the Parmesan on the prepared baking sheet into 4 mounds, spreading each mound out so it is flat but not touching the others.
3. Bake until brown and crisp, 3 to 5 minutes.
4. Cool for 5 minutes. Use a spatula to remove to a plate to continue cooling.

Per Serving
Calories: 216 | fat: 14.1g | protein: 19.1g | carbs: 2.0g | fiber: 0g | sugar: 1.5g | sodium: 765mg

Homemade Jack Cheese Snack with Salsa

Prep time: 5 minutes | Cook time: 10 minutes | Serves 4

4 slices pepper Jack cheese, quartered
4 slices Colby Jack

cheese, quartered
4 slices cheddar cheese, quartered

1. Heat oven to 400ºF (205ºC). Line a cooking sheet with parchment paper.
2. Place cheese in a single layer on prepared pan and bake 10 minutes, or until cheese gets firm.
3. Transfer to paper towel line surface to absorb excess oil. Let cool, cheese will crisp up more as it cools.
4. Store in airtight container, or Ziploc bag. Serve with your favorite dip or salsa.

Per Serving
Calories: 254 | fat: 19.9g | protein: 15.1g | carbs: 1.1g | fiber: 0g | sugar: 0g | sodium: 475mg

Buttery Almond Biscuits

Prep time: 10 minutes | Cook time: 15 minutes | Serves 4 biscuits

¼ cup Low-fat Greek yogurt
2 tablespoons unsalted butter, melted

Pinch salt
1½ cups finely ground almond flour

1. Preheat the oven to 375ºF (190ºC).
2. Combine the yogurt, butter, and salt in a bowl. Stir to mix well.
3. Fold the almond flour in the mixture. Keep stirring until a dough without lumps forms.
4. Divide the dough into 4 balls, and then bash the balls into 1-inch biscuits with your hands.
5. Arrange the biscuits on a baking pan lined with parchment paper. Bake in the preheated oven for 14 minutes or until well browned.
6. Remove the biscuits from the oven and serve warm.

Per Serving
Calories: 312 | fat: 27.9g | protein: 10.2g | carbs: 8.9g | fiber: 5.1g | sugar: 2.1g | sodium: 31mg

Diabetic Friendly Vanilla Granola Bars

Prep time: 10 minutes | Cook time: 35 minutes | Makes 36 Bars

1 egg, beaten
⅔ cup margarine, melted
3½ cup quick oats
1 cup almonds, chopped
½ cup sunflower kernels
½ cup coconut,
unsweetened
½ cup dried apples
½ cup dried cranberries
1 teaspoon vanilla
1 tablespoon honey
½ teaspoon cinnamon
Nonstick cooking spray

1. Heat oven to 350ºF (180ºC). Spray a large baking sheet with cooking spray.
2. Spread oats and almonds on prepared pan. Bake for 12 to 15 minutes until toasted, stirring every few minutes.
3. In a large bowl, combine egg, margarine, honey, and vanilla. Stir in remaining.
4. Stir in oat mixture. Press into baking sheet and bake for 13 to 18 minutes, or until edges are light brown.
5. Cool on a wire rack. Cut into bars and store in an airtight container.

Per Serving (1 Bar)
Calories: 120 | fat: 5.9g | protein: 2.1g | carbs: 13.1g | fiber: 1.0g | sugar: 7.0g | sodium: 8mg

Best Cinnamon Apple Ever

Prep time: 5 minutes | Cook time: 10 minutes | Serves 2

1 medium apple, sliced thin
¼ teaspoon cinnamon
¼ teaspoon nutmeg
Nonstick cooking spray

1. Heat oven to 375ºF (190ºC). Spray a baking sheet with cooking spray.
2. Place apples in a mixing bowl and add spices. Toss to coat.
3. Arrange apples, in a single layer, on prepared pan. Bake 4 minutes, turn apples over and bake 4 minutes more.
4. Serve immediately or store in airtight container.

Per Serving
Calories: 60 | fat: 0g | protein: 0g | carbs: 15.1g | fiber: 3.1g | sugar: 11.2g | sodium: 1mg

Most Delicious Margarine Apple Popcorn

Prep time: 30 minutes | Cook time: 50 minutes | Serves 11

4 tablespoons margarine, melted
10 cup plain popcorn
2 cup dried apple rings, unsweetened and chopped
½ cup walnuts, chopped
2 tablespoons honey
1 teaspoon cinnamon
½ teaspoon vanilla

1. Heat oven to 250ºF (121ºC).
2. Place chopped apples in a baking dish and bake 20 minutes. Remove from oven and stir in popcorn and nuts.
3. In a small bowl, whisk together margarine, honey, vanilla, Splenda, and cinnamon. Drizzle evenly over popcorn and toss to coat.
4. Bake 30 minutes, stirring quickly every 10 minutes. If apples start to turn a dark brown, remove immediately.
5. Pout onto waxed paper to cool at least 30 minutes. Store in an airtight container. Serving size is 1 cup.

Per Serving
Calories: 135 | fat: 8.1g | protein: 3.0g | carbs: 14.1g | fiber: 3.1g | sugar: 6.9g | sodium: 2mg

3 Ingredient Low Carb Almond Cookies

Prep time: 5 minutes | Cook time: 15 minutes | Serves 8

½ cup coconut oil, melted
1½ cups almond flour
¼ cup Stevia

1. Heat oven to 350ºF (180ºC). Line a cookie sheet with parchment paper.
2. In a mixing bowl, combine all and mix well.
3. Spread dough onto prepared cookie sheet, ¼-inch thick. Use a paring knife to score into 24 crackers.
4. Bake for 10 to 15 minutes or until golden brown.
5. Separate and store in airtight container.

Per Serving
Calories: 282 | fat: 22.9g | protein: 4.1g | carbs: 16.1g | fiber: 2.1g | sugar: 12.9g | sodium: 0mg

Buffalo Chicken Celery Rolls

Prep time: 10 minutes | Cook time: 0 minutes | Serves 4

1 teaspoon Buffalo hot sauce
¼ cup chunky blue cheese dressing
1 cup rotisserie

chicken meat, shredded
8 celery stalks, cut into halves lengthwise

1. Combine the hot sauce and blue cheese dressing in a bowl, then dunks the shredded rotisserie chicken in the bowl to coat well.
2. Divide the mixture in the celery stalks and serve.

Per Serving
Calories: 148 | fat: 11.9g | protein: 9.1g | carbs: 2.8g | fiber: 1.2g | carbs: 1.6g | sodium: 461mg

No Bake Chocolate Peanut Butter Balls

Prep time: 10 minutes | Cook time: 0 minutes | Serves 16 balls

½ cup sugar-free peanut butter
2 tablespoons unsweetened cocoa powder

2 tablespoons canned coconut milk or more as needed
¼ cup sugar-free peanut butter powder

1. Combine all the ingredients in a large bowl. Stir to mix well.
2. Divide the mixture into 16 balls with a spoon, and then arrange the balls on a baking sheet lined with parchment paper.
3. Place the sheet in the refrigerator to chill the balls for 1 to 2 hours or until the balls are firm
4. Remove the peanut butter balls from the refrigerator and serve chilled.

Per Serving
Calories: 65 | fat: 5.1g | protein: 4.1g | carbs: 2.0g | fiber: 0.8g | carbs: 1.2g | sodium: 18mg

Oven baked Stevia Almonds

Prep time: 5 minutes | Cook time: 15 minutes | Serves 4

1 cup almonds
2 packets powdered stevia

1 tablespoon cocoa powder

1. Preheat the oven to 350ºF (180ºC).
2. Arrange the almonds in a single layer in a baking pan lined with parchment paper.
3. Bake in the preheated oven for 5 minutes.
4. Meanwhile, combine the stevia and cocoa powder in a small bowl.
5. Dunk the almonds in the bowl of mixture. Toss to coat well.
6. Put the almonds back to the baking pan, and bake for an additional 5 minutes or until soft.
7. Remove the almonds from the oven and serve warm.

Per Serving
Calories: 210 | fat: 18.1g | protein: 8.1g | carbs: 8.9g | fiber: 5.1g | carbs: 3.8g | sodium: 1mg

Easy Cinnamon Roasted Pumpkin Seeds

Prep time: 5 minutes | Cook time: 45 minutes | Serves 4

1 cup pumpkin seeds
1 teaspoon cinnamon
2 (0.04-ounce / 1 g)

packets stevia
1 tablespoon canola oil
¼ teaspoon sea salt

1. Preheat the oven to 300°F (150°C).
2. Combine the pumpkin seeds with cinnamon, stevia, canola oil and salt in a bowl. Stir to mix well.
3. Pour the seeds in the single layer on a baking sheet, and then arrange the sheet in the preheated oven.
4. Bake for 45 minutes or until well toasted and fragrant. Shake the sheet twice to bake the seeds evenly.
5. Serve immediately.

Per Serving
Calories: 202 | fat: 18.0g | protein: 8.8g | carbs: 5.1g | fiber: 2.3g | sugar: 0.4g | sodium: 151mg

Instant Bacon Shrimps Lettuce Wraps

Prep time: 10 minutes | Cook time: 6 minutes | Serves 10

20 shrimps, peeled and deveined
7 slices bacon, cut into

3 strips crosswise
4 leaves romaine lettuce

1. Preheat the oven to 400ºF (205ºC).
2. Wrap each shrimp with each bacon strip, and then arrange the wrapped shrimps in a single layer on a baking sheet, seam side down.
3. Broil in the preheated oven for 6 minutes or until the bacon is well browned. Flip the shrimps halfway through the cooking time.
4. Remove the shrimps from the oven and serve on lettuce leaves.

Per Serving
Calories: 70 | fat: 4.5g | protein: 7.0g | carbs: 0g | fiber: 0g | sugar: 0g | sodium: 150mg

Classic Peppery Eggs

Prep time: 5 minutes | Cook time: 8 minutes | Serves 12

6 large eggs
⅛ teaspoon mustard powder

Salt and freshly ground black pepper, to taste

1. Sit the eggs in a saucepan, and then pour in enough water to cover the egg. Bring to a boil, and then boil the eggs for another 8 minutes. Turn off the heat and cover, then let sit for 15 minutes.
2. Transfer the boiled eggs in a pot of cold water and peel under the water.
3. Transfer the eggs on a large plate, and then cut in half. Remove the egg yolks and place them in a bowl, then mash with a fork.
4. Add the mustard powder, salt, and pepper to the bowl of yolks, and then stir to mix well.
5. Spoon the yolk mixture in the egg white on the plate. Serve immediately.

Per Serving
Calories: 45 | fat: 3.0g | protein: 3.0g | carbs: 1.0g | fiber: 0g | sugar: 0g | sodium: 70mg

Cheesy Tomato with Italian Vinaigrette

Prep time: 5 minutes | Cook time: 0 minutes | Serves 2

12 cherry tomatoes
8 (1-inch) pieces Mozzarella cheese

12 basil leaves
¼ cup Italian Vinaigrette, for serving

Special Equipment:
4 wooden skewers, soaked in water for at least 30 minutes

1. Thread the tomatoes, cheese, and bay leaves alternatively through the skewers.
2. Place the skewers on a large plate and baste with the Italian Vinaigrette.
3. Serve immediately.

Per Serving
Calories: 230 | fat: 12.6g | protein: 21.3g | carbs: 8.5g | fiber: 1.9g | sugar: 4.9g | sodium: 672mg

Crispy Garlic Kale Chips

Prep time: 5 minutes | Cook time: 15 minutes | Serves 1

¼ teaspoon garlic powder
Pinch cayenne, to taste
1 tablespoon extra-virgin olive oil
½ teaspoon sea salt,

or to taste
1 (8-ounce / 227-g) bunch kale, trimmed and cut into 2-inch pieces, rinsed

1. Preheat the oven to 350ºF (180ºC). Line two baking sheets with parchment paper.
2. Combine the garlic powder, cayenne pepper, olive oil, and salt in a large bowl, and then dunk the kale in the bowl. Toss to coat well.
3. Place the kale in the single layer on one of the baking sheet.
4. Arrange the sheet in the preheated oven and bake for 7 minutes. Remove the sheet from the oven and pour the kale in the single layer of the other baking sheet.
5. Move the sheet of kale back to the oven and bake for another 7 minutes or until the kale is crispy.
6. Serve immediately.

Per Serving
Calories: 136 | fat: 14.0g | protein: 1.0g | carbs: 3.0g | fiber: 1.1g | sugar: 0.6g | sodium: 1170mg

Delicious Splenda Almond Berry Granola Bars

Prep time: 15 minutes | Cook time: 20 minutes | Makes 12 Bars

1 egg	¼ cup almonds, chopped
1 egg white	2 tablespoons Splenda
2 cup low-fat granola	1 teaspoon almond extract
¼ cup dried cranberries, sweetened	½ teaspoon cinnamon

1. Heat oven to 350ºF (180ºC). Line the bottom and sides of a baking dish with parchment paper.
2. In a large bowl, combine dry including the cranberries.
3. In a small bowl, whisk together egg, egg white and extract. Pour over dry and mix until combined.
4. Press mixture into the prepared pan. Bake 20 minutes or until light brown.
5. Cool in the pan for 5 minutes. Then carefully lift the bars from the pan onto a cutting board.
6. Use a sharp knife to cut into 12 bars. Cool completely and store in an airtight container.

Per Serving (1 Bar)
Calories: 86 | fat: 3.1g | protein: 3.0g | carbs: 14.1g | fiber: 1.1g | sugar: 4.9g | sodium: 10mg

The Best Low Fat Cream Bars Ever

Prep time: 15 minutes | Cook time: 0 minutes | Makes 20 Bars

8 ounces (227 g) low fat cream cheese, soft	1 package lemon gelatin, sugar free
⅓ cup butter, melted	1½ cup graham cracker crumbs
3 tablespoons fresh lemon juice	1 cup boiling water
12 ounces (340 g) evaporated milk	¾ cup Splenda
	1 teaspoon vanilla

1. Pour milk into a large, metal bowl, place beaters in the bowl, cover and chill 2 hours.
2. In a small bowl, combine cracker crumbs and butter, reserve 1 tablespoon. Press the remaining mixture on the bottom of a baking dish. Cover and chill until set.
3. In a small bowl, dissolve gelatin in boiling water. Stir in lemon juice and let cool.
4. In a large bowl, beat cream cheese, Splenda and vanilla until smooth. Add gelatin and mix well.
5. Beat the chilled milk until soft peaks form. Fold into cream cheese mixture.
6. Pour over chilled crust and sprinkle with reserved crumbs. Cover and chill 2 hours before serving.

Per Serving (1 Bar)
Calories: 125 | fat: 5.1g | protein: 3.0g | carbs: 15.1g | fiber: 0g | sugar: 9.9g | sodium: 50mg

Coconut Almond Margarine Cookies

Prep time: 5 minutes | Cook time: 50 minutes | Serves 16

1 egg, room temperature	coconut, grated
1 egg white, room temperature	¾ cup almonds, sliced
½ cup margarine, melted	⅔ cup Splenda
2½ cup flour	2 teaspoons baking powder
1⅓ cup unsweetened	1 teaspoon vanilla
	½ teaspoon salt

1. Heat oven to 350ºF (180ºC). Line a baking sheet with parchment paper.
2. In a large bowl, combine dry.
3. In a separate mixing bowl, beat other together. Add to dry and mix until thoroughly combined.
4. Divide dough in half. Shape each half into a loaf measuring 8x2 ¾-inches. Place loaves on pan 3 inches apart.
5. Bake for 25 to 30 minutes or until set and golden brown. Cool on wire rack 10 minutes.
6. With a serrated knife, cut loaf diagonally into ½-inch slices. Place the cookies, cut side down, back on the pan and bake another 20 minutes, or until firm and nicely browned. Store in airtight container. Serving size is 2 cookies.

Per Serving
Calories: 235 | fat: 17.9g | protein: 5.1g | carbs: 13.1g | fiber: 3.1g | sugar: 8.9g | sodium: 84mg

Low Carb Butter Milk Cauliflower Cake

Prep time: 15 minutes | Cook time: 10 minutes | Makes 16 hush puppies

1 whole cauliflower, including stalks and florets, roughly chopped
¾ cup buttermilk
¾ cup low-fat milk
1 medium onion, chopped
2 medium eggs
2 cups yellow cornmeal
1½ teaspoons baking powder
½ teaspoon salt

1. In a blender, combine the cauliflower, buttermilk, milk, and onion and purée. Transfer to a large mixing bowl.
2. Crack the eggs into the purée, and gently fold until mixed.
3. In a medium bowl, whisk the cornmeal, baking powder, and salt together.
4. Gently add the dry ingredients to the wet ingredients and mix until just combined, taking care not to over mix.
5. Working in batches, place ⅓-cup portions of the batter into the basket of an air fryer.
6. Set the air fryer to 390ºF (199ºC), close, and cook for 10 minutes. Transfer the hush puppies to a plate. Repeat until no batter remains.
7. Serve warm with greens.

Per Serving
Calories: 180 | fat: 8.1g | protein: 4.1g | carbs: 27.9g | fiber: 6.1g | sugar: 11.0g | sodium: 251mg

Buttery Mashed Cauliflower Puree

Prep time: 7 minutes | Cook time: 20 minutes | Serves 4

1 head cauliflower, cored and cut into large florets
½ teaspoon kosher salt
½ teaspoon garlic pepper
2 tablespoons Low-fat
Greek yogurt
¾ cup freshly grated Parmesan cheese
1 tablespoon unsalted butter or ghee (optional)
Chopped fresh chives

1. Pour 1 cup of water into the electric pressure cooker and insert a steamer basket or wire rack.
2. Place the cauliflower in the basket.

3. Close and lock the lid of the pressure cooker. Set the valve to sealing.
4. Cook on high pressure for 5 minutes.
5. When the cooking is complete, hit Cancel and quick release the pressure.
6. Once the pin drops, unlock and remove the lid.
7. Remove the cauliflower from the pot and pour out the water. Return the cauliflower to the pot and add the salt, garlic pepper, yogurt, and cheese. Use an immersion blender or potato masher to purée or mash the cauliflower in the pot.
8. Spoon into a serving bowl, and garnish with butter (if using) and chives.

Per Serving
Calories: 141 | fat: 6.1g | protein: 12.1g | carbs: 11.9g | fiber: 4.1g | sugar: 5.0g | sodium: 591mg

Appetizing Buttery Tomato Waffles

Prep time: 15 minutes | Cook time: 40 minutes | Serves 8 waffles

Dry:
½ cup almond flour
½ cup coconut flour
½ teaspoon baking soda
½ teaspoon dried chives
1 cup gluten-free all-purpose flour
2 teaspoons baking powder

Wet:
1 tablespoon olive oil
½ cup tomato, crushed
1 medium egg
2 medium egg whites
2 cups low-fat buttermilk

1. Preheat a waffle iron. Grease the waffle iron with olive oil.
2. Combine all the dry ingredients in a bowl. Stir to mix well.
3. Combine all the remaining wet ingredients in a separate bowl. Stir to mix well.
4. Gently stir the dry ingredients in the wet ingredients until well combined.
5. Pour ¼- to ½-cup of the mixture in the waffle iron and cook for 5 minutes or until the waffle is golden brown. Repeat with remaining mixture.
6. Transfer the waffles onto several serving plates and serve warm.

Per Serving
Calories: 142 | fat: 4.1g | protein: 6.9g | carbs: 20.8g | fiber: 5.1g | sugar: 2.8g | sodium: 167mg

Chapter 13: Desserts

Grandma's Best Ambrosia Salad Recipe

Prep time: 10 minutes | Cook time: 0 minutes | Serves 8

3 oranges, peeled, sectioned, and quartered
2 (4-ounce / 113-g) cups diced peaches in water, drained

1 cup shredded, unsweetened coconut
1 (8-ounce / 227-g) container fat-free crème fraîche

1. In a large mixing bowl, combine the oranges, peaches, coconut, and crème fraîche.
2. Gently toss until well mixed. Cover and refrigerate overnight.

Per Serving
Calories: 113 | fat: 5.1g | protein: 2.1g | carbs: 12.1g | fiber: 2.9g | sugar: 8.1g | sodium: 8mg

Healthy Cinnamon Brown Rice Dessert

Prep time: 5 minutes | Cook time: 35 minutes | Serves 6

2 cups short-grain brown rice
6 cups fat-free milk
1 teaspoon ground nutmeg, plus more for serving
1 teaspoon ground

cinnamon, plus more for serving
¼ teaspoon orange extract
Juice of 2 oranges (about ¾ cup)
2 tablespoon honey

1. In an electric pressure cooker, stir the rice, milk, nutmeg, cinnamon, orange extract, orange juice, and erythritol together.
2. Close and lock the lid, and set the pressure valve to sealing.
3. Select the Manual/Pressure Cook setting, and cook for 35 minutes.
4. Once cooking is complete, quick-release the pressure. Carefully remove the lid.
5. Stir well and spoon into serving dishes. Enjoy with an additional sprinkle of nutmeg and cinnamon.

Per Serving
Calories: 321 | fat: 2.1g | protein: 12.9g | carbs: 60.9g | fiber: 2.1g | sugar: 15g | sodium: 131mg

Easy Healthy Strawberry Rhubarb Bowl

Prep time: 10 minutes | Cook time: 15 minutes | Serves 2

1 cup sliced strawberries

1 cup chopped rhubarb
½ teaspoon cinnamon

1. In a medium pot, combine the strawberries, rhubarb and cinnamon. Bring to a simmer on medium heat, stirring.
2. Reduce the heat to medium-low. Simmer, stirring frequently, until the rhubarb is soft, about 15 minutes. Allow to cool slightly.

Per Serving
Calories: 86 | fat: 2g | protein: 3g | carbs: 16g | fiber: 3g | sugar: 8.41g | sodium: 37mg

Chilled Chocolate Almond Squares

Prep time: 10 minutes | Cook time: 0 minutes | Makes 9 pieces

2 ounces unsweetened baking chocolate
½ cup almond butter
1 can coconut milk, refrigerated overnight,

thickened cream only
1 teaspoon vanilla extract
4 (1-gram) packets stevia (or to taste)

1. Line a 9-inch square baking pan with parchment paper.
2. In a small saucepan over medium-low heat, heat the chocolate and almond butter, stirring constantly, until both are melted. Cool slightly.
3. In a medium bowl, combine the melted chocolate mixture with the cream from the coconut milk, vanilla, and stevia. Blend until smooth. Taste and adjust sweetness as desired.
4. Pour the mixture into the prepared pan, spreading with a spatula to smooth. Refrigerate for 3 hours. Cut into squares.

Per Serving
Calories: 200 | fat: 20g | protein: 4g | carbs: 6g | fiber: 2g | sugar: 16.9g | sodium: 8mg

Ultimate Maple Apple Pecan Bake

Prep time: 10 minutes | Cook time: 15 minutes | Serves 4

2 apples, peeled, cored, and chopped
½ teaspoon cinnamon
½ teaspoon ground ginger
2 tablespoons pure maple syrup
¼ cup pecans, chopped

1. Preheat the oven to 350ºF (180ºC).
2. Combine all the ingredients, except for the pecans, in a bowl. Stir to mix well.
3. Pour the mixture in a baking dish, and spread the pecans over the mixture.
4. Bake in the preheated oven for 15 minutes or until the apples are soft.
5. Remove them from the oven and serve warm.

Per Serving
Calories: 124 | fat: 5.1g | protein: 1.1g | carbs: 20.8g | fiber: 3.2g | sugars: 18.6g | sodium: 1mg

Vanilla flavored Pistachio Stuffed Peaches

Prep time: 5 minutes | Cook time: 10 minutes | Serves 4

2 peaches, halved and pitted
1 teaspoon pure vanilla extract
½ cup Low-fat Greek yogurt
2 tablespoons unsalted pistachios, shelled and broken into pieces
¼ cup unsweetened dried coconut flakes

1. Preheat the broiler to high.
2. Place the peach halves on a baking sheet, cut side down, and broil for 7 minutes or until soft and lightly browned.
3. Meanwhile, combine the vanilla and yogurt in a bowl.
4. Divide the mixture among the pits of peach halves, and then scatter the pistachios and coconut flakes on top before serving.

Per Serving
Calories: 103 | fat: 4.9g | protein: 5.1g | carbs: 10.8g | fiber: 2.1g | sugars: 7.8g | sodium: 10mg

Healthy Cardamom Almond Date Balls

Prep time: 15 minutes | Cook time: 0 minutes | Serves 36 Balls

1 pound (454 g) pitted dates
½ pound (227 g) blanched almonds
¼ cup water
¼ cup butter, at room temperature
1 teaspoon ground cardamom
1 teaspoon vanilla extract
½ teaspoon ground cinnamon
2 tablespoons ground flaxseed
1 cup toasted sesame seeds

1. In a food processor, add the pitted dates, almonds, water, butter, cardamon, vanilla, and cinnamon, and pulse until the mixture has broken down into a smooth paste.
2. Scoop out the paste and form into 36 equal-sized balls with your hands.
3. Spread out the flaxseed and sesame seeds on a baking sheet. Roll the balls in the seed mixture until they are evenly coated on all sides.
4. Serve immediately or store in an airtight container in the fridge for 2 days.

Per Serving (1 Ball)
Calories: 113 | fat: 7.1g | protein: 2.9g | carbs: 12.0g | fiber: 2.0g | sugar: 7.8g | sodium: 10mg

Chilled Blackberry Yogurt bowl

Prep time: 10 minutes | Cook time: 0 minutes | Serves 4

12 ounces Low-fat Greek yogurt
1 cup blackberries
1 Pinch nutmeg to
taste
¼ cup milk
2 (1-gram) packets stevia

1. In a blender, combine all of the ingredients. Blend until smooth.
2. Pour the mixture into 4 ice pop moulds. Freeze for 6 hours before serving.

Per Serving
Calories: 75 | fat: 6g | protein: 9g | carbs: 9g | fiber: 2g | sugar: 10.1g| sodium: 7mg

Iced Coffee Coconut Pops

Prep time: 10 minutes | Cook time: 5 minutes | Serves 4

2 teaspoons espresso powder (or to taste)
2 cups raw coconut milk
½ teaspoon vanilla extract
½ teaspoon cinnamon
3 (1-gram) packets stevia

1. In a medium saucepan over medium-low heat, heat all of the ingredients, stirring constantly, until the espresso powder is completely dissolved, about 5 minutes.
2. Pour the mixture into 4 ice pop moulds. Freeze for 6 hours before serving.

Per Serving
Calories: 225 | fat: 24g | protein: 2g | carbs: 7g | fiber: 3g | sugar: 16.6g| sodium: 15mg

Margarine Apricot Bake

Prep time: 5 minutes | Cook time: 30 minutes | Serves 6

4 egg whites
3 egg yolks, beaten
3 tablespoons margarine
¾ cup sugar free apricot fruit spread
⅓ cup dried apricots, diced fine
¼ cup warm water
2 tablespoons flour
¼ teaspoon cream of tartar
⅛ teaspoon salt

1. Heat oven to 325ºF (163ºC).
2. In a medium saucepan, over medium heat, melt margarine. Stir in flour and cook, stirring, until bubbly.
3. Stir together the fruit spread and water in a small bowl and add it to the saucepan with the apricots. Cook, stirring, 3 minutes or until mixture thickens.
4. Remove from heat and whisk in egg yolks. Let cool to room temperature, stirring occasionally.
5. In a medium bowl, beat egg whites, salt, and cream of tartar on high speed until stiff peaks form. Gently fold into cooled apricot mixture.
6. Spoon into a 1½–quart soufflé dish. Bake 30 minutes, or until puffed and golden brown. Serve immediately.

Per Serving
Calories: 116 | fat: 8.1g | protein: 4.0g | carbs: 7.1g | fiber: 0g | sugar: 1.1g | sodium: 95mg

Healthy Cinnamon Baked Apple Chips

Prep time: 10 minutes | Cook time: 2 hours | Serves 4

2 medium apples, sliced
1 teaspoon ground cinnamon

1. Preheat the oven to 200ºF (93ºC). Line a baking sheet with parchment paper.
2. Arrange the apple slices on the prepared baking sheet, then sprinkle with cinnamon.
3. Bake in the preheated oven for 2 hours or until crispy. Flip the apple chips halfway through the cooking time.
4. Allow to cool for 10 minutes and serve warm.

Per Serving
Calories: 50 | fat: 0g | protein: 0g | carbs: 13.0g | fiber: 2.0g | sugar: 9.0g | sodium: 0mg

Mom's Special Banana Cake with Walnuts

Prep time: 10 minutes | Cook time: 1 minutes | Serves 1

½ ripe banana, mashed
3 tablespoons egg white
1 teaspoon oat flour
½ tablespoon vanilla protein powder
1 teaspoon rolled oats
1 teaspoon cocoa powder
½ teaspoon baking powder
2 tablespoons stevia
1 teaspoon olive oil
2 teaspoons chopped walnuts

1. Whisk together the banana and egg whites in a bowl.
2. Add the flour, vanilla protein powder, rolled oats, cocoa powder, baking powder, and stevia to the bowl. Stir to mix well.
3. Grease a microwave-safe mug with olive oil.
4. Pour the mixture in the bowl, and then scatter with chopped walnuts.
5. Microwave them for 1 minute or until puffed.
6. Serve immediately.

Per Serving
Calories: 211 | fat: 12.0g | protein: 11.3g | carbs: 46.7g | fiber: 2.8g | sugar: 6.6g | sodium: 97mg

Coconut Milk Pineapple Bowl

Prep time: 5 minutes | Cook time: 5 minutes | Serves 2

2 large slices fresh pineapple
2 tablespoons coconut milk

2 tablespoons unsweetened shredded coconut
¼ teaspoon sea salt

1. Preheat the oven broiler on high.
2. On a rimmed baking sheet, arrange the pineapple in a single layer. Brush lightly with the coconut milk and sprinkle with the coconut.
3. Broil until the pineapple begins to brown, 3 to 5 minutes.
4. Sprinkle with the sea salt.

Per Serving
Calories: 78 | fat: 4g | protein: 3g | carbs: 13g | fiber: 2g | sugar: 9.35g| sodium: 148mg

Tender Cinnamon Pecans and Apples

Prep time: 10 minutes | Cook time: 15 minutes | Serves 4

2 apples, peeled, cored, and chopped
½ tablespoons pure maple syrup

½ teaspoon cinnamon
½ teaspoon ground ginger
¼ cup chopped pecans

1. Preheat the oven to 350°F(177°C).
2. In a bowl, mix the apples, syrup, cinnamon, and ginger. Pour the mixture into a 9-inch square baking dish. Sprinkle the pecans over the top.
3. Bake until the apples are tender, about 15 minutes.

Per Serving
Calories: 122 | fat: 5g | protein: 1g | carbs: 21g | fiber: 3g | sugar: 41.9g| sodium: 2mg

Almond Pumpkin Smoothie

Prep time: 10 minutes | Cook time: 0 minutes | Serves 1

2 tablespoons cream cheese, at room temperature
½ cup canned pumpkin purée (not pumpkin

pie mix)
1 cup almond milk
1 teaspoon pumpkin pie spice
½ cup crushed ice

1. In a blender, combine all of the ingredients. Blend until smooth.

Per Serving
Calories: 186 | fat: 14g | protein: 5g | carbs: 14g | fiber: 5g | sugar: 16.6g| sodium: 105mg

Instant Chocolate Avocado Bowl

Prep time: 5 minutes | Cook time: 0 minutes | Serves 2

1 avocados, mashed
¼ cups canned coconut milk
2 tablespoons unsweetened cocoa powder

½ tablespoons pure maple syrup
½ teaspoon espresso powder
½ teaspoon vanilla extract

1. In a blender, combine all of the ingredients. Blend until smooth.
2. Pour the mixture into 4 small bowls and serve.

Per Serving
Calories: 203 | fat: 17g | protein: 2g | carbs: 15g | fiber: 6g | sugar: 15g| sodium: 11mg

Lemony Raspberry Dessert

Prep time: 1 hours | Cook time: 0 minutes | Serves 4

1 cup unsweetened vanilla almond milk
2 cup plus ½ cup raspberries, divided
¼ cup chia seeds

1½ teaspoons lemon juice
½ teaspoon lemon zest
1 tablespoon honey

1. Stir together the almond milk, 2 cups of raspberries, chia seeds, lemon juice, lemon zest, and honey in a small bowl.
2. Transfer the bowl to the fridge to thicken for at least 1 hour, or until a pudding-like texture is achieved.
3. When the pudding is ready, give it a good stir. Scatter with the remaining ½ cup raspberries and serve immediately.

Per Serving
Calories: 122 | fat: 5.2g | protein: 3.1g | carbs: 17.9g | fiber: 9.0g | sugar: 6.8g | sodium: 51mg

Sugarless Vanilla Peanut Cookies

Prep time: 10 minutes | Cook time: 0 minutes | Makes 12 cookies

¾ cup unsweetened shredded coconut
½ cup peanut butter
2 tablespoons cream cheese, at room temperature
2 tablespoons unsalted butter, melted

2 tablespoons unsweetened cocoa powder
½ tablespoons pure maple syrup
½ teaspoon vanilla extract

1. In a medium bowl, mix all of the ingredients until well combined.
2. Spoon into 12 cookies on a platter lined with parchment paper. Refrigerate to set, about 2 hours.

Per Serving
Calories: 143 | fat: 12g | protein: 4g | carbs: 6g | fiber: 2g | sugar: 12.2g| sodium: 13mg

Perfect Orange Almond Cake

Prep time: 15 minutes | Cook time: 30 minutes | Serves 24

Unsalted non-hydrogenated plant-based butter, for greasing the pan
1½ cups gluten-free baking flour, plus more for dusting
1½ cups almond flour
½ teaspoon baking soda

½ teaspoon baking powder
9 medium eggs, at room temperature
1 cup coconut sugar
Zest of 3 oranges
Juice of 1 orange
1 cup extra-virgin olive oil

1. Preheat the oven to 325ºF (163ºC).
2. Grease two bundt pans with butter and dust with the baking flour.
3. In a medium bowl, whisk the baking flour, almond flour, baking soda, and baking powder together.
4. In a large bowl, whip the eggs with the coconut sugar until they double in size.
5. Add the orange zest and orange juice.
6. Add the dry ingredients to the wet ingredients, stirring to combine.
7. Add the olive oil, a little at a time, until incorporated.
8. Divide the batter between the two prepared bundt pans.

9. Transfer the bundt pans to the oven, and bake for 30 minutes, or until browned and a toothpick inserted into the center comes out clean.
10. Remove the bundt pans from the oven, and let cool for 15 minutes.
11. Invert the bundt pans onto plates, and gently tap the cakes out of the pan.

Per Serving
Calories: 180 | fat: 12.1g | protein: 4.1g | carbs: 14.9g | fiber: 1.1g | sugar: 8.1g | sodium: 51mg

Cinnamon Pumpkin Muffins

Prep time: 20 minutes | Cook time: 25 minutes | Serves 12 Muffins

¾ cup blanched almond flour
½ cup coconut flour
3 tablespoons tapioca
1 tablespoon cinnamon
1 tablespoon baking powder
Pinch of nutmeg
½ cup stevia in raw
¼ teaspoon salt

1 cup puréed pumpkin
4 large eggs, whites and yolks separated
1½ teaspoons vanilla extract
½ cup coconut oil
10 drops liquid stevia
1½ cups frozen raspberries

1. Preheat the oven to 350ºF (180ºC). Line a 12-cup muffin pan with paper muffin cups.
2. Combine the flours, tapioca, cinnamon, baking powder, nutmeg, stevia in raw, and salt in a large bowl. Stir to mix well.
3. Mix in the puréed pumpkin, egg yolks, vanilla extract, coconut oil, and liquid stevia until a batter forms. Divide the batter into the muffin cups.
4. Whip the egg whites in a separate large bowl until it forms the stiff peaks.
5. Top the batter with the beaten egg whites and raspberries.
6. Place the muffin pan in the preheated oven and bake for 25 minutes or until a toothpick inserted in the center of the muffins comes out clean.
7. Remove the muffins from the oven and allow to cool for 5 minutes before serving.

Per Serving (1 Muffin)
Calories: 223 | fat: 15.6g | protein: 4.4g | carbs: 29.3g | fiber: 2.9g | sugar: 7.7g | sodium: 76mg

Best Air Fried Banana Almond Peach Bowl

Prep time: 15 minutes | Cook time: 15 minutes | Serves 7

4 ripe bananas, peeled
2 cups chopped peaches
1 medium egg

2 medium egg whites
¾ cup almond meal
¼ teaspoon almond extract

1. In a large bowl, mash the bananas and peaches together with a fork or potato masher.
2. Blend in the egg and egg whites.
3. Stir in the almond meal and almond extract.
4. Working in batches, place ¼-cup portions of the batter into the basket of an air fryer.
5. Set the air fryer to 390ºF (199ºC), close, and cook for 12 minutes.
6. Once cooking is complete, transfer the fritters to a plate. Repeat until no batter remains.

Per Serving
Calories: 163 | fat: 7.1g | protein: 5.9g | carbs: 21.9g | fiber: 4.1g | sugar: 12.0g | sodium: 24mg

Delicious Watermelon Avocado Mousse

Prep time: 10 minutes | Cook time: 10 minutes | Serves 8

1 small, seedless watermelon, halved and cut into 1-inch rounds
2 ripe avocados, pitted

and peeled
½ cup fat-free plain yogurt
¼ teaspoon cayenne pepper

1. On a hot grill, grill the watermelon slices for 2 to 3 minutes on each side, or until you can see the grill marks.
2. To make the avocado mousse, in a blender, combine the avocados, yogurt, and cayenne and process until smooth.
3. To serve, cut each watermelon round in half. Top each with a generous dollop of avocado mousse.

Per Serving
Calories: 127 | fat: 3.9g | protein: 3.1g | carbs: 24.1g | fiber: 2.9g | sugar: 16.9g | sodium: 15mg

Honeyed Blackberry Bowl

Prep time: 10 minutes | Cook time: 15 minutes | Serves 4

1 cup blackberries, sliced
1 cup rhubarb, chopped

½ tablespoon honey
½ teaspoon cinnamon
2 tablespoons water

1. Combine all the ingredients, in a pot.
2. Bring to a boil over medium heat, and then turn down the heat to medium-low. Simmer for 15 minutes or until the rhubarb is tender. Stir constantly.
3. Serve.

Per Serving
Calories: 88 | fat: 2.1g | protein: 3.1g | carbs: 15.8g | fiber: 3.2g | sugars: 12.6g| sodium: 35mg

Homemade Coconut Chocolate Hazelnut Bites

Prep time: 10 minutes | Cook time: 0 minutes | Makes 12 cookies

¼ cup hazelnuts, crumbled
½ cup peanut butter
½ teaspoon vanilla extract
¾ cup unsweetened shredded coconut
2 tablespoons pure maple syrup

2 tablespoons unsalted butter, melted
2 tablespoons unsweetened cocoa powder
2 tablespoons cream cheese, at room temperature

1. Line a baking sheet with parchment paper.
2. Combine all the ingredients in a bowl. Stir to mix well.
3. Drop 12 equal portions of the mixture on the baking sheet, then arrange the sheet in the refrigerator to chill for 2 hours or until the cookies are firm.
4. Remove the cookies from the refrigerator and serve chilled.

Per Serving
Calories: 145 | fat: 11.9g | protein: 4.1g | carbs: 6.1g | fiber: 2.2g | sugars: 3.9g | sodium: 12mg

Tender Coconut Chocolate Milk Shake

Prep time: 5 minutes | Cook time: 0 minutes | Serves 2

1½ cup vanilla ice cream	2½ tablespoons coconut flakes
½ cup coconut milk, unsweetened	1 teaspoon unsweetened cocoa

1. Heat oven to 350ºF (180ºC).
2. Place coconut on a baking sheet and bake, 2 to 3 minutes, stirring often, until coconut is toasted.
3. Place ice cream, milk, 2 tablespoons coconut, and cocoa in a blender and process until smooth.
4. Pour into glasses and garnish with remaining toasted coconut. Serve immediately.

Per Serving
Calories: 324 | fat: 24.0g | protein: 3.0g | carbs: 23.1g | fiber: 4.0g | sugar: 18.1g | sodium: 107mg

Creamy Chocolate Pudding with Toasted Coconut

Prep time: 5 minutes | Cook time: 0 minutes | Serves 4

2 cup heavy whipping cream	flakes, toasted
½ cup reduced-fat cream cheese, soft	2 tablespoons stevia, divided
½ cup hazelnuts, ground	½ teaspoon of vanilla
4 tablespoons unsweetened coconut	½ teaspoon of hazelnut extract
	½ teaspoon of cacao powder, unsweetened

1. In a medium bowl, beat cream, vanilla, and 1 tablespoon stevia until soft peaks form.
2. In another mixing bowl, beat cream cheese, cocoa, remaining stevia, and hazelnut extract until smooth.
3. In 4 glasses, place ground nuts on the bottom, add a layer of the cream cheese mixture, then the whip cream, and top with toasted coconut. Serve immediately.

Per Serving
Calories: 397 | fat: 35.0g | protein: 6.0g | carbs: 12.1g | fiber: 1.0g | sugar: 9.1g | sodium: 210mg

Broiled Peach Bowl with Whipped Topping

Prep time: 5 minutes | Cook time: 5 minutes | Serves 2

1 peach	free whipped topping
1 nectarine	1 tablespoon Honey
2 tablespoons sugar	Nonstick cooking spray

1. Heat oven to broil. Line a shallow baking dish with foil and spray with cooking spray.
2. Cut the peach and nectarine in half and remove pits. Place cut side down in prepared dish. Broil 3 minutes.
3. Turn fruit over and pour Honey. Broil another 2 to 3 minutes.
4. Transfer 1 of each fruit to a dessert bowl and top with 1 tablespoon of whipped topping. Serve.

Per Serving
Calories: 100 | fat: 1.0g | protein: 1.0g | carbs: 22.1g | fiber: 2.0g | sugar: 19.1g | sodium: 0mg

Citrus Blueberry Coconut Cakes

Prep time: 5 minutes | Cook time: 10 minutes | Serves 5

4 eggs	melted
½ cup coconut milk	1 teaspoon baking soda
½ cup blueberries	½ teaspoon lemon extract
2 tablespoons lemon zest	¼ teaspoon stevia extract
½ cup plus 1 teaspoon coconut flour	Pinch salt
¼ cup Splenda	
¼ cup coconut oil,	

1. In a small bowl, toss berries in the 1 teaspoon of flour.
2. In a large bowl, stir together remaining flour, Splenda, baking soda, salt, and zest.
3. Add the remaining and mix well. Fold in the blueberries.
4. Divide batter evenly into 5 coffee cups. Microwave, one at a time, for 90 seconds, or until they pass the toothpick test.

Per Serving
Calories: 264 | fat: 20.0g | protein: 5.0g | carbs: 14.1g | fiber: 2.0g | sugar: 12.1g | sodium: 87mg

Cranberry Almond Cake

Prep time: 10 minutes | Cook time: 30 minutes | Serves 10

3 eggs, room temperature
1 cup of fresh cranberries
4 ounces (113 g) cream cheese, soft
3 tablespoons fat free sour cream
2 tablespoons butter, melted
2 cup of almond flour, sifted
¾ cup Splenda
¾ cup pumpkin purée
1½ tablespoons baking powder
2 teaspoons cinnamon
1 teaspoon pumpkin spice
1 teaspoon ginger
¼ teaspoon nutmeg
¼ teaspoon salt
Nonstick cooking spray

1. Heat oven to 350ºF (180ºC). Spray a cast iron skillet or cake pan with cooking spray.
2. In a large bowl, beat Splenda, butter and cream cheese until thoroughly combined. Add eggs, one at a time, beating after each.
3. Add pumpkin and spices and combine. Add the dry and mix well. Stir in the sour cream. Pour into prepared pan.
4. Sprinkle cranberries over the batter and with the back of a spoon; push them halfway into the batter.
5. Bake 30 minutes or the cake passes the toothpick test. Cool completely before serving.

Per Serving
Calories: 280 | fat: 17.1g | protein: 7.0g | carbs: 23.1g | fiber: 3.0g | sugar: 16.1g | sodium: 166mg

Vanilla flavored Maple Custard

Prep time: 5 minutes | Cook time: 1 hour 15 minutes | Serves 6

2½ cup half-and-half
½ cup egg substitute
3 cup boiling water
¼ cup Splenda
2 tablespoons sugar
free maple syrup
2 teaspoons vanilla
Dash nutmeg
Nonstick cooking spray

1. Heat oven to 325ºF (163ºC). Lightly spray 6 custard cups or ramekins with cooking spray.
2. In a large bowl, whisk together half-and-half, egg substitute, Splenda, vanilla, and nutmeg. Pour evenly into prepared custard cups. Place cups in a baking dish.

3. Pour boiling water around, being careful not to splash it into, the cups. Bake 1 hour 15 minutes, centers will not be completely set.
4. Remove cups from pan and cool completely. Cover and chill overnight.
5. Just before serving, drizzle with the maple syrup.

Per Serving
Calories: 191 | fat: 12.1g | protein: 5.0g | carbs: 15.1g | fiber: 0g | sugar: 8.1g | sodium: 152mg

Pear Apple Yogurt Dessert

Prep time: 10 minutes | Cook time: 25 minutes | Makes 24 Squares

1 Granny Smith apple, sliced, leave peel on
1 Red Delicious apple, sliced, leave peel on
1 ripe pear, sliced, leave peel on
3 eggs
½ cup plain fat-free yogurt
1 tablespoon lemon juice
1 tablespoon margarine
1 package spice cake mix
1¼ cup water, divided
½ cup pecan pieces
1 tablespoon Splenda
1 teaspoon cinnamon
½ teaspoon vanilla
¼ teaspoon nutmeg
Nonstick cooking spray

1. Heat oven to 350ºF (180ºC). Spray jelly-roll pan with nonstick cooking spray.
2. In a large bowl, beat cake mix, 1 cup water, eggs and yogurt until smooth. Pour into prepared pan and bake 20 minutes or it passes the toothpick test. Cool completely.
3. In a large nonstick skillet, over medium-high heat, toast the pecans, stirring, about 2 minutes or until lightly browned. Remove to a plate.
4. Add the remaining ¼ cup water, sliced fruit, juice and spices to the skillet. Bring to a boil. Reduce heat to medium and cook 3 minutes or until fruit is tender crisp.
5. Remove from heat and stir in Splenda, margarine, vanilla, and pecans. Spoon evenly over cooled cake. Slice into 24 squares and serve.

Per Serving (1 Square)
Calories: 131 | fat: 5.1g | protein: 2.0g | carbs: 20.1g | fiber: 1.0g | sugar: 9.9g | sodium: 158mg

Delicious Blackberry Egg Baked Dish

Prep time: 15 minutes | Cook time: 30 minutes | Serves 4

12 ounces (340 g) blackberries	1 tablespoon water
4 egg whites	1 tablespoon Swerve powdered sugar
1/3 cup Splenda	Nonstick cooking spray

1. Heat oven to 375ºF (190ºC). Spray 4 1-cup ramekins with cooking spray.
2. In a small saucepan, over medium-high heat, combine blackberries and 1 tablespoon water, bring to a boil. Reduce heat and simmer until berries are soft. Add Splenda and stir over medium heat until Splenda dissolves, without boiling.
3. Bring back to boiling, reduce heat and simmer 5 minutes. Remove from heat and cool 5 minutes.
4. Place a fine meshed sieve over a small bowl and push the berry mixture through it using the back of a spoon. Discard the seeds. Cover and chill 15 minutes.
5. In a large bowl, beat egg whites until soft peaks form. Gently fold in berry mixture. Spoon evenly into prepared ramekins and place them on a baking sheet.
6. Bake 12 minutes, or until puffed and light brown. Dust with powdered Swerve and serve immediately.

Per Serving
Calories: 142 | fat: 0g | protein: 5.0g | carbs: 26.1g | fiber: 5.0g | sugar: 20.1g | sodium: 56mg

Blackberry Splenda Pie

Prep time: 10 minutes | Cook time: 20 minutes | Serves 6

1 (9-inch) pie crust, unbaked	2 tablespoons butter, soft
2 cup fresh blackberries	3 tablespoons Splenda, divided
Juice and zest of 1 lemon	2 tablespoons cornstarch

1. Heat oven to 425ºF (220ºC). Line a large baking sheet with parchment paper and unroll pie crust in pan.
2. In a medium bowl, combine blackberries, 2 tablespoons Splenda, lemon juice and zest, and cornstarch. Spoon onto crust leaving a 2-inch edge. Fold and crimp the edges.
3. Dot the berries with 1 tablespoon butter. Brush the crust edge with remaining butter and sprinkle crust and fruit with remaining Splenda.
4. Bake for 20 to 22 minutes or until golden brown. Cool before cutting and serving.

Per Serving
Calories: 207 | fat: 11.1g | protein: 2.0g | carbs: 24.1g | fiber: 3.0g | sugar: 9.1g | sodium: 226mg

Fat free Blueberry Cheesecake

Prep time: 5 minutes | Cook time: 0 minutes | Serves 8

1 pound (454 g) fat free cream cheese, softened	margarine, melted
	8 zwieback toasts
	1 cup boiling water
1 cup sugar free frozen whipped topping, thawed	1/3 cup Splenda
	1 envelope unflavored gelatin
3/4 cup blueberries	1 teaspoon vanilla
1 tablespoon	

1. Place the toasts and margarine in a food processor. Pulse until mixture resembles coarse crumbs. Press on the bottom of a spring form pan.
2. Place gelatin in a medium bowl and add boiling water. Stir until gelatin dissolved completely.
3. In a large bowl, beat cream cheese, Splenda, and vanilla on medium speed until well blended. Beat in whipped topping.
4. Add gelatin, in a steady stream, while beating on low speed. Increase speed to medium and beat 4 minutes or until smooth and creamy.
5. Gently fold in berries and spread over crust. Cover and chill 3 hours or until set.

Per Serving
Calories: 315 | fat: 23.0g | protein: 6.0g | carbs: 20.1g | fiber: 0g | sugar: 10.1g | sodium: 417mg

Appetizing Vanilla flavored Butter Cake

Prep time: 10 minutes | Cook time: 35 minutes | Serves 14

4 eggs
3.25 ounces (92 g) cream cheese, soft
4 tablespoons butter, soft
1¼ cup almond flour
¾ cup Splenda

1 teaspoon baking powder
1 teaspoon of vanilla
¼ teaspoon salt
Butter flavored cooking spray

1. Heat oven to 350ºF (180ºC). Spray a loaf pan with cooking spray.
2. In a medium bowl, combine flour, baking powder, and salt.
3. In a large bowl, beat butter and Splenda until light and fluffy. And cream cheese and vanilla and beat well.
4. Add the eggs, one at a time, beating after each one. Stir in the dry until thoroughly combined.
5. Pour into prepared pan and bake for 30 to 40 minutes or cake passes the toothpick test. Let cool 10 minutes in the pan, then invert onto serving plate. Slice and serve.

Per Serving
Calories: 203 | fat: 13.0g | protein: 5.0g | carbs: 15.1g | fiber: 1.0g | sugar: 13.1g | sodium: 84mg

Vanilla flavored Loaf Cake

Prep time: 15 minutes | Cook time: 25 minutes | Serves 10

6 eggs, separated
1 cup skim milk
1 cup fat free whipped topping
2 tablespoons butter, soft
½ cup Splenda
⅓ cup molasses
¼ cup flour

2 teaspoons pumpkin pie spice
2 teaspoons vanilla
1 teaspoon ginger
¼ teaspoon salt
⅛ teaspoon cream of tartar
Butter flavored cooking spray

1. Heat oven to 350ºF (180ºC). Spray 10 ramekins with cooking spray and sprinkle with Splenda to coat, shaking out excess. Place on a large baking sheet.
2. In a large saucepan, over medium heat, whisk together milk, Splenda, flour and salt until smooth.

3. Bring to a boil, whisking constantly. Pour into a large bowl and whisk in molasses, butter, vanilla, and spices. Let cool 15 minutes.
4. Once spiced mixture has cooled, whisk in egg yolks.
5. In a large bowl, beat egg whites and cream of tartar on high speed until stiff peaks form.
6. Fold into spiced mixture, a third at a time, until blended completely. Spoon into ramekins.
7. Bake for 25 minutes until puffed and set. Serve immediately with a dollop of whipped topping.

Per Serving
Calories: 171 | fat: 5.0g | protein: 4.0g | carbs: 24.1g | fiber: 0g | sugar: 18.1g | sodium: 289mg

Individual Cinnamon Bread Muffins

Prep time: 5 minutes | Cook time: 35 minutes | Serves 12

6 slices cinnamon bread, cut into cubes
1¼ cup skim milk
½ cup egg substitute
1 tablespoon

margarine, melted
⅓ cup Splenda
1 teaspoon vanilla
⅛ teaspoon salt
⅛ teaspoon nutmeg

1. Heat oven to 350ºF (180ºC). Line 12 medium-size muffin cups with paper baking cups.
2. In a large bowl, stir together milk, egg substitute, Splenda, vanilla, salt and nutmeg until combined. Add bread cubes and stir until moistened. Let rest 15 minutes.
3. Spoon evenly into prepared baking cups. Drizzle margarine evenly over the tops.
4. Bake for 30 to 35 minutes or until puffed and golden brown. Remove from oven and let cool completely.

Per Serving
Calories: 106 | fat: 2.0g | protein: 4.0g | carbs: 16.1g | fiber: 1.0g | sugar: 9.1g | sodium: 118mg

Homemade Macadamia Coconut Cream Pie

Prep time: 5 minutes | Cook time: 10 minutes | Serves 8

2 cup raw coconut, grated and divided
2 cans coconut milk, full fat and refrigerated for 24 hours
½ cup raw coconut, grated and toasted

2 tablespoons margarine, melted
1 cup Splenda
½ cup macadamia nuts
¼ cup almond flour

1. Heat oven to 350ºF (180ºC).
2. Add the nuts to a food processor and pulse until finely ground. Add flour, ½ cup Splenda, and 1 cup grated coconut. Pulse until are finely ground and resemble cracker crumbs.
3. Add the margarine and pulse until mixture starts to stick together. Press on the bottom and sides of a pie pan. Bake 10 minutes or until golden brown. Cool
4. Turn the canned coconut upside down and open. Pour off the water and scoop the cream into a large bowl.
5. Add remaining ½ cup Splenda and beat on high until stiff peaks form.
6. Fold in remaining 1 cup coconut and pour into crust. Cover and chill at least 2 hours. Sprinkle with toasted coconut, slice, and serve.

Per Serving
Calories: 330 | fat: 23.0g | protein: 4.0g | carbs: 15.1g | fiber: 11.0g | sugar: 4.1g | sodium: 24mg

Perfect Margarine Baked Bread Pudding

Prep time: 10 minutes | Cook time: 45 minutes | Serves 6

4 cups day-old French or Italian bread, cut into ¾-inch cubes
2 cups skim milk
2 egg whites
1 egg
4 tablespoons

margarine, sliced
5 teaspoons Splenda
1½ teaspoons cinnamon
¼ teaspoon salt
⅛ teaspoon ground cloves

1. Heat oven to 350ºF (180ºC).

2. In a medium sauce pan, heat milk and margarine to simmering. Remove from heat and stir till margarine is completely melted. Let cool 10 minutes.
3. In a large bowl, beat egg and egg whites until foamy. Add Splenda, spices and salt. Beat until combined, and then add in cooled milk and bread.
4. Transfer mixture to a 1½ quart baking dish. Place on rack of roasting pan and add 1 inch of hot water to roaster.
5. Bake until pudding is set and knife inserted in center comes out clean, about 40 to 45 minutes.

Per Serving
Calories: 363 | fat: 10.0g | protein: 14.0g | carbs: 25.1g | fiber: 2.0g | sugar: 10.1g | sodium: 1090mg

Vegan Almond Banana Pancakes

Prep time: 15 minutes | Cook time: 15 minutes | Serves 7

2 cups peaches, chopped
4 ripe bananas, peeled
2 medium egg whites

1 medium egg
¼ teaspoon almond extract
¾ cup almond meal

1. Preheat the oven to 400ºF (205ºC).
2. Put all the ingredients in a food processor, and pulse until mix well and it has a thick consistency.
3. Pour the mixture in a baking dish lined with parchment paper.
4. Bake in the preheated oven for 10 minutes or until a toothpick inserted in the center of the pancakes comes out clean.
5. Remove the pancakes from the oven and slice to serve.

Per Serving
Calories: 166 | fat: 6.9g | protein: 6.1g | carbs: 21.8g | fiber: 4.2g | sugars: 11.8g | sodium: 22mg

Creamy Pineapple Peanut Butter Dessert

Prep time: 10 minutes | Cook time: 0 minutes | Serves 6

1 cup peanut butter
2 cups frozen pineapple

½ cup unsweetened almond milk

1. Put the peanut butter and pineapple in a food processor, and then pour the almond milk in the food processor.
2. Pulse until creamy and smooth, then pour the mixture into 6 glasses and serve.

Per Serving
Calories: 303 | fat: 21.8g | protein: 14.1g | carbs: 14.8g | fiber: 4.2g | sugars: 7.8g | sodium: 37mg

Apple Cinnamon Tortillas

Prep time: 15 minutes | Cook time: 15 minutes | Serves 4

2 apple, cored and chopped
3 tablespoons splenda, divided
¼ cup water

½ teaspoon ground cinnamon
4 (8-inch) whole-wheat flour tortillas
Nonstick cooking spray

Special Equipment:
4 toothpicks, soaked in water for at least 30 minutes

1. Preheat the oven to 400ºF (205ºC). Line a baking sheet with parchment paper and set aside.
2. Add the apples, 2 tablespoons of splenda, water, and cinnamon to a medium saucepan over medium heat.
3. Stir to combine and allow the mixture to boil for 5 minutes, or until the apples are fork-tender, but not mushy.
4. Remove the apple filling from the heat and let it cool to room temperature.
5. Place the tortillas on a lightly floured surface.
6. Spoon 2 teaspoons of prepared apple filling onto each tortilla and fold the tortilla over to enclose the filling.
7. Roll each tortilla up and run the toothpicks through to secure. Spritz the tortillas lightly with nonstick cooking spray.
8. Arrange the tortillas on the prepared baking sheet, seam-side down. Scatter the remaining splenda all over the tortillas.
9. Bake in the preheated oven for 10 minutes, flipping the tortillas halfway through, or until they are crispy and golden brown on each side.
10. Remove from the oven to four plates and serve while warm.

Per Serving
Calories: 201 | fat: 6.2g | protein: 3.9g | carbs: 32.8g | fiber: 5.0g | sugar: 7.9g | sodium: 241mg

Lime Tarts with Homemade Whipped Cream

Prep time: 5 minutes | Cook time: 10 minutes | Serves 8

4 sheets phyllo dough
¾ cup skim milk
¾ cup fat-free whipped topping, thawed
½ cup egg substitute
½ cup fat free sour cream

6 tablespoons fresh lime juice
2 tablespoons cornstarch
½ cup Splenda
Butter-flavored cooking spray

1. In a medium saucepan, combine milk, juice, and cornstarch. Cook, stirring, over medium heat 2 to 3 minutes or until thickened. Remove from heat.
2. Add egg substitute and whisk 30 seconds to allow it to cook. Stir in sour cream and Splenda. Cover and chill until completely cool.
3. Heat oven to 350ºF (180ºC). Spray 8 muffin cups with cooking spray.
4. Lay 1 sheet of the phyllo on a cutting board and lightly spray it with cooking spray. Repeat this with the remaining sheets so they are stacked on top of each other.
5. Cut the phyllo into 8 squares and gently place them in the prepared muffin cups, pressing firmly on the bottom and sides. Bake for 8 to 10 minutes or until golden brown. Remove them from the pan and let cool.
6. To serve: spoon the lime mixture evenly into the 8 cups and top with whipped topping. Garnish with fresh lime slices if desired.

Per Serving
Calories: 83 | fat: 1.0g | protein: 3.0g | carbs: 13.1g | fiber: 1.0g | sugar: 10.1g | sodium: 111mg

Chapter 14: Sauces, Dips, and Dressing

Best Garlic Basil Paprika Blend

Prep time: 10 minutes | Cook time: 40 minutes | Makes ¾ cup

2 tablespoons garlic powder
2 tablespoons dried basil
1 tablespoon sweet paprika
1 tablespoon smoked paprika
1 tablespoon freshly ground black pepper

1 tablespoon onion powder
1 tablespoon cayenne pepper
1 tablespoon dried thyme
1 tablespoon dried oregano
1 teaspoon ground red sweet pepper

1. In an airtight container, combine the garlic powder, basil, sweet paprika, smoked paprika, black pepper, onion powder, cayenne, thyme, oregano, and sweet pepper.

Per Serving
Calories: 15 | fat: 0g | protein: 1.1g | carbs: 2.9g | fiber: 1.1g | sugar: 1.0g | sodium: 4mg

Creamy Butter Lemon Sauce

Prep time: 5 minutes | Cook time: 3 to 5 minutes | Makes 2 cups

1 cup half-and-half
1 tablespoon unsalted butter
2 tablespoons Parmesan cheese,

shredded
1 teaspoon freshly squeezed lemon juice
¼ teaspoon garlic powder

1. Add all ingredients to a saucepan and cook over medium-low heat for about 3 to 5 minutes, stirring frequently, or until the sauce is heated through.
2. Remove from the heat to a bowl. Let it cool for a few minutes before serving.

Per Serving
Calories: 55 | fat: 5.2g | protein: 3g | carbs: 1g | fiber: 0g | sugar: 0g | sodium: 40mg

The Best Homemade Butter Milk Garlic salad

Prep time: 10 minutes | Cook time: 0 minutes | Serves 8 to 10

8 ounces (227 g) fat-free Low-fat Greek yogurt
¼ cup low-fat buttermilk
1 tablespoon garlic powder
1 tablespoon dried dill

1 tablespoon dried chives
1 tablespoon onion powder
1 tablespoon dried parsley
Pinch freshly ground black pepper

1. In a shallow, medium bowl, combine the Greek yogurt and buttermilk.
2. Stir in the garlic powder, dill, chives, onion powder, parsley, and pepper and mix well.
3. Serve with animal protein or vegetable of your choice, or place in an airtight container.

Per Serving
Calories: 30 | fat: 0g | protein: 3.0g | carbs: 3.0g | fiber: 0g | sugar: 2.0g | sodium: 24mg

Instant Garlic Cucumber Dip

Prep time: 10 minutes | Cook time: 0 minutes | Makes 1½ cups

1 medium cucumber, peeled and grated
¼ teaspoon salt
1 cup Low-fat Greek yogurt
2 garlic cloves, minced

1 tablespoon freshly squeezed lemon juice
1 tablespoon extra-virgin olive oil
¼ teaspoons freshly ground black pepper

1. Put the cucumber in a colander, and then sprinkle with salt. Set aside.
2. Combine the remaining ingredients in a bowl. Stir to mix well.
3. Wrap the cucumber in a muslin cloth and squeeze the liquid out as much as possible.
4. Put the cucumber in the bowl of mixture, and then stir to mix well.
5. Wrap the bowl in plastic and refrigerate to marinate for 2 hours.

Per Serving
Calories: 50 | fat: 3.0g | protein: 4.0g | carbs: 3.0g | fiber: 0g | sugars: 2.0g | sodium: 102mg

Tasty Thyme Garlic Chicken Gravy

Prep time: 5 minutes | Cook time: 15 minutes | Makes 1½ cup

2 cups low-sodium chicken broth, divided
4 tablespoons whole-wheat flour, divided
1 medium yellow onion, chopped
½ bunch fresh thyme, roughly chopped
2 garlic cloves, minced
1 bay leaf
½ teaspoon celery seeds
Freshly ground black pepper, to taste
1 teaspoon Worcestershire sauce

1. In a shallow stockpot, combine ½ cup of broth and 1 tablespoon of whole-wheat flour and cook over medium-low heat, whisking until the flour is dissolved.
2. Continue to add about ½ cup of broth and the remaining 3 tablespoons of flour in increments for about 2 minutes, or until a thick sauce is formed.
3. Add the onion, thyme, garlic, bay leaf, and ½ cup of broth, stirring well.
4. Add the celery seeds, pepper, Worcestershire sauce, and remaining ½ cup of broth. Stir and cook for 2 to 3 minutes, or until the gravy is thickened. Discard the bay leaf.
5. Serve spooned over Baked Chicken Stuffed with Collard Greens or your protein of choice.

Per Serving
Calories: 17 | fat: 0g | protein: 1.1g | carbs: 3.0g | fiber: 0g | sugar: 1.0g | sodium: 17mg

So Easy Peanut Butter Puree

Prep time: 5 minutes | Cook time: 0 minutes | Serves 4

¼ cup peanut butter
Juice of 1 lime
1 tablespoon peeled and grated fresh ginger
½ tablespoon honey
1 garlic clove, minced
Pinch red pepper flakes

1. In a small bowl, whisk all of the ingredients together until well combined.

Per Serving
Calories: 118 | fat: 8g | protein: 4g | carbs: 9g | fiber: 1g | sugar: 35.78g| sodium: 137mg

Absolutely Fabulous Greek Vinaigrette Bowl

Prep time: 5 minutes | Cook time: 0 minutes | Serves 4

Greek:
¼ cup extra virgin olive oil
3 garlic cloves, minced
1 tablespoon freshly squeezed lemon juice
1 tablespoon red wine vinegar
1 teaspoon dried marjoram
1 teaspoon dried oregano
½ teaspoon lemon zest
¼ teaspoon sea salt

Italian:
¼ cup extra-virgin olive oil
2 tablespoons red wine vinegar
1 teaspoon Dijon mustard
2 teaspoons Italian seasoning
1 garlic clove, finely minced
1 tablespoon minced shallot
¼ teaspoon sea salt
⅛ teaspoon freshly ground black pepper

1. Stir together all ingredients in a medium bowl until completely mixed and emulsified.

Per Serving
Calories: 129 | fat: 14.3g | protein: 0g | carbs: 1.1g | fiber: 0.8g | sugar: 0.2g | sodium: 76mg

Creamy Tahini Honeyed Bowl

Prep time: 5 minutes | Cook time: 0 minutes | Makes 1 cup

½ cup water
¾ cup unsalted tahini
⅓ cup freshly squeezed lemon juice
1 teaspoon honey
½ teaspoon salt

1. Mix together the water, tahini, lemon juice, honey, and salt in a medium bowl, and stir vigorously until well incorporated.
2. Store the leftover dressing in an airtight container in the fridge for up to 2 weeks and shake before using.

Per Serving (2 Tablespoons)
Calories: 168 | fat: 13.1g | protein: 4.7g | carbs: 10.3g | fiber: 2.8g | sugar: 8.0g | sodium: 148mg

Garlic Dill Yogurt Bowl

Prep time: 5 minutes | Cook time: 0 minutes | Makes ⅔ cup

1 teaspoon freshly squeezed lemon juice
1 teaspoon fresh dill, chopped
½ cup Low-fat Greek yogurt
¼ teaspoon garlic powder
¼ teaspoon salt

1. Combine all the ingredients in a bowl. Stir to mix well.

Per Serving
Calories: 36 | fat: 1.0g | protein: 3.2g | carbs: 3.1g | fiber: 0g | sugars: 1.9g | sodium: 176mg

Basil Pesto Sauce

Prep time: 5 minutes | Cook time: 0 minutes | Serves 4

⅓ cup raw pine nuts, almonds, walnuts, pecans or pepitas
2 cups packed fresh basil leaves
¼ cup grated Parmesan cheese
1 tablespoon lemon juice
2 cloves garlic, roughly chopped
½ teaspoon fine sea salt
½ cup extra-virgin olive oil

1. Toast the nuts or seeds for extra flavour: In a medium skillet, toast the nuts/seeds over medium heat, stirring frequently until nice and fragrant, 3 to 5 minutes.
2. Pour them into a bowl to cool for a few minutes.
3. To make the pesto, combine the basil, cooled nuts/seeds, Parmesan, lemon juice, garlic and salt in a food processor or blender. With the machine running, slowly drizzle in the olive oil.
4. Continue processing until the mixture is well blended but still has some texture, pausing to scrape down the sides as necessary.
5. Taste, and adjust if necessary. Add a pinch of salt if the basil tastes too bitter or the pesto needs more zing. Add more Parmesan if you'd like a creamier/cheesier pesto.
6. If desired, you can thin out the pesto with more olive oil.

7. Store leftover pesto in the refrigerator, covered, for up to 1 week. You can also freeze pesto—my favourite way is in an ice cube try.
8. Once frozen, transfer to a freezer bag, and then you can thaw only as much as you need later.

Per Serving
Calories: 200 | fat: 21g | protein: 4g | carbs: 2g | fiber: 1g | sugar: 5.3g| sodium: 254mg

Quick and Easy Dipping Sauce

Prep time: 5 minutes | Cook time: 0 minutes | Makes ½ cup

1 to 2 teaspoons hot sauce, to your liking
2 teaspoons rice vinegar
1 teaspoon sesame oil

1. Stir together the hot sauce, rice vinegar, and oil in a small bowl until thoroughly smooth.
2. Chill for at least 30 minutes to blend the flavors.

Per Serving (2 Tablespoons)
Calories: 54 | fat: 4.7g | protein: 0g | carbs: 1.7g | fiber: 0g | sugar: 1.0g | sodium: 190mg

5 Minutes Asian Salad Dressing

Prep time: 5 minutes | Cook time: 0 minutes | Serves 2

¼ cup extra-virgin olive oil
3 tablespoons apple cider vinegar
1 tablespoon peeled and grated fresh ginger
1 tablespoon freshly squeezed lime juice
1 tablespoon chopped fresh cilantro
1 garlic clove, minced
½ teaspoon sriracha

1. In a small bowl, whisk all of the ingredients together until well combined.

Per Serving
Calories: 252 | fat: 27g | protein: 0g | carbs: 2g | fiber: 1g | sugar: 0.57g| sodium: 3mg

Best Ever Lemony Soy Peanut Sauce

Prep time: 10 minutes | Cook time: 0 minutes | Makes ²/₃ cup

½ cup natural peanut butter
2 tablespoons rice vinegar
4 teaspoons sesame oil
2 to 4 teaspoons freshly squeezed lime

juice, to your liking
2 to 2½ teaspoons hot sauce (optional)
1 teaspoon low-sodium soy sauce
1 teaspoon chopped peeled fresh ginger
1 teaspoon honey

1. Mix together the peanut butter, rice vinegar, sesame oil, lime juice, hot sauce (if desired), soy sauce, ginger, and honey in a small bowl, and whisk to combine well.
2. You can store it in an airtight container in the fridge for up to 2 weeks.

Per Serving (2½ Tablespoons)
Calories: 206 | fat: 16.7g | protein: 7.9g | carbs: 8.2g | fiber: 3.1g | sugar: 3.0g | sodium: 113mg

Drink your Veggie Smoothie

Prep time: 10 minutes | Cook time: 5 minutes | Serves 4

1 red bell pepper, seeded and chopped
1 red onion, chopped
1 tomato, chopped
4 garlic cloves, minced
1 red chile, seeded and chopped
2 tablespoons extra-

virgin olive oil
Juice of 1 lemon
1 tablespoon smoked paprika
1 tablespoon dried oregano
1 teaspoon sea salt

1. In a blender or food processor, combine all of the ingredients. Process until smooth.
2. In a small saucepan over medium-high heat, bring the mixture to a simmer, stirring constantly. Reduce heat to medium and simmer for 5 minutes and serve.

Per Serving
Calories: 99 | fat: 7g | protein: 1g | carbs: 8g | fiber: 3g | sugar: 12.32g| sodium: 296mg

5 Minute Lemony Avocado Bowl

Prep time: 5 minutes | Cook time: 0 minutes | Makes 1 cup

1 large avocado, peeled and pitted
½ cup Low-fat Greek yogurt
¾ cup fresh cilantro
1 tablespoon water

2 teaspoons freshly squeezed lime juice
⅛ teaspoon garlic powder
Pinch salt to taste

1. Process the avocado, yogurt, cilantro, water, lime juice, garlic powder, and salt in a blender until creamy and emulsified.
2. Chill for at least 30 minutes in the refrigerator to let the flavors blend.

Per Serving
Calories: 92 | fat: 6.8g | protein: 4.1g | carbs: 4.9g | fiber: 2.3g | sugar: 1.0g | sodium: 52mg

Homemade Spicy Tomato Sauce

Prep time: 5 minutes | Cook time: 15 minutes | Makes 3 cups

1¼ cup tomato purée
1½ cup white vinegar
1 tablespoon yellow mustard
1 teaspoon mustard seeds
1 teaspoon ground turmeric
1 teaspoon sweet paprika

1 teaspoon garlic powder
1 teaspoon celery seeds
½ teaspoon cayenne pepper
½ teaspoon onion powder
½ teaspoon freshly ground black pepper

1. In a medium pot, combine the tomato purée, vinegar, mustard, mustard seeds, turmeric, paprika, garlic powder, celery seeds, cayenne, onion powder, and black pepper.
2. Simmer over low heat for 15 minutes, or until the flavors come together.
3. Remove the sauce from the heat, and let cool for 5 minutes. Transfer to a blender and purée until smooth.

Per Serving
Calories: 10 | fat: 0g | protein: 0.3g | carbs: 1.5g | fiber: 0.3g | sugar: 1.0g | sodium: 14mg

Authentic Italian Olive Oil Parsley Condiment

Prep time: 5 minutes | Cook time: 0 minutes | Serves 4

½ cup Italian parsley
¼ cup extra-virgin olive oil
¼ cup fresh cilantro stems removed
Zest of 1 lemon

2 tablespoons red wine vinegar
½ teaspoon sea salt
1 garlic clove, minced
¼ teaspoon red pepper flakes

1. Process all the ingredients in a food processor until smooth.
2. Store in an airtight container in the fridge for up to 2 days or in the freezer for 6 months.

Per Serving
Calories: 124 | fat: 13.7g | protein: 0g | carbs: 0.8g | fiber: 0g | sugar: 0.5g | sodium: 150mg

7 Ingredients Peanut Sauce

Prep time: 5 minutes | Cook time: 0 minutes | Serves 4

¼ cup peanut butter
Juice of 1 lime
¼ tablespoon honey
1 minced garlic clove
1 tablespoon reduced-

sodium soy sauce
1 tablespoon peeled fresh ginger, grated
Pinch red pepper flakes

1. Put all ingredients in a medium bowl and whisk until well blended.

Per Serving
Calories: 120 | fat: 8.3g | protein: 4.2g | carbs: 9.2g | fiber: 1.1g | sugar: 7.3 | sodium: 138mg

Tomato Oregano Sauce

Prep time: 5 minutes | Cook time: 30 minute s| Serves 15

¼ cup extra virgin olive oil
3 cloves garlic finely diced
128 (3.6 kg) ounce can dice tomatoes

½ teaspoon dried oregano
1 teaspoon white vinegar
½ teaspoon sea salt

1. In a small saucepan over medium-high heat, sauté the garlic in the olive oil.

2. Sauté for a minute until the garlic is fragrant. Make sure the garlic doesn't brown and become burnt.
3. Turn the heat down and add the tomatoes, oregano, vinegar, and salt to the saucepan.
4. Bring to a simmer and allow cooking for 30 – 40 minutes, allowing the sauce to reduce and thicken.

Per Serving
Calories: 80 | fat: 3.2g | protein: 2.9g | carbs: 12.9g | fiber: 6.9g | sugar: 8.3g| sodium: 580mg

One Pot Veggie Green peas Smoothie

Prep time: 5 minutes | Cook time: 0 minutes | Serves 2

½ cup fresh green peas
½ cup grated Parmesan cheese
¼ cup fresh basil leaves

¼ cup extra-virgin olive oil
¼ cup pine nuts
2 garlic cloves, minced
¼ teaspoon sea salt

1. In a blender or food processor, combine all of the ingredients. Process until smooth.

Per Serving
Calories: 248 | fat: 23g | protein: 7g | carbs: 5g | fiber: 1g | sugar: 3.92g| sodium: 338mg

Savory Parsley Smoothie

Prep time: 5 minutes | Cook time: 0 minutes | Serves 4

½ cup Italian parsley
¼ cup fresh cilantro stems removed
¼ cup extra-virgin olive oil
2 tablespoons red wine

vinegar
1 garlic clove, minced
Zest of 1 lemon
½ teaspoon sea salt
¼ teaspoon red pepper flakes

1. In a blender or food processor, combine all the ingredients. Process until smooth.

Per Serving
Calories: 125 | fat: 14g | protein: 0g | carbs: 1g | fiber: 0g | sugar: 2.11g| sodium: 151mg

Conclusion

You may worry that having diabetes means going without foods you enjoy. The good news is that you can still eat your favorite foods, but you might need to eat smaller portions or enjoy them less often. Your health care team will help create a diabetes meal plan for you that meet your needs and likes. Eat a wide range of foods – including fruit, vegetables and some starchy foods like pasta. Keep sugar, fat and salt to a minimum. Eat breakfast, lunch and dinner every day – do not skip meals.

Nutrition and physical activity are important parts of a healthy lifestyle when you have diabetes. Along with other benefits, following a healthy meal plan and being active can help you keep also called blood sugar, in your target range. To manage your blood glucose, you need to balance what you eat and drink with physical activity and diabetes medicine, if you take any. What you choose to eat, how much you eat, and when you eat are all important in keeping your blood glucose level in the range that your health care team recommends.

For diabetes, a healthy diet may just be the best medicine. In fact, a diabetes diet, which is really just an overall healthy diet with good portion control, can go beyond helping you achieve blood sugar control; Lowering your risk for serious health conditions, from heart disease to cancer, are among the benefits.

Resources

- Centers for Disease Control and Prevention
- National Agricultural Library
- [1] Greger, M., Stone, G. How not to die. (2015) Flatiron Books.

Appendix 1: Measurement Conversion Chart

US STANDARD	METRIC (APPROXIMATE)
1/8 teaspoon	0.5 mL
1/4 teaspoon	1 mL
1/2 teaspoon	2 mL
3/4 teaspoon	4 mL
1 teaspoon	5 mL
1 tablespoon	15 mL
1/4 cup	59 mL
1/2 cup	118 mL
3/4 cup	177 mL
1 cup	235 mL
2 cups	475 mL
3 cups	700 mL
4 cups	1 L

US STANDARD	US STANDARD (OUNCES)	METRIC (APPROXIMATE)
2 tablespoons	1 fl.oz.	30 mL
1/4 cup	2 fl.oz.	60 mL
1/2 cup	4 fl.oz.	120 mL
1 cup	8 fl.oz.	240 mL
1 1/2 cup	12 fl.oz.	355 mL
2 cups or 1 pint	16 fl.oz.	475 mL
4 cups or 1 quart	32 fl.oz.	1 L
1 gallon	128 fl.oz.	4 L

WEIGHT EQUIVALENTS

US STANDARD	METRIC (APPROXIMATE)
1 ounce	28 g
2 ounces	57 g
5 ounces	142 g
10 ounces	284 g
15 ounces	425 g
16 ounces (1 pound)	455 g
1.5 pounds	680 g
2 pounds	907 g

TEMPERATURES EQUIVALENTS

FAHRENHEIT(F)	CELSIUS(C) (APPROXIMATE)
225 °F	107 °C
250 °F	120 °C
275 °F	135 °C
300 °F	150 °C
325 °F	160 °C
350 °F	180 °C
375 °F	190 °C
400 °F	205 °C
425 °F	220 °C
450 °F	235 °C
475 °F	245 °C
500 °F	260 °C

Appendix 2: The Dirty Dozen and Clean Fifteen

The Environmental Working Group (EWG) is a nonprofit, nonpartisan organization dedicated to protecting human health and the environment Its mission is to empower people to live healthier lives in a healthier environment. This organization publishes an annual list of the twelve kinds of produce, in sequence, that have the highest amount of pesticide residue-the Dirty Dozen-as well as a list of the fifteen kinds ofproduce that have the least amount of pesticide residue-the Clean Fifteen.

THE DIRTY DOZEN

- The 2016 Dirty Dozen includes the following produce. These are considered among the year's most important produce to buy organic:

Strawberries	Spinach
Apples	Tomatoes
Nectarines	Bell peppers
Peaches	Cherry tomatoes
Celery	Cucumbers
Grapes	Kale/collard greens
Cherries	Hot peppers

- *The Dirty Dozen list contains two additional itemskale/collard greens and hot peppers-because they tend to contain trace levels of highly hazardous pesticides.*

THE CLEAN FIFTEEN

- The least critical to buy organically are the Clean Fifteen list. The following are on the 2016 list:

Avocados	Papayas
Corn	Kiw
Pineapples	Eggplant
Cabbage	Honeydew
Sweet peas	Grapefruit
Onions	Cantaloupe
Asparagus	Cauliflower
Mangos	

- *Some of the sweet corn sold in the United States are made from genetically engineered (GE) seedstock. Buy organic varieties of these crops to avoid GE produce.*

Appendix 3: Glycemic Index and Glycemic Load Food Lists

FOOD	GLYCEMIC INDEX	SERVING SIZE (GRAMS)	GLYCEMIC LOAD (PER SERVING)
BAKERY PRODUCTS			
Bagel, white	72	70	25
Baguette, white	95	30	15
Barley bread	34	30	7
Corn tortilla	52	50	12
Croissant	67	57	17
Doughnut	76	47	17
Pita bread	68	30	10
Sourdough rye	48	30	6
Soya and linseed bread	36	30	3
Sponge cake	46	63	17
Wheat tortilla	30	50	8
White wheat flour bread	71	30	10
Whole-wheat bread	71	30	9
SNACK FOODS			
Cashews, salted	27	50	3
Corn chips, salted	42	50	11
Fruit Roll-Ups	99	30	24
Graham crackers	74	25	14
Honey	61	25	12
Hummus	6	30	0
M&M's, peanut	33	30	6
Microwave popcorn, plain	55	20	6
Muesli bar	61	30	13
Nutella	33	20	4
Peanuts	7	50	0
Potato chips	51	50	12
Pretzels	83	30	16
Rice cakes	82	25	17
Rye crisps	64	25	11
Shortbread	64	25	10
Vanilla wafers	77	25	14

BEVERAGES			
Apple juice, unsweetened	44	250mL	30
Coca-Cola	63	250mL	16
Gatorade	78	250mL	12
Lucozade	95	250mL	40
Orange juice, unsweetened	50	250mL	12
Tomato juice, canned	38	250mL	4
BREAKFAST CEREALS			
All-Bran	55	30	12
Coco Pops	77	30	20
Cornflakes	93	30	23
Muesli	66	30	16
Oatmeal	55	50	13
Special K	69	30	14
DAIRY			
Ice cream, regular	57	50	6
Milk, full fat	41	250mL	5
Milk, skim	32	250mL	4
Reduced-fat yogurt with fruit	33	200	11
FRUITS			
Apple	39	120	6
Banana, ripe	62	120	16
Cherries	22	120	3
Dates, dried	42	60	18
Grapefruit	25	120	3
Grapes	59	120	11
Mango	41	120	8
Orange	40	120	4

Peach	42	120	5
Pear	38	120	4
Pineapple	51	120	8
Raisins	64	60	28
Strawberries	40	120	1
Watermelon	72	120	4
GRAINS			
Brown rice	50	150	16
Buckwheat	45	150	13
Bulgur	30	50	11
Corn on the cob	60	150	20
Couscous	65	150	9
Fettucini	32	180	15
Gnocchi	68	180	33
Macaroni	47	180	23
Quinoa	53	150	13
Spaghetti, white	46	180	22
Spaghetti, whole-wheat	42	180	26
Vermicelli	35	180	16
White rice	89	150	43
LEGUMES			
Baked beans	40	150	6
Black beans	30	150	7
Butter beans	36	150	8
Chickpeas	10	150	3
Kidney beans	29	150	7
Lentils	29	150	5
Navy beans	31	150	9
Soybeans	50	150	1
VEGETABLES			
Beetroot	64	80	4
Carrot	35	80	2
Green peas	51	80	4
Parsnip	52	80	4
Sweet potato	70	150	22
White potato, boiled	81	150	22
Yam	54	150	20

Sources: Harvard Health Publications (http://www.health.harvard.edu/healthy-eating/glycemic_index_and_glycemic_load_for_100_foods) and Mendosa.com (http://www.mendosa.com/gilists.htm).

Appendix 4: Recipe Index

CPSIA information can be obtained
at www.ICGtesting.com
Printed in the USA
BVHW010603250721
612416BV00033B/582